Minor
Veterinary
Surgery

A Handbook
for Veterinary Nurses

For Elsevier:

Commissioning Editor: *Mary Seager*
Development Editor: *Rebecca Nelemans*
Project Manager: *Jane Dingwall*
Designer: *Andy Chapman*
Illustration Manager: *Bruce Hogarth*
Illustrations: *Samantha Elmhurst*

Minor Veterinary Surgery

A Handbook for Veterinary Nurses

Julian Hoad BSc(Hons) BVetMed MRCVS

Veterinary Surgeon, Wingrave Veterinary Hospital, Surrey, UK

Foreword by

Margaret Moore MA VN CertEd FETC MIScT

Principal, Cerberus Training & Consultancy, Henley-on-Thames, Oxon, UK

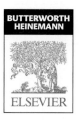

Edinburgh   London   New York   Oxford   Philadelphia   St Louis   Sydney   Toronto   2006

BUTTERWORTH
HEINEMANN
ELSEVIER

First published 2006

ISBN 0 7506 8807 6

British Library Cataloguing in Publication Data
A catalogue record for this book is available from the British Library

Library of Congress Cataloging in Publication Data
A catalog record for this book is available from the Library of Congress

Knowledge and best practice in this field are constantly changing. As new research and experience broaden our knowledge, changes in practice, treatment and drug therapy may become necessary or appropriate. Readers are advised to check the most current information provided (i) on procedures featured or (ii) by the manufacturer of each product to be administered, to verify the recommended dose or formula, the method and duration of administration, and contraindications. It is the responsibility of the practitioner, relying on their own experience and knowledge of the patient, to make diagnoses, to determine dosages and the best treatment for each individual patient, and to take all appropriate safety precautions.
To the fullest extent of the law, neither the publisher nor the author assumes any liability for any injury and/or damage.

The Publisher

Printed in China

Working together to grow
libraries in developing countries

www.elsevier.com | www.bookaid.org | www.sabre.org

 ELSEVIER   BOOK AID International   Sabre Foundation

ELSEVIER your source for books, journals and multimedia in the health sciences

www.elsevierhealth.com

The
Publisher's
policy is to use
**paper manufactured
from sustainable forests**

Contents

Foreword

At last – a book on minor surgical techniques written for veterinary nurses by a veterinary surgeon who clearly views his nurses as valuable members of the veterinary team. This book should enthuse veterinary nurses and surgeons alike to embrace the notion of honing the surgical and related nursing skills of listed veterinary nurses. This can only contribute to job satisfaction and of course increase the revenue of the practice.

I can highly recommend this excellent tome to all listed veterinary nurses interested in expanding their skills and underpinning knowledge of minor acts of veterinary surgery.

Taken as a whole, the chapters are sequential and guide the reader through each stage in a logical order from assessment of the minor surgical case, premedication and preparation, and anaesthesia, through to suitable dressings and bandages for wounds arising from surgery. Each chapter is, in itself, also a useful reference for these individual topics.

The principles of common surgical and dental procedures are also detailed in full followed by advice on care of the postoperative patient.

The contents are illustrated by colour photographs which support the text where needed, making the information easier to understand and use.

In conclusion, I consider this book to be an essential addition to any veterinary practice or college library.

Margaret C Moore

Preface

Veterinary nursing as a profession has changed much in the last few years, with changes to the Veterinary Surgeons' Act (schedule 3 amendments) and an increasing number of diploma-holders. The role of the veterinary nurse is moving away from the outdated 'kennel-maid'/anaesthetic assistant to encompass a wider range of activities, including nursing consultations and health care clinics, in order to utilise more fully the excellent knowledge and training of the veterinary nurse.

Minor surgery is one such role. Allowing nurses to perform minor surgical techniques such as intravenous catheter placement, suturing wounds and even lumpectomies makes for a much more efficient use of practice time and increases team-building and job satisfaction, reducing staff turn-over and improving practice profits.

This book is aimed at those veterinary nurses who want to learn more about surgical techniques and those who are already performing minor surgery but who want to improve. Other than providing information regarding the reasoning behind minor surgical techniques, there are easy-to-follow instructions for performing many minor surgical techniques. It is hoped that veterinary students and recent graduates may also find the book a useful source of reference.

Wherever possible, I have included colour photographs to help clarify certain procedures and to provide examples of different techniques. Wherever relevant, dosages are given for standard or useful drug combinations for average-sized dogs and cats.

Preoperative examination and preparation of patients are discussed in detail, as well as the procedure for admitting surgical patients, advice to owners and suggestions for organising surgery lists.

Any pitfalls or potential complications of procedures are detailed, together with relevant aftercare. Handy hints are widespread throughout. Each procedure is dealt with separately, allowing this book to be used either as a 'patient-side' reference, or as a textbook.

Much discussion is given to wound care and advances in dressing compounds, as well as practical advice on dealing with most types of wound.

Dental medicine and surgery are dealt with in some detail, including a review of dental instrumentation and techniques for cleaning and polishing dog and cat teeth; rabbit dental care is also covered.

Postoperative care and pain management form the bulk of the last chapter, with a section on dealing with client concerns and complaints, giving practical advice for improving client communication.

I hope this book will encourage veterinary nurses to develop their surgical skills and knowledge; I also hope that it will encourage practices to appreciate more fully the abilities of their veterinary nurses, and to provide support and help for them to become proficient in various minor surgical techniques.

Julian Hoad

Acknowledgements

There are many people who have encouraged and supported me in the course of writing this book, and my heartfelt thanks go to all my friends and co-workers. In particular, I must thank my uncle, Robert Hutchinson, for encouraging me to start writing, and my employer, Nic Dodds, for allowing me continually to disrupt the working day to gather photographs, and in granting me a generous amount of time off for writing. My computer would like to thank Adrian Ward for debugging it several times.

My family have been very patient with me and I would like to thank my mother, Alicia, my brother, Marcel, and my sister, Giselle, for tolerating my ratty moods whilst I was writing.

The many hands and faces that appear in the book holding patients or instruments belong to Giselle Hoad, Josey Killner, Kerry Mead, Nicky Cole and Sandy Griffith. Special thanks also to Minky Broad for consenting to be photographed in dozens of bandages!

This book would not have been written without the love and encouragement of Sylvia, my fiancée, to whom this book is dedicated.

Abbreviations

ACh	acetylcholine	IV	intravenous
ACP	acepromazine	IVFT	intravenous fluid therapy
AIPMMA	antibiotic-impregnated polymethylmethacrylate	LDS	ligating and dividing system stapler
		MAC	minimum alveolar concentration
BID	(of dosing) twice daily	MCT	mast-cell tumour
CBA	cat-bite abscess	MRSA	methicillin-resistant *Staphylococcus aureus*
CO_2	carbon dioxide	N_2O	nitrous oxide
CoSHH	Control of Substances Hazardous to Health Act 1988	NaCl	sodium chloride
		NSAID	non-steroidal anti-inflammatory drug
CPD	continuing professional development	O_2	oxygen
CRT	capillary refill time (less than 2–3 s normally)	OCRL/OCL	odontoclastic resorption lesions/odontoclastic lesions
CVP	central venous pressure	OD	outside diameter
ECG	electrocardiogram	PDS II	polydioxanone sulphate (suture material, Ethicon)
E-collar	Elizabethan collar		
ET	endotracheal	PO	orally
FeLV/FIV	feline leukaemia virus/feline immuno-deficiency virus	PVC	polyvinyl chloride
		RCVS	Royal College of Veterinary Surgeons
FNAB	fine-needle aspiration biopsy	RTA	road traffic accident
G	gauge (thickness) of needle	SC	subcutaneous
GIA/ILA	gastrointestinal anastomosis	SID	(of dosing) once daily
HMSO	Her Majesty's Stationery Office (publishers of government documents)	SpO_2	arterial haemoglobin saturation
		TA	thoracoabdominal
IC	intracardiac	TID	(of dosing) three times daily
IM	intramuscular	VDS	Veterinary Defence Society
IPPV	intermittent positive-pressure ventilation	VN	(listed) veterinary nurse
IT	intratracheal		

Part 1:
General principles

The veterinary nurse and minor surgery

1

DEFINITION AND SCOPE OF MINOR VETERINARY SURGERY

Minor veterinary surgery includes procedures ranging from removing skin masses and suturing minor wounds to certain dental procedures. Specifically, minor veterinary surgery:
- Does not involve any procedure considered to be life-threatening or risky
- Does not involve any complex procedure
- Is carried out on a patient that is otherwise healthy
- Does not involve entry into a body cavity

- Is covered by the Royal College of Veterinary Surgeons (RCVS) Veterinary Surgeons' Act (1966) with schedule 3 amendments (see later)

Thus, suturing a skin laceration on the tarsus of a healthy 6-year-old cat would be considered minor surgery, whereas placement of a chest drain and closing the thoracic cavity clearly would not be. Similarly, a small skin tear on an eyelid margin may require precise repair utilising magnification – certainly not minor surgery. However, closing the subcutaneous tissue and skin after **laparotomy** or thoracic surgery would be considered to be within the scope of minor surgery.

Lumpectomies are usually considered minor surgery. However, there is considerable difference between a grape-sized flank lipoma and a football-sized lipoma in the axilla – the size of lump for which a dog needs to be treated for separation anxiety after its removal!

For example, a mast-cell **tumour** with high **metastatic** potential will need to be removed with a large margin and may require complex skin reconstruction techniques to close the wound. None of this procedure would be considered to be minor surgery. However, removal of a 1–2-cm cutaneous mass, which has been

3

demonstrated to be benign and is not in an area of the body where skin closure is likely to cause any problem, would fall into the definition of minor surgery.

It is therefore difficult to produce a definitive list of minor surgical procedures. The decision of what constitutes minor surgery will depend on:

- Size, depth and position of wound (Figures 1.1 and 1.2)
- Condition of underlying tissue
- Complexity of surgery, including incision and repair
- Competence and experience of surgeon/ nurse
- Overall health of the patient
- Proximity of surgical area to delicate or important organs
- Specific limitations under the schedule 3 amendments
- Practice policies

ROLE OF THE VETERINARY NURSE

Increasingly, the role of the veterinary nurse (VN) in practice is changing. More practices are

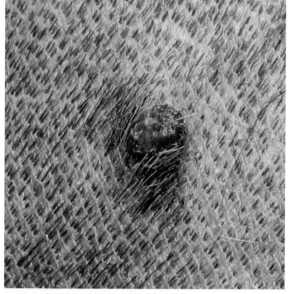

Figure 1.1 This small mass was shown by fine-needle aspiration biopsy to be benign. Removal would constitute minor surgery.

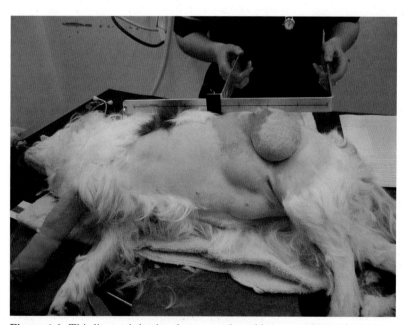

Figure 1.2 This lipoma is benign, but removal would not constitute minor surgery.

utilising their nursing staff to the full, taking advantage of the excellent training the VN course provides.

In addition to more basic nursing duties, many nurses now:

- Run various nursing clinics (weight, dental, worming)
- Regularly perform minor veterinary surgery
- Take part in client education programmes within the practice
- Perform radiographic procedures

Specific to surgery, nurses should:

- Organise the operating-room schedule, taking into account the numbers and types of clean, **contaminated** and dirty procedures to be performed
- Ensure that staffing levels are adequate for the number of procedures (arrange nursing rotas)
- Ensure that the correct levels of equipment, materials and drugs are available

Of course, it depends on the nature of the practice whether it is feasible or efficient for the nurse to be performing surgery, but there are strong reasons to allow this in many settings:

- Efficient use of personnel: in a hospital setting, a nurse can perform a **lumpectomy** or suture a wound, thus allowing the vet more time to undertake diagnosis
- More procedures can be performed: the number of personnel is effectively increased
- A trained, scrubbed assistant can be invaluable during a complex procedure for retraction of organs, passing instruments and applying hand pressure over haemorrhages
- There is less waiting time for surgery – benefiting pet and owner
- It increases the overall knowledge and practical ability of the team
- Permitting VNs to take part in minor surgery encourages personal development
- It can lead to increased job satisfaction

It is not intended that nurses become 'mini vets', rather the nurses' education and training are utilised more fully, allowing for a better use of personnel. It would not be acceptable, for example,

for a small practice to budget on a nurse-only team performing surgery whilst the veterinary surgeon consults in a distant room. Nor would it be acceptable for a nurse to act as both anaesthetist and surgeon at the same time. This clearly falls outside the RCVS requirement for constant monitoring.

THE RCVS SCHEDULE 3 AND ITS APPLICATION TO MINOR SURGERY WITHIN THE PRACTICE

The Veterinary Surgeons' Act 1966 (schedule 3 amendment) order 2002/2004 dictates what procedures a VN may carry out. This schedule is constantly revised and amended, and is open to an extraordinary amount of interpretation. However, the main points are that it only applies to listed qualified VNs, or to student VNs who are enrolled at an approved training and assessment centre or an approved veterinary practice.

A VN may perform any medical treatment or minor surgery to any animal (pet or domestic), provided that:

- The animal is, for the time being, under the care of a registered veterinary surgeon or veterinary practitioner and the medical treatment or minor surgery is carried out by the VN at the surgeon's/practitioner's direction
- The registered veterinary surgeon or veterinary practitioner is the employer or is acting on behalf of the employer of the VN
- The registered veterinary surgeon or veterinary practitioner directing the medical treatment or minor surgery is satisfied that the VN is qualified to carry out the treatment or surgery

A student VN may perform any medical treatment or minor surgery to any animal (pet or domestic), provided that:

- The animal is, for the time being, under the care of a registered veterinary surgeon or veterinary practitioner and the medical treatment or minor surgery is carried out by the student VN at the surgeon's/practitioner's direction and in the course of the student VN's training

- The treatment or surgery is supervised by a registered veterinary surgeon, veterinary practitioner or VN and, in the case of surgery, the supervision is direct, continuous and personal
- The registered veterinary surgeon or veterinary practitioner is the employer or is acting on behalf of the employer of the student VN

Confusion always occurs over what constitutes minor surgery. The RCVS is fairly vague over this, but stipulates that it should not involve entry into a body cavity. Some discretion is left to the veterinary surgeon to decide whether the nurse is competent to perform the surgery, or whether it is appropriate for that procedure to be performed by a nurse.

Dentistry has also caused confusion in the profession under the terms of schedule 3, as the oral cavity is a body cavity under the terms of the Act. At the time of writing:

- A VN may not extract teeth with instruments unless the teeth are already mobile
- A VN may not perform work under the gum margin

- A VN may not create flaps for **periodontal** surgery

However, nurses may still:
- Examine teeth for evidence of lesions
- Use instruments such as ultrasonic scalers and mechanical scrapers to clean teeth
- Use instruments to remove loose teeth
- Polish teeth

Although more amendments to schedule 3 will undoubtedly be made, it is unlikely that substantial changes will occur to prevent nurses from carrying out the above procedures.

What is certain, though, is that competence plays a very important role in the decision to allow or forbid certain procedures (Figure 1.3). Thus it is up to individual nurses, and to the profession as a whole, to gain experience and competence in minor surgery (Box 1.1).

ENSURING PROFESSIONAL SUPPORT

With increased surgical competence, the number and variety of procedures assigned to a nurse will

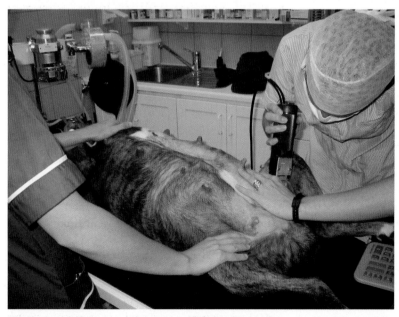

Figure 1.3 Efficient use of time: a qualified nurse monitors the anaesthetic while a trainee nurse prepares the surgical site. The veterinary surgeon can be scrubbing ready for the caesarean section.

Box 1.1

The inclusion of a specific procedure in this book does not necessarily suggest that it is a minor surgical technique nor that it is appropriate for a veterinary nurse to perform such a procedure. In most cases the procedure is included for completeness. For example, it makes little sense to discuss dental treatment without discussing extractions.

The decision to allow a veterinary nurse to perform a specific procedure is made on the basis of current schedule 3 legislation, individual practice policy and the surgical experience and competence of the nurse

increase. So, inevitably, will the pressure and accountability placed on that nurse. Performing a surgical technique that is within one's 'comfort zone' of ability should be enjoyable. However, it can take some time to reach that level of ability. It is very important to have the support of the rest of the practice team whilst gaining experience. The level of support may vary from practice to practice, but here are a few guidelines to help reduce the stress of learning:

- Under the terms of the RCVS schedule 3, a qualified veterinary surgeon must be on hand at all times during a procedure under anaesthetic
- There is no strict requirement for this during non-anaesthetic procedures, but it would seem sensible to ensure that advice and support are available for most procedures, certainly when they are being performed for the first time
- Everybody has to learn – don't make extravagant claims about your abilities. This will only lead to disappointment and lack of trust if the procedure is not successful
- Discuss all cases with your colleagues before starting: this way a clear plan can be made, and any alternative ways of treating may be discussed
- Learn to take criticism – well-structured criticism can be very helpful for the future

- Try to adopt a mentor within the practice – this may be a more experienced nurse, or a vet – who will undertake to allow you to perform minor surgery under his/her guidance. This is a way of quickly building up trust and experience

PERSONAL LEARNING, DEVELOPMENT AND SELF-ASSESSMENT

At the time of writing, there is no strict requirement for nurses to complete minimum hours of continuing professional development (CPD). The RCVS does make the point that surgical treatments can become outdated: the implication is that one should keep up to date with techniques. It is recommended that nurses keep a record of their CPD.

Personal learning can be achieved in several ways:

- Revising anatomy and surgical approaches before each procedure
- Reading review articles in journals
- Attending CPD courses
- Attending other practices and centres of excellence
- Discussing cases with colleagues
- Practising (where appropriate) on cadavers or suture dummies
- Being self-critical about cases

The last point is most important: unfortunately, mistakes can occur. Learning from those mistakes requires that you:

- Recognise the mistake and how it occurred
- Ask your colleagues (veterinary surgeons, nurses) whether they have had the same problem
- Listen to their advice and act positively on it

Ultimately, only practice and dedication to detail will allow development. At first, surgical instruments will feel clumsy and awkward. With time, however, familiarity with instruments will come and confidence will follow.

Do not rush: surgery is not a race and haste is a bad thing! Nor is it acceptable to spend too long over a procedure, as this will extend anaesthetic time and occupy theatre time. Competence and confidence will increase speed and safety.

2 The minor surgical patient

OWNER COMMUNICATION

Every year, the Veterinary Defence Society (VDS) handles complaints from owners; these complaints arise as a result of lack of proper communication between the practice and the client.

Owners typically want:

- Reassurance that their pet will be all right
- An estimate of costs, together with an understanding of when payment is due
- Reassurance that there is a full understanding of the pet's problems and a detailed plan of the procedures
- To be kept up to date with their pet's progress

On the other hand, the practice wants from the owner:

- Reassurance that the owner understands what procedures are being carried out
- Understanding of the likely costs
- Any changes in the animal's condition since the appointment was made
- Written permission to perform the procedures and deal with any emergency that may arise
- Contact details in case of emergency

All of the above need to be addressed and, where appropriate, notarised.

Effective owner communication is the best way of avoiding misunderstandings that lead to complaints.

Costs are often a big issue and veterinary bills are often very high. It is up to the owner to decide whether he or she can afford the recommended veterinary treatment, and there should be no embarrassment or shyness over discussing estimates. There should be enough pride in the quality of work carried out at the practice to justify the fee charged.

- The owner should be fully aware of the procedure being undertaken

- Some owners have an unrealistic expectation of surgery: they may assume an instant diagnosis or cure following treatment
- Make certain that the owner understands the need for any patient preparation: some owners, for example, are more upset about fur being shaved than about a large surgical wound
- Be careful to avoid certainties (of diagnosis, treatment costs and prognosis) – some owners will press for an answer where it may be inappropriate to give one
- Make sure the owner is aware of who is performing the surgery – any note should be made of requests for particular surgeons
- Any concerns should be addressed before admission

It is common practice in a human hospital to have a wound attended to by a nurse. The doctor may merely examine the wound and decide on the nature of treatment. Unfortunately, at present, the public perception is that the vet will carry out all procedures, with the veterinary nurse (VN) acting in a more ancillary capacity. That perception will change in time, but only through excellent owner communication and education.

ADMITTING THE PATIENT

Very often, it is the nurse who admits surgical patients to the practice or hospital. It is thus the nurse's responsibility to ensure all of the above points are met. The simple question: 'do you have any questions regarding today's procedure?' is not enough.
- The plan for the patient should be discussed openly, together with any requirements or suggestion for preoperative fluids or blood tests
- Any optional extras such as microchip placement should be discussed (Box 2.1)

Individual appointments should be made for admission wherever possible.
- This focuses attention on the owner and the patient and makes it less likely that anything will be overlooked
- Appointments also highlight the importance of a surgical procedure and make admissions more formal

Box 2.1

Admission of the patient is taken as the effective start of any minor surgical procedure, since it consists of some very important aspects that could affect the subsequent management of the patient.

- This creates an atmosphere of professionalism, which is of benefit to the owner and practice
- Appointments also allow time for the consent form to be completed fully

THE CONSENT FORM

Since a consent form must be signed by the owner when admitting any surgical patient, it makes a great deal of sense for that form to act as a checklist to ensure all points are covered. An example of a consent form is shown in Figure 2.1.

A consent form should clearly have the owner's details, including address and contact numbers.

The pet name, together with the species and breed, should be written, and it is a good idea to have a description of the animal. This becomes especially important if an owner brings in more than one animal! The planned procedures should be written clearly on the form and an estimate should always be given. If the owner declines an estimate, a note should be made on the consent form.

There should be some statement of risk on the consent form: this is often glossed over or ignored by the person admitting the animal, perhaps because it is feared that mentioning risk may alarm or worry the owner. However, this is the most critical part of the form and it is vital that the owner understands the implications of accepting the risk of anaesthesia, surgery or medical treatment.

Anaesthetic deaths in healthy animals are uncommon: recent studies suggest a figure in the order of 1 death in 1000 anaesthetics, and other studies put the figure lower than that in practices with excellent monitoring. Thus, for a minor

The PetScan Clinic

Veterinary Surgery
1 Halstead Street
Lembert
Surrey

19th April 2005

FORM OF CONSENT FOR ANAESTHETIC AND OPERATION

Mr B Smith
Punters Lane
Homeville
Surrey

Contact numbers: 0208 1234567
07973 1234567

Patient: Alfie
Species: Canine
Breed: Labrador
Age: 8 years 5 months
Colour: Yellow
Sex: Male (neutered)
Weight: 25kg
Vaccination status: Vaccinated February 2005
Insurance: Legit, Grabbit and Runn

Operation/procedure: Lumpectomy and histology
Pre-anaesthetic sheet sent: Yes
Last meal: Last night
Pre-anaesthetic blood sample: Yes
IV fluids: Yes (Hartmanns)
Any current medication: Rimadyl 50mg BID
Last given: Last night
Any items left: Collar and lead

Pre GA profile	GHP	PCV	WBC and Diff	Other Urine

Cost estimate: £350 a guide: ✓ detailed:

I hereby give permission for the above animal to be admitted for inpatient tests, treatment, observation and any other procedures that may prove necessary.

I understand that while very care and attention will be given to Alfie, the Practice cannot be held responsible for any untoward events that may occur.

I also understand that while every effort will be made to contact me in the event of unplanned procedures being necessary, the Practice must be permitted to perform any procedures they feel necessary to maintain the well being of Alfie. In extreme cases, this may include euthanasia if undue suffering is occurring and the chances of recovery are thought to be poor.

I understand that the full fee will be payable on release of the animal.

Signed: Bernie Smith (Owner/authorised agent)

Date: 19/4/05

Figure 2.1 Example of a consent form.

surgical procedure on a young animal, it would be reasonable to say something along the lines that, although there is always a risk with any procedure, the risk is small and the practice makes every effort to reduce that risk still further.

Any changes to the planned treatment must be noted on the consent form, along with requirements for intravenous fluids and preanaesthetic blood or urine tests.

- The owner should be given ample time to read the consent form
- Informed consent is crucial, so ensure that the owner understands what he or she is signing
- It may be a good idea to read the consent form out loud after the client has read it
- The consent form should make some reference to the postoperative care of the patient: whether it is expected that the pet will be going home after the surgery, or whether it is intended, or possible, that hospitalisation for one or several days will be required
- The consent form serves not only as a legal document, but also as an aide-mémoire to ensure all treatments are carried out
- Any relevant previous drug reactions should be noted on the form

Once the owner has signed the consent form, it is not advisable to make any alterations or additions to the form.

Also note that it is not acceptable for anyone less than 16 years of age to sign a consent form.

PREANAESTHETIC HISTORY REVIEW, NURSE EXAMINATION AND HEALTH CHECK

During the admission appointment, a review of the clinical history should be performed, to ensure that:

- Any previous anaesthetic problems or drug reactions are noted
- Relevant blood or lab tests are rechecked
- Any change in the clinical condition can be noted (for example, increase or decrease in size of lump, change in position, increase in number)

- Any concurrent illness is considered (for example, diabetes, epilepsy)
- Any prescribed current medication is noted

A full clinical examination should be performed, to include:

- Examination of mucous membranes and evaluation of capillary refill time
- Temperature, pulse and respiration
- Any sign of dehydration
- Any sign of clotting disorder (petechiae, ecchymoses)
- Any concurrent disease (dental disease, skin infections, etc.)
- Any sign of cardiopulmonary disorder (heart murmur, cough, etc.)
- The position of skin masses or wounds should be noted on the consent form

The owner should be questioned as to the pet's current health: has there been any recent diarrhoea or vomiting, lethargy or inappetance, increased or decreased thirst?

If the owner has not previously been informed or advised about preoperative blood or urine tests, or intraoperative intravenous fluids, now is a good time to discuss these. Many practices send out a preanaesthetic leaflet to owners once surgery has been booked: these leaflets discuss the benefits of preanaesthetic testing and intravenous fluids and are to be encouraged.

However, the fact that a leaflet was sent is no guarantee that the client read it! Be prepared to spend time going over any advice given in the leaflet. Remember, what is routine to you may be a highly stressful and unique experience to the client.

Any qualms should be noted and veterinary advice sought either before or after admission, as appropriate. Any concerns which may lead to postponement of surgery are obviously best addressed before admission.

PLANNING OPERATING-THEATRE LISTS AND TIME

Whether the practice is a small, one-vet practice or a large hospital, theatre lists should be prioritised on the basis of:

- Sterility: clean, clean **contaminated**, **contaminated** surgery should be performed in that order
- Health status of patient: aged patients should be operated on before young, healthy patients

There are several reasons for scheduling geriatric patients before young patients:

- Anaesthetic patients will have been starved for several hours, frequently overnight: older patients may have a more catabolic metabolism and require feeding more frequently. Scheduling their surgery early on will mean that they will be able to eat sooner
- The same is true of drinking – water should be left down for geriatric patients until an hour or so before surgery
- Older patients may be more susceptible to stress due to leaving their home environment. Stressed patients should be scheduled early in the day in order to be allowed home as soon as they have recovered properly
- Older or geriatric patients often take longer to recover than young ones. Scheduling an early anaesthetic allows for recovery to take place during the morning and reduces the chance that the patient may need to be hospitalised for an extra night

Other considerations are:

- Arranging a time when more staff will be on duty for long procedures
- Whether to get quick operations out of the way before starting complex ones
- Ensuring that there will be enough kits (or personnel) available for the required number of procedures
- If more than one theatre is available, then one should be designated for **contaminated** procedures, such as dentals
- What postoperative treatment or care is required for a patient? for example, scheduling a routine thoracotomy for a Friday may be a bad idea if there is going to be a reduced staffing level at the weekend to provide aftercare
- What order of surgery will make the most of available personnel?

In any case, when first performing minor surgical procedures, it is important to leave enough time not to feel rushed. Better to reschedule, or allow a more experienced surgeon to perform the surgery, than to panic and operate under pressure. Wherever possible, ensure that when attempting a novel procedure, the rest of the team is experienced and competent within their role (for example, the anaesthetist). In this way, there will be fewer distractions.

3 Premedication and patient preparation

RATIONALE AND REVIEW OF COMMON SEDATIVE/PREMEDICATION DRUGS

General anaesthesia is commonly preceded by premedication with one or, more usually, several drugs. Premedication drugs:
- Reduce the amount of anaesthetic required (injectable and inhalant), so reducing side-effects (and costs!)
- Relax muscles
- Provide analgesia
- Provide sedation
- Suppress vomit reflexes

- May help calm a stressed animal – this makes hospitalisation prior to surgery more comfortable
- May help make the animal easier to handle
- Improve recovery (fewer tremors and less vocalising) – this may be largely due to the analgesic action

The choice of premedication drugs varies according to:
- Practice/vet preference, depending on experience of the drugs: it is always safest to use a drug or a combination of drugs with which the vet is familiar and knows the effects. It is much easier to note any adverse reactions to medication if there is experience of the normal response
- Age or health status of the patient: some drugs may not be licensed for use in immature animals. Conversely, there may be contraindications for the use of certain drugs in an older or unwell animal. For example, acepromazine (ACP) should not be used in animals with epilepsy, as it is may reduce the threshold at which seizures can occur. Morphine should not be used in patients with severe **uraemia**
- Pregnancy: ACP and **opioids** can cause a reduction in fetal blood supply or blood

pressure. Other drugs may have specific contraindications in pregnancy
- Route of injection: it may be difficult or risky attempting to administer an intravenous (IV) injection to a nervous or fractious cat
- Species or breed: ACP should be used with caution in boxers and should be used at reduced dose in greyhounds
- Procedure planned: one should take into account any specific contraindications for certain procedures (for example, ACP should not be administered to patients undergoing myelography). Consideration should also be given to the suitability of drug combinations for specific procedures. For example, using morphine before radiography may be excessive and needlessly extend the **soporific** effect of the anaesthetic. Alternatively, using butorphanol before ligament surgery is unlikely to provide sufficient analgesia
- Concurrent drug usage: butorphanol may antagonise (reverse the effects of) metoclopramide; the use of atropine in patients on long-term corticosteroid treatment may result in increased **intraocular pressure**
- Planned postoperative treatment: if the animal is going to require morphine postoperatively, then including buprenorphine in the premed may cause antagonism of the analgesic effects

COMMONLY USED PREMEDICATION DRUGS

The following list is not exhaustive: it is merely intended as an overview of the most commonly used premedication drugs. Suggestions for preanaesthetic or sedative combinations are shown in Table 3.1. Where a standard proprietary formulation is given, the dose in millilitres per 4-kg cat or 10-kg dog is stated. For convenience, and to avoid unnecessary repetition, the analgesic properties of the drugs are discussed alongside their sedative properties. Doses for analgesia rather than premedication are suggested in Table 3.2.

Acepromazine maleate

- Phenothiazine: the full chemical name is 2-acetyl-10-(3-dimethylaminopropyl)phenothiazine

- It is used extensively as a **tranquilliser** to calm aggressive and apprehensive animals
- Use as a premedicant reduces the amount of injectable and inhalant anaesthetics required
- Often used alone or in combination to provide sedation for minor procedures (ultrasound, dressing changes) or for home medication as a sedative, e.g. for travelling
- Also often used for the management of sound phobias, including fireworks, but this use is contraindicated
- ACP has little or no analgesic action: this must be borne in mind when using it as a sedative for minor procedures
- ACP causes a reduction in arterial pressure: increased doses do not seem to decrease pressure further, but increase the duration of hypotension
- ACP should not be used in animals that are hypovolaemic
- Increased doses do not appear to increase sedation either, but do increase duration
- On occasion, ACP has been seen to increase aggression in dogs and cats, presumably by removing fear of the aggressor
- The IV, IM, SC or oral dose may be used in the dog or cat
- Doses: dogs: 0.01–0.1 mg/kg IV, intramuscularly (IM), subcutaneously (SC), 1–3 mg/kg oral; cats: 0.05–1.0 mg/kg IV, IM, SC, 1–3 mg/kg oral

Atropine

- Atropine is a **parasympatholytic**, blocking acetylcholine (ACh)
- Historically, it was used to decrease salivary and airway secretions during anaesthetics
- Modern inhalant anaesthetics are less irritating to the airways, and so there is little rationale for the routine use of atropine preoperatively these days
- Atropine can increase the occurrence of cardiac dysrrhythmias
- The main uses of atropine now are to facilitate ophthalmic examination by dilating the pupil (mydriasis) or to treat or prevent certain types of **bradycardia** or bradyarrhythmias

Table 3.1 Preanaesthetic or sedative combinations

Drug combination	Proprietary name, concentration supplied	Suggested sedative, preanaesthetic or anaesthetic doses (all IM unless otherwise stated)	Dose/ 10-kg dog (ml)	Dose/ 4-kg cat (ml)
ACP, buprenorphine	ACP (Novartis Animal Health) 2 mg/ml Vetergesic (Alstoe Animal Health) 0.3 mg/ml	**Sedative** ACP: dogs, cats 0.05 mg/kg Vetergesic: 0.01 mg/kg **Preanaesthetic** ACP: dogs 0.02 mg/kg cats 0.05 mg/kg Vetergesic: 0.01 mg/kg	0.25 0.33 0.1 0.13	0.1 0.13 0.1 0.13
Diazepam, ketamine	Diazepam injection (Phoenix Pharma) 5 mg/ml Ketaset (Fort Dodge) 100 mg/ml	**Sedative** Valium: dogs 0.2 mg/kg cats 0.5 mg/kg Ketaset: dogs 11 mg/kg cats 20 mg/kg **Preanaesthetic** Valium: dogs 0.2 mg/kg cats 0.2 mg/kg Ketaset: cats 5 mg/kg	0.4 1.1 0.4	0.4 0.8 0.16 0.2
Midazolam, ketamine	Hypnovel (Roche) 5 mg/ml Ketaset 100 mg/ml	**Sedative** Hypnovel: 0.25 mg/kg Ketaset: dogs 11 mg/kg cats 20 mg/kg	0.5 1.1	0.2 0.8
ACP, morphine	ACP 2 mg/ml Morphine (Evans Pharmaceutical) 10 mg/ml	**Preanaesthetic** ACP: dogs 0.02 mg/kg cats 0.05 mg/kg Morphine: dogs 0.25 mg/kg cats 0.2 mg/kg	0.1 0.25	0.1 0.08
ACP, butorphanol	ACP 2 mg/ml Torbugesic (Fort Dodge) 10 mg/ml	**Sedative/preanaesthetic** ACP: dogs 0.02 mg/kg cats 0.05 mg/kg Torbugesic: dogs 0.1 mg/kg cats 0.4 mg/kg	0.1 0.1	0.1 0.16
Medetomidine, butorphanol (reverse with atipamezole)	Domitor (Pfizer) 1 mg/ml Torbugesic 10 mg/ml Antisedan (Pfizer) 5 mg/ml	**Sedative** Domitor: dogs 0.025 mg/kg cats 0.05 mg/kg Torbugesic: dogs 0.1 mg/kg cats 0.4 mg/kg Reverse with Antisedan **Preanaesthetic** Domitor: dogs only 0.01 mg/kg Torbugesic: dogs 0.1 mg/kg cats 0.4 mg/kg (IM, SC)	0.25 0.1 0.10 0.10	0.2 0.16 0.10 0.16
Medetomidine, butorphanol, ketamine	Domitor 1 mg/ml Torbugesic 10 mg/ml Ketaset 100 mg/ml	**Anaesthetic** Domitor: dogs 0.025 mg/kg cats 0.08 mg/kg Torbugesic: dogs 0.1 mg/kg cats 0.4 mg/kg Ketaset: dogs 5 mg/kg (15 min later in dogs) cats 5 mg/kg Reverse with Antisedan (cats only, after 45 min)	0.25 0.1 0.5	0.32 0.16 0.2 0.16

ACP, acepromazine; IM, intramuscular; SC, subcutaneously.

Table 3.2 Analgesics: dosages and frequency

Drug (generic and trade name, concentration)	Dose and frequency			
	Cats (mg/kg)	ml/4-kg cat	Dogs (mg/kg)	ml/10-kg dog
Morphine (morphine, Evans Pharmaceutical, 10mg/ml)	0.1mg/kg IV 0.1–0.5mg/kg IM SC q 6–8h	0.04ml 0.04–0.2ml	0.1–0.25mg/kg IV IM SC q 4–6h	0.1–0.25ml
Buprenorphine (Vetergesic, Alstoe, 0.3mg/ml)	0.006–0.03mg/kg IV IM SC q 3–6h	0.08–0.39ml	0.006–0.03mg/kg IV IM SC q 3–6h	0.2–1ml
Pethidine (pethidine injection, Arnolds Veterinary Products, 50mg/ml)	2–10mg/kg IM SC q 4–6h	0.16–0.8ml	2–10mg/kg IM SC q 4–6h	0.4–2ml
Fentanyl (fentanyl patch, Durogesic, Janssen-Cilag)	0.004mg/kg transdermally q 3–5 days	25µg/h for cats between 3.2 and 6.8kg	0.004mg/kg transdermally q 3–5 days	25µg/h (3.2–6.8kg) 50µg/h (6.8–18.2kg) 75µg/h (18.2–27.3kg) 100µg/h (> 27.3kg)
Carprofen (Rimadyl small-animal injection, Pfizer, 50mg/ml, Rimadyl tablets 20mg, 50mg)	4mg/kg IV SC prior to anaesthesia Ongoing use contraindicated	0.32ml –	4mg/kg IV SC prior to anaesthesia 4mg/kg PO once daily	0.8ml 2 × 20-mg tablets
Meloxicam (Metacam solution for injection, Boehringer Ingelheim, 5mg/ml, oral suspension 1.5mg/ml)	0.3mg/kg SC prior to surgery. Ongoing use not recommended	0.24ml –	0.2mg/kg IV SC prior to surgery 0.1mg/kg PO once daily	0.4ml 0.75ml
Tepoxalin (Zubrin, Schering-Plough Animal Health, 50mg, 100mg, 200mg oral lyophilisates)	N/A	–	10mg/kg PO once daily	One tablet
Ketoprofen (Ketofen, Merial Animal Health, 10mg/ml, Ketofen tablets 5mg, 20mg)	2mg/kg SC once daily. Not recommended prior to anaesthesia 1mg/kg PO once daily	0.8ml 1 × 5-mg tablet	2mg/kg IV IM SC once daily. Not recommended prior to anaesthesia 1mg/kg PO once daily	2ml $^{1}/_{2}$ × 20-mg tablet
Medetomidine (Domitor, Pfizer, 1mg/ml)	50–100µg/kg IM SC every 3h (sedation outlasts analgesia)	0.2–0.4ml	30–80µg/kg IV IM SC every 3h (sedation outlasts analgesia)	0.3–0.8ml
Ketamine (Ketaset, Fort Dodge Animal Health, 100mg/ml)	0.5–1mg/kg IM SC every 3–4h	0.02–0.04ml	0.5–1mg/kg IM SC every 3–4h	0.05–0.1ml

IV, intravenously; IM, intramuscularly; SC, subcutaneously; PO, orally.

- Doses: dogs/cats: 0.02 mg/kg IV, 0.045 mg/kg IM or SC

Diazepam

- Diazepam is a benzodiazepine
- It has various uses, including as a sedative, **tranquilliser**, anticonvulsant, skeletal muscle relaxant and appetite stimulant (in cats)
- When used alone, diazepam occasionally results in excitation rather than sedation, so it is most often used in combination with another sedative, usually ketamine
- The amount of sedation may vary considerably from patient to patient: an increased dose usually results in an increased duration of action as well as an increased effect
- It is especially useful as a premedicant in epileptic patients, or in patients undergoing myelography
- The oral presentation appears to be quite successful in managing sound phobias such as fireworks
- Care should be used when injecting diazepam IV: **phlebitis** can occur. Extravasation may result in local necrosis and a good deal of pain
- Little or no **analgesia** is provided, although in humans diazepam has an amnesic effect, so that no pain is remembered
- In the author's experience, IV administration of diazepam and ketamine results in a variable degree of sedation in dogs and cats and is usually sufficient for minor procedures such as dressing changes, ultrasound or radiographs (5–20 min of sedation: addition of incremental half-doses of diazepam may extend sedation for a further 20–40 min)
- Dose: dogs/cats: 0.1–0.5 mg/kg IV

Ketamine

- Ketamine is unrelated to any other anaesthetic/sedative agent
- It is effective if administered by any route (IV, SC, IM, oral), making it especially useful for fractious cats (the author has induced anaes-

thesia orally from 10 paces in the case of an extremely aggressive cat, by careful aim)
- There may be some pain with IM injection
- Little cardiac depression is seen with ketamine, although it should be used with caution in patients with severe cardiac disease as it increases the heart muscle's oxygen demand
- Similarly, ketamine results in little or no respiratory depression
- Ketamine is a potent analgesic, even below anaesthetic doses, making it a useful premedicant prior to painful surgery
- A disadvantage of ketamine is that it results in hypertonicity of muscles: patients are quite plastic. This can be offset by concurrent use of a second agent
- Doses: dogs: 11–22 mg/kg IM, IV, SC; cats: 1.0–33 mg/kg IM, SC, IV

Medetomidine

- Medetomidine is an α_2-adrenergic **agonist**
- Good skeletal muscle relaxation, sedation and **analgesia** are induced by administration
- The **analgesia** is more potent against visceral than skeletal pain and is reversed by the **antagonist** (atipamezole)
- There is a great deal of controversy over the cardiovascular effects: there is a dose-dependent reduction in arterial pressure. Cardiac output is at first reduced, then normalises. In general, it should not be used in animals with cardiac dysfunction
- Although IM or IV routes are preferred, absorption from SC injection is good, meaning that intra-animal injection in difficult patients is possible
- Sedation is reversed by administration of atipamezole, making it a very popular drug for quick procedures, especially minor surgical procedures during evening surgery! However, the convenience of a reversible sedative should not result in a slipshod technique: normal precautions of preanaesthetic evaluation, including blood tests and IV fluid therapy, should be observed as appropriate
- Although sedation is generally very good, even apparently well-sedated dogs can, on

occasion, waken extremely rapidly, and bite without warning
- Doses: dogs: 0.01–0.08 mg/kg IV, IM, SC; cats: 0.05–0.15 mg/kg IV, IM, SC

Midazolam

- Midazolam is similar to diazepam; it is another member of the benzodiazepine group of drugs
- As with diazepam, there is little or no analgesic action
- Less irritant to tissues than diazepam, it is unlikely to cause tissue damage if extravasation occurs during IV administration
- Midazolam is shorter-acting than diazepam, but when used in combination with ACP or ketamine, seems to provide a deeper sedation
- Doses: dogs/cats: 0.06–0.3 mg/kg IV, IM, SC

Non-steroidal anti-inflammatory drugs (NSAIDs)

NSAIDs should be administered before anaesthesia in any minor or major surgical procedure unless there are clear contraindications to their use (such as renal impairment or hepatic failure). The increase in **analgesia** perioperatively following the use of a non-steroidal is considerable.

Several NSAIDs are licensed for pre- or postoperative administration in dogs and cats (e.g. carprofen, meloxicam, ketoprofen).

However, NSAIDs do have the potential for severe adverse reactions, including, most notably: gastric ulceration, liver or kidney failure. These side-effects are seen most commonly when NSAIDs are used inappropriately, or outside the data sheet recommendations. Preoperative blood and urine tests, accurate dosing and use of IV fluids all help reduce the risks.

Opioids

- **Opioids** include buprenorphine, butorphanol, fentanyl, morphine and pethidine

- **Opioids** are all related to opium, the drug obtained from a certain type of poppy, *Papaver somniferum*
- **Opioids** work by interacting with opiate receptors present within the central nervous system and throughout the body
- There are various receptor types (μ, δ, κ, σ) which mediate **analgesia**, respiratory depression, **emesis** and other **psychotropic** effects. Different **opioids** are more or less specific for different receptor types, making them stronger or weaker analgesics and respiratory depressants. In general, μ_1-receptors are most important for **analgesia**
- **Opioids** are increasingly used in **epidural** injections to provide very effective prolonged **analgesia** for surgery of the hind limbs, tail and perineum
- All **opioids** tend to cause respiratory depression to some extent, and morphine and butorphanol are very effective cough suppressants
- Although most **opioids** cause **emesis**, butorphanol is a mild antiemetic and may be used before chemotherapeutic administration to reduce vomiting
- **Opioids** tend to reduce gut movement and can cause constipation
- Effects on the cardiovascular system are dose-dependent and generally of little consequence at usual doses

Buprenorphine

- Buprenorphine is a partial μ-opioid **agonist/antagonist**
- It is moderately analgesic
- It is fairly long-acting: between 3 and 8 h
- It is a schedule 3 controlled drug, so must be kept in a locked cupboard, but the dangerous drugs book does not need to be signed each time it is used
- It is rarely used as a premedicant on its own, but it enhances the sedative effect of ACP at low doses of both drugs (the combination of an **opioid** with a **tranquilliser** is known as neuroleptanalgesia)
- The much-maligned bell-shaped curve of dosage suggests that topping up buprenorphine may lead to a reduction in **analgesia**

due to self-antagonism. In fact, this is unlikely to happen at usual doses

- SC injection may markedly reduce the analgesic effect, so IM or IV administration is preferred
- Doses: dogs/cats: 0.006–0.3 mg/kg IV, IM, SC. Can be repeated every 3–6 h

Butorphanol

- Butorphanol is a partial **opioid agonist/antagonist**
- Analgesic action is not as effective as other **opioids**
- It provides good sedation when used with other agents and is commonly used with medetomidine and/or ketamine for dog and cat sedation
- It is not a schedule 3 controlled drug, which has increased its popularity
- It has a quicker onset of action than buprenorphine (15 min or so compared to 30 min for buprenorphine), but a shorter duration of action (around 3 h)
- Doses: dogs/cats: 0.05–0.6 mg/kg IV, IM, SC every 6–8 h

Fentanyl

- Fentanyl is a schedule 2 controlled drug
- It has a very rapid onset of activity (2 min after IV injection), but very short duration of activity (15–20 min). This has made it less popular as a premedication drug, but increasingly popular as an analgesic in a balanced anaesthetic protocol
- It gives approximately 1000 times more potent **analgesia** than morphine
- Fentanyl has a more marked respiratory depressive effect than morphine, and so intermittent positive-pressure ventilation precautions must be on hand
- Slow-release patches are available for ongoing **analgesia** (see later)
- Dose: dogs/cats: 2–10 μg/kg IV

Morphine

- Morphine is the first of the **opioid** alkaloids to be isolated and regarded to be the standard analgesic against which others are measured

- It is a schedule 2 controlled drug, meaning that it must be kept in a locked dangerous drug cupboard to which only veterinary surgeons may have access. The dangerous drugs book must be signed each time morphine is dispensed
- The minor inconvenience this causes, and the concerns for misuse or drug abuse, discourage a lot of practices from using morphine
- It is a powerful analgesic and provides reasonable sedation: sedation is improved when used with ACP
- It is very inexpensive
- The onset of action is much more rapid when administered IM or IV (10–15 min) than when the SC route is used (30–45 min), although the analgesic action appears to be similar with either route
- The duration of activity is fairly short (1–2 h), thus requiring more frequent dosing than buprenorphine or butorphanol
- IV injection should be performed slowly as histamine release (with rapid IV injection) can cause collapse or hyperactivity – these effects are reduced if ACP is used
- Doses: dogs: 0.1–0.25 mg/kg IV, IM, SC every 4–6 h; cats: 0.1 mg/kg IV, 0.1–0.5 mg/kg IM, SC every 6–8 h

Pethidine

- Pethidine is a pure μ-agonist derived from morphine
- It is a schedule 2 controlled drug, thus subject to the same controls as morphine
- It is quick-acting (10 min) but short-lasting (30–45 min)
- It is a fairly strong analgesic, with less of a sedative effect than morphine
- The IV route can cause marked histamine release, so this route is not generally used
- It is probably less useful than some of the other **opioids** due to the short duration of action, although it provides good sedation when used with ACP
- Dose: dogs/cats: 2–10 mg/kg IM, SC every 4–6 h

RECORDING PREANAESTHETIC DRUG ADMINISTRATION

Clear notes should be made of the drug given and the time and route of administration, and any notes made of difficulty or pain on administration. In addition to this, it is good practice to record any visual effects of administration. For example:

'0.1 ml ACP, 0.3 ml buprenorphine administered IM at 9.45 a.m.

10 a.m.: third eyelids protruding, patient appears wobbly.'

INJECTION ROUTES AND TECHNIQUES FOR PREMEDICATION

Generally, IM or IV routes should be used for most premedication combinations. SC routes frequently result in drug absorption or distribution that is too low or slow to provide reasonable sedation and/or **analgesia**. Exceptions are rabbits, where the SC route appears as effective as the IM route for many drugs.

If the IM route is to be used, then:

- Ensure the combination can be given in the same syringe, or else use separate syringes
- Use a fresh needle for each drug to be drawn up
- In deciding which drug to draw up first, as a general rule, draw from a multi-use bottle before a single-use vial, or else draw the larger volume of drug first
- Palpate the injection site to ensure there are no lesions or wounds which may allow for contamination of the injection or be painful
- I prefer to inject over the lumbar area: in my experience this site elicits less pain response from the animals
- If injecting into the hind limb, then use the quadriceps (cranial to the femur): there is a risk of damaging the sciatic nerve if injection into the **caudal** muscle groups is attempted

If the IV route is used, then:

- The skin overlying the vein should be close-clipped and a brief surgical scrub performed
- An IV cannula should be placed: this reduces the risk of extravasation of the drug during administration. It provides a portal for easy access for incremental doses of anaesthetic, or for other drugs. An IV cannula also provides emergency venous access and allows for addition of a fluid administration set

- Have some **sterile** saline at hand in case of accidental perivascular administration (for example, of diazepam). If this occurs, then inject 2–15 ml of **sterile** saline into the injection site. Be very wary of injecting lidocaine to numb the site, as IV injection can have severe or fatal consequences. The application of a local anaesthetic cream (such as Emla cream (*e*utectic *m*ix of *l*ocal *a*nalgesics, AstraZeneca) 5% (lidocaine 25 mg/g, prilocaine 25 mg/g), AstraZeneca) can be very soothing
- If an IV administration set is not to be placed at this stage, the cannula should be flushed with heparinised saline after administration of the premed and an injection bung or stylet placed
- Be careful not to inject too rapidly, as with some drugs this can cause a sudden drop in vasovagal tone, resulting in fainting or collapse. If this happens, then follow standard resuscitation procedures (see Appendix 2)

Having given the premedication, allow sufficient time for it to work before attempting to induce anaesthesia. Most premedication drugs begin to show clinical effects of sedation (ataxia, third eyelid protrusion) 15–20 min after IM injection, 5–10 min after IV injection and up to 45 min after SC injection. However, full analgesic effect may not be achieved until some time after sedation is noted. In general, at least 20–30 min should be allowed after IV or IM injection, and about 1 h following SC injection.

The animal should be left quietly during that time, preferably in a slightly darkened room.

Placement of intravenous cannulae

For a minor surgical patient, a peripheral vein such as the cephalic vein is usually suitable and convenient.

You will need:

- Clippers
- Emla cream

- Cotton wool/swabs
- Surgical scrub solution (chlorhexidine, tri-closan, povidone-iodine)
- 23 G hypodermic needle (for cut-down: optional)
- IV cannula
- Sticky tape (e.g. Durapore tape, 3M) pre-cut into strips of about 10–15 cm (depending on size of patient)
- Bandaging material: OpSite dressing, or Soffban, K-Band, Co-flex
- 2-ml syringe containing heparin flush (1 unit heparin per ml of 0.9% sodium chloride (NaCl))
- **Sterile** bung or stylet

The skin overlying the proposed catheter site should be close-clipped and a small amount of Emla cream applied. Having allowed 20 min for the local anaesthetic cream to take effect, a surgical scrub is performed. An optional step here is to use the end of a 23 G needle to make a small incision over the vein. This has the benefit of reducing the amount of force necessary to insert the catheter and reduces the chance of the sleeve becoming caught or crumpled on the skin.

The catheter is secured in place with a strip of sticky tape (Figure 3.1) and the catheter is flushed with 0.5 ml heparinised saline. If the IV fluid administration set is not due to be connected at this stage, a **sterile** bung or stylet is placed. The catheter is covered with a dressing.

Care of indwelling catheters

Various problems can occur with catheters, even if they are only in place for a relatively short time. The most common problem is for the catheter to become kinked or blocked due to positional placement. To avoid this:

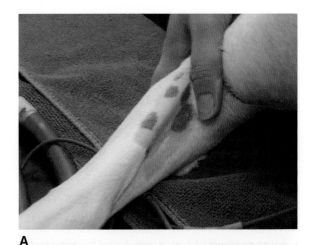
A

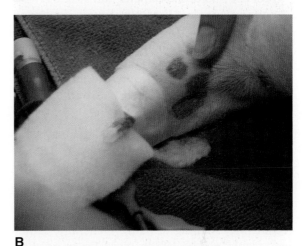
B

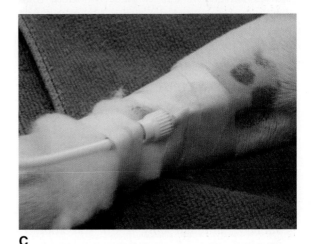
C

Figure 3.1 Placement of cephalic catheter. (A) The skin overlying the catheter site is clipped and a brief surgical prep performed. The vein is raised by an assistant.
(B) The catheter is passed and taped in place. The catheter is flushed with heparinised saline. A pad (Soffban) is placed under the connector site to increase comfort.
(C) The intravenous line is attached and taped into place. Finally, a bandage is placed.

- Always use an appropriately sized catheter for the patient – there is rarely a need to use a 25 G catheter on any but the smallest of kittens or puppies; they will block much more readily than a 23 G
- Always ensure the catheter is placed in the distal third of the limb, if a cephalic catheter, and away from a joint. Most cephalic catheters block because they are placed too close to the elbow. If necessary, a catheter splint may be used, but in the author's experience these are rarely needed if the catheter is correctly placed
- Make sure that the catheter is securely taped over the hub of the catheter and at one or two points along the IV administration set. Avoid using very sticky tapes, as this can irritate skin and be tricky to remove
- Make sure the tape and the overlying bandage are not too tight: rely on padding holding things in place rather than pressure!

The bandage should be checked regularly (at least four times daily) to make sure it has not slipped and is clean and dry.

The catheter should be flushed with heparinised saline four times daily and the catheter site should be checked daily for any signs of **phlebitis** (reddening, swelling or pain). Generally, catheters should not be left in place for more than 3 days, but provided the site is clean and free from inflammation this rule can be stretched a little to spare the patient's other limbs!

BASICS OF SURGICAL FLUID ADMINISTRATION

Although our minor surgical patients should be otherwise healthy, and we would hope that the anaesthetic time is short, it is good practice to administer IV fluids to all anaesthetised patients. There are various reasons for this:

- The patient will have been starved prior to surgery: although only 4–6 h starvation is required, many of our patients will have been starved for much longer, often for 17 h or so. It is not necessary to withhold water from

anaesthetic patients, but most cats and many dogs will not drink adequate quantities of water at home without eating and may not drink at all in the veterinary practice
- The premedication and the anaesthetic will reduce cardiovascular function to some degree, often reducing cardiac output and renal perfusion
- IV fluid administration during surgery ensures the presence of a patent venous access at all times, should emergencies occur, or for routine administration of IV drugs during surgery
- Although most minor surgery patients are expected to go home the same day, maintaining IV fluid administration during their recovery ensures that the patient does not become dehydrated postoperatively and is prepared for ongoing hospitalisation if that becomes necessary

Which fluids? What rate?

Table 3.3 lists the most common IV fluids and suggested usage. For most minor surgery patients, 0.9% NaCl or lactated Ringer's (Hartmann's solution) will be most appropriate.

Fluids should be administered at maintenance rate (2 ml/kg per h) until anaesthesia, and increased to 5–10 ml/kg per h during anaesthesia. Depending on length of surgery and recovery of patient, the fluid rate should then be reduced back to maintenance until the patient is eating. An easy calculation chart is presented in Table 3.4.

As with any patient on IV fluid therapy, minor surgical patients should be monitored for urine production: cats may not use a litter tray in a cage, in which case regular palpation (every 3 h or so) of the bladder is recommended. Dogs should be taken out to urinate regularly (every 3–4 h) and the bladder palpated if not urinating.

If reduced urine output is suspected, the patient should be catheterised and urine production monitored. Urine output lower than 1 ml/kg per h suggests renal perfusion is reduced.

Table 3.3 Common fluids for intravenous administration

Fluid type	Main composition	Application
NaCl 0.9% (Aqupharm No. 1, AnimalCare)	Na^+ 154 mmol/l Cl^- 154 mmol/l K^+ 0 mmol/l	Correction of water and electrolyte depletion, especially after vomiting. Not suitable for prolonged administration
NaCl 0.9%, glucose 5% (Aqupharm No. 3, AnimalCare)	Na^+ 154 mmol/l Cl^- 154 mmol/l Glucose 50 g/l	Correction of water and electrolyte depletion, where there has also been reduction in carbohydrate intake. Indicated for addisonian crisis and urethral obstruction. Not suitable for prolonged administration
Ringer's solution (Aqupharm No. 9, AnimalCare)	Na^+ 147 mmol/l Cl^- 155 mmol/l K^+ 4 mmol/l Ca^{2+} 2 mmol/l	Correction of water and electrolyte depletion, especially after prolonged vomiting, where loss of potassium is likely to have occurred
Hartmann's solution (Ringer's lactate) (Aqupharm No. 11, AnimalCare)	Na^+ 131 mmol/l Cl^- 111 mmol/l K^+ 5 mmol/l Ca^{2+} 2 mmol/l HCO_3^- (lactate) 29 mmol/l	As above, but more suitable for prolonged use and for treatment of metabolic acidosis. This is the most versatile of crystalloids and can be used in most fluid therapy cases
NaCl 0.18%, glucose 4% (Aqupharm No. 18, AnimalCare)	Na^+ 30 mmol/l Cl^- 30 mmol/l Glucose 40 g/l	Maintenance therapy, having already corrected water and electrolyte depletion
Hypertonic saline (7.5%) Sanofi Animal Health	Na^+ 1283 mmol/l Cl^- 1283 mmol/l	Management of severe shock. Not suitable for prolonged administration. Must only be administered intravenously
Haemaccel (Intervet UK)	Na^+ 147 mmol/l Cl^- 155 mmol/l K^+ 5 mmol/l Ca^{2+} 5 mmol/l Gelatin (average molecular weight 30 000) 35 g/l	As a plasma volume expander in cases of shock. Not suitable for prolonged use
Oxyglobin (Arnolds Veterinary Products)	Bovine haemoglobin 130 g/l	To improve clinical signs of anaemia in cats and dogs. Not suitable for prolonged use

NaCl, sodium chloride.

Table 3.4 Intravenous fluid rates

Weight of patient (kg)	Rate of fluid administration: 1 drop every ____ seconds (AnimalCare burette set 60 drops/ml) (drops/second)		Weight of patient (kg)	Rate of fluid administration: 1 drop every ____ seconds (AnimalCare giving set 20 drops/ml) (drops/second)	
	2 ml/kg per h	10 ml/kg per h		2 ml/kg per h	10 ml/kg per h
1	30	6			
2	15	3			
3	10	2			
4	7.5	1.5			
5	6	1.2			
6	5	1	6	15	3
7	4.3	0.86 (1.2)	7	12.8	2.6
8	3.8	0.75 (1.3)	8	11.3	2.2
9	3.3	0.67 (1.5)	9	10	2
10	3	0.6 (1.7)	10	9	1.8
			12	7.5	1.5
			14	6.4	1.3
			16	5.6	1.1
			18	5	1
			20	4.5	0.9 (1.1)
			25	3.6	0.7 (1.4)
			30	3	0.6 (1.7)
			35	2.6	0.5 (2)
			40	2.2	0.45 (2.2)
			45	2	0.4 (2.5)
			50	1.8	0.35 (2.9)
			55	1.6	0.33 (3)
			60	1.5	0.3 (3.3)

ANALGESIC DRUGS AND PAIN MANAGEMENT

Table 3.2 lists analgesic drug dosages and frequencies.

Balanced analgesia

The perception of pain evolved as a protective measure: it allows the body to realise injury has occurred and to avoid using and thus further damaging the traumatised region. Pain in our patients is unnecessary, as in general we have corrected the trauma.

In response to clinically induced pain, the peripheral and central nervous systems become sensitised (the so-called 'wind-up' of pain). This leads to increased perception of pain and reduces the efficacy of analgesics. Pre-emptive **analgesia** counters this sensitisation. By using more than one form of analgesic we can suppress several pain pathways (sequential **analgesia**) and increase analgesic effect tremendously. It is not acceptable to assume that dogs or cats feel pain any differently from ourselves and so we should not deny them any pain relief.

Recognition of pain in animals

In order to manage pain, it is necessary to recognise pain in our minor surgical patients. Clearly, any wound or trauma must be considered painful: this includes any wound that we may inflict through surgery.

Animals in pain may:
- Vocalise when touched over a painful area or when moving a painful limb or part of the body
- Pant or have an increased respiratory rate or heart rate
- Become aggressive or fearful: try to attack or to hide
- Become inappetent
- Sit hunched, reluctant to move, or else become restless and not settle

Apart from being unpleasant for the patient, pain slows healing, both directly and by reducing food intake or creating disuse atrophy of operated limbs.

It is a good idea to use some sort of scoring system for pain, so that individual patients can be more effectively assessed and monitored. Pain monitoring should be an integral part of the hospitalisation chart.

Very young or very old patients may have reduced pain thresholds: they will also have reduced drug metabolism and excretion. In these patients it may be best to use stronger and more rapidly metabolised drugs such as pethidine, rather than buprenorphine. Some breeds may feel pain more than others (e.g. labradors appear more stoical than greyhounds).

An outdated argument for withholding analgesic is that a small amount of pain will result in the animal restricting its movement postsurgery, thus preventing disruption of the wound site or fracture. This is not to be recommended for several reasons:
- How can a small amount of pain be quantified? It is likely that a reduction in **analgesia** will leave the patient in agony or severe discomfort at the very least
- A repair should be strong or stable enough that the patient's own movement will not damage the repair. If not, then the technique of repair should come under question

There is overwhelming evidence that pain reduces healing: this is likely to occur through metabolic/physiologic mechanisms, and also through disuse atrophy, of an affected limb, for example.

Other forms of pain management

The use of sequential pain blockade has already been mentioned, using several drugs that interact at different stages along the pain pathways to prevent the build-up of pain. In addition to NSAIDs and **opioids**, local anaesthetics, **epidurals**, bandages and good old tender loving care may be used to manage pain.

Fentanyl patches

Continuous absorption of fentanyl from transdermal patches is a useful way of providing prolonged **analgesia** postoperatively. The patches are available in a variety of sizes (Table 3.2) and can give approximately 3 days of **analgesia** in dogs and cats. A drawback is that it can take 24h to reach therapeutic concentrations in dogs. Guidelines for use are:

- Hair over the lateral thorax or neck should be clipped, but not cleaned with alcohol or surgical scrub as this may affect the absorption
- Gloves should be worn to apply the patch
- Bandages may be applied to help hold the patch in place. Tissue adhesives can affect the absorption of the patch and should not be used
- Patches must be stored in the dangerous drugs cupboard and signed out. Used patches should be flushed down a toilet in the presence of a witness
- Patients should be regularly assessed for adequate **analgesia**, respiratory depression and sedation
- Due to the risk of accidental contact, care must be exercised when allowing patients with patches to go home

Local anaesthesia

Local anaesthetics are underused in small-animal practice, although they are a fundamental component of large-animal and equine surgery.

Local anaesthetics may be used in minor veterinary surgery in several ways: topical or surface, infiltration, nerve block/paravertebral blocks, **epidural** and IV regional.

Topical anaesthesia
- This involves direct application of a local anaesthetic to skin or mucous membrane. Emla cream is most commonly applied direct to skin: in general, however, penetration through cornified epidermis is poor
- Eye drops containing tetracaine are used to examine or perform minor corneal surgery: the penetration through the cornea is good
- Local anaesthetic can be applied directly to wounds to numb them before surgery, or whilst preparing the patient or theatre for surgery. It is questionable how successful this is, as the

anaesthetic is fairly rapidly removed from the area by the circulatory system
- The application of local anaesthetic (Emla cream or an injectable trickled on) to a patch of wet eczema seems to provide moderate relief to the patient
- Topical application of local anaesthetic is most often used before taking blood samples or placing IV cannulae or naso-oesophageal tubes

Infiltration anaesthesia
- This is the most usual way of using local anaesthesia and involves injecting small amounts (1–2 ml in 0.1–0.2-ml blebs) around a wound or a surgical site
- Local anaesthetics often sting on injection and can cause quite a strong pain response. It is recommended that local anaesthetic injection be performed after general anaesthesia is induced
- Injecting local anaesthetic before making an incision seems to be quite effective at decreasing postoperative pain in the area (Figure 3.2). There is little point in injecting local anaesthetic after the incision has been made
- A specific form of infiltration anaesthesia may be used when amputating tails in cases of tail tip trauma (see Chapter 8). Especially in cats,

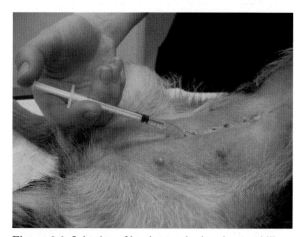

Figure 3.2 Injection of local anaesthesia prior to midline bitch spay.

use of local anaesthetic in this way reduces postoperative self trauma

- Care must be taken not to inject the local anaesthetic intravenously, nor to inject too much. This is of particular importance when dealing with very young or very small patients (the maximum dose for lidocaine is 10 mg/kg)
- The presence of local anaesthetic in a wound can retard healing or reduce blood supply. This is rarely of anything other than theoretical importance with small doses of local anaesthetic, but may become a problem if adrenaline (epinephrine) is present in the local anaesthetic, resulting in necrosis of the wound edges due to vasoconstriction

Nerve blocks/paravertebral blocks
- Local anaesthetic is injected into the area directly surrounding a nerve in a distal limb or a spinal nerve as it exits the intervertebral foramen
- This approach is of more use in cattle or horses, where local anaesthesia is used instead of general anaesthesia
- It is used most routinely in thoracic surgery in small animals, where the intercostal nerves running along the **caudal** surface of the ribs may be blocked dorsally, providing 3–4 h of good **analgesia** following paracostal incisions
- It may be useful in digit amputations, although infiltration anaesthesia is easier to perform in small animals

Epidural anaesthesia
- This approach involves administration of local anaesthetic into the **epidural** space in the lumbar region
- Injection must be performed on an anaesthetised or sedated patient to reduce the risk of damage to the spinal cord
- This procedure is becoming more popular and affords a prolonged numbing period for the hind limbs, tail and perineum
- It must be performed by a veterinary surgeon
- Addition of morphine to the **epidural** mix (0.1 mg/kg) may extend **analgesia** to around 24 h

Intravenous regional anaesthesia
- Local anaesthesia is injected intravenously into a distal limb, having temporarily occluded circulation in the limb with a tourniquet
- This achieves surgical anaesthesia in that limb for as long as the tourniquet remains in place, usually 30–120 min
- Care must be taken not to allow the tourniquet to loosen before about 30 min, as there is a risk of IV local anaesthetic then entering systemic circulation and stabilising the cardiac neuronal pathways
- After 30 min or so, most of the local anaesthetic has diffused from the blood vessels and the tourniquet may be safely removed
- The technique is popular in human surgery, but is probably more applicable to large-animal surgery where general anaesthesia is avoided wherever possible

Although local anaesthetics can and may be used to improve **analgesia** perioperatively in small animals, it should rarely be used instead of general anaesthesia. Although it is tempting to avoid the need for a full general anaesthesia in some cases, small animals are difficult to restrain adequately for a reasonable amount of time, and movement can compromise asepsis and lead to poor technique and a rushed job.

Veterinary acupuncture

Increasingly, acupuncture is being used in companion animals to supplement western medication. One of the major applications is in controlling chronic pain in conditions such as arthritis or **neoplasia**. Although not used extensively for postoperative pain, it seems likely that acupuncture may provide further **analgesia** in these cases. However, considerable training is required to become proficient at acupuncture, since its correct use requires knowledge of highly specific anatomical points and combinations of needle placements. Acupuncture in animals is considered an act of veterinary surgery and as such can only be performed by qualified and registered veterinary surgeons.

PRE- AND POSTOPERATIVE ANTIBIOTICS

The aim of perioperative antibiosis is to prevent the growth of contaminating bacteria from the patient's skin or environment from multiplying to high enough numbers to cause infection. Another aim is to reduce bacterial numbers prior to surgery to levels where contamination of surgical wounds is unlikely to occur.

This is a contentious issue, as there are often strong feelings about whether or not to administer antibiotics pre- or postoperatively.

- For routine clean surgery (castration, spay, **lumpectomy**): as long as strict aseptic technique is followed, and the patient is not immunocompromised, there is no requirement for perioperative antibiotics
- For clean surgery where there has been a breach in aseptic technique (for example, drape slippage): antibiotics should be administered intraoperatively and postoperatively
- For clean surgery that takes an appreciable amount of time (usually over 120 min): perioperative antibiotics should be administered
- For clean surgery where any infection would be catastrophic (spinal surgery, joint surgery): perioperative antibiotics should be administered
- For clean **contaminated** surgery (surgery of the gastrointestinal tract, urinary tract): perioperative antibiotics should be administered
- For **contaminated** surgery (**abscess**-lancing, dental surgery): perioperative antibiotics should be administered, plus a follow-up course of antibiotics

Which antibiotic to use?

Antibiotic choice is influenced by:
- The type of bacteria expected
- Distribution of antibiotic to the surgical area
- Any known or suspected contraindications to that antibiotic, with regard to type of surgery

(for example, gentamicin is known to retard corneal healing and so would be a poor choice following corneal surgery)
- Any history of hypersensitivity or adverse reaction to that antibiotic or a related one (for example, do not use any β-lactam antibiotic in a patient known or suspected to be allergic to penicillin). Similarly, do not send the patient home on a β-lactam antibiotic if the owner is known or suspected to be allergic to penicillin
- Other factors such as palatability of tablets if an ongoing course of antibiotics is to be prescribed, known breed sensitivities to antibiotics (avoid trimethoprim/sulfonamide combinations in breeds prone to dry eye (**keratoconjunctivitis sicca**))

Bearing in mind that wounds in small animals tend to culture *Escherichia coli* or coagulase-positive *Staphylococcus* spp., it is recommended that an antibiotic that targets these organisms be used.

A good choice is a second-generation cephalosporin, such as cefuroxime (Zinacef, Glaxo) 20–50 mg/kg IV, IM.

Administration intravenously at the time of induction is recommended. Due to perioperative reduction in skin vasculature perfusion, SC administration is likely not to result in a rapid enough absorption of antibiotic to be of any benefit during the surgery.

It is often tempting to administer intralesional antibiotics (intra-abdominal during exploratory **laparotomy** or intra-articular during joint surgery) as one feels that delivering antibiotics right where they are required must be helpful. However, there is little evidence to suggest that antibiotics are of much benefit as they are usually absorbed from the site fairly rapidly. Nevertheless, slow-release antibiotic formulations such as gentamicin-soaked beads can be very useful in controlling or treating some chronically infected wounds.

4 General anaesthesia

THE ROLE OF THE VETERINARY NURSE IN ANAESTHESIA

There are various laws concerning the use of anaesthesia in veterinary practice:

- Protection of Animals (Anaesthetics) Act 1964 – very few procedures can be carried out without anaesthesia: castration in some species below a certain age, tail docking, dewclaw removal, disbudding of < 1-week-old calves
- Misuse of Drugs Act 1971 – this restricts storage and use of various anaesthetic and analgesic agents

- Control of Substances Hazardous to Health (CoSHH) 1988 – restricts the use and storage of various anaesthetic and analgesic agents
- Veterinary Surgeons Act 1966 – with schedule 3 amendments. As discussed in Chapter 1, this dictates the role of veterinary nurses (VNs) in anaesthesia and allows that, provided the veterinary surgeon is physically present during induction and otherwise immediately on hand, a qualified, listed VN may:
  - Administer the selected pre- and postoperative analgesic or sedative
  - Administer prescribed non-incremental anaesthetic agents on the instruction of the directing veterinary surgeon (in other words, induce anaesthesia: for this, the veterinary surgeon must be physically present)
  - Monitor clinical signs and maintain an anaesthetic record
  - Maintain anaesthesia. This may be by repeating injection of intravenous (IV) anaesthetic or by adjusting the volatile anaesthetic concentration. In either case, it should be done under the direct supervision of the veterinary surgeon

The role of the VN in anaesthesia is therefore to administer anaesthetics when directed by a veterinary surgeon, to monitor the anaesthetic and make adjustments to the level of anaesthesia, and, importantly, to maintain an anaesthetic record. This chapter aims to address that role and to provide a brief, practical summary of anaesthetic drugs and monitoring.

RATIONALE AND REVIEW OF COMMONLY USED DRUGS

Most small-animal surgical patients require a general anaesthetic. General anaesthetics fall into two main categories:

1. Injectable. IV administration of the agent results in loss of consciousness of the patient for a period. Depending on the agent, repeated injections may be given to maintain anaesthesia, or else it may be continued by the addition of an inhalant (volatile) agent
2. Inhalant anaesthetic. With some agents or patients it is possible to induce anaesthesia in this way; it is more usual, however, to induce with an injectable and maintain with an inhalant (or volatile) agent

The choice of anaesthetic or anaesthetic technique depends on:
- Practice facilities, equipment, drugs and personal experience
- Skill and experience of the team: in a small-practice situation it may be wiser to keep to a simple anaesthetic protocol than a complex one involving many different drugs
- Postoperative recovery facilities
- Temperament of patient, ease of handling
- Species and breed of animal: some breeds may be less tolerant to some anaesthetics than others: for example, greyhounds take a much longer time to recover from thiopental anaesthesia than labradors
- Age and general health of patient: for example, methohexitone should not be used in patients with epilepsy as it can reduce the seizure threshold
- Site of surgery proposed: oral surgery may necessitate the use of different anaesthetics than abdominal surgery. Thoracic surgery will

demand circuits that enable intermittent positive-pressure ventilation (IPPV)
- Type of surgery: for example, the practice's usual choice of anaesthetic may not be ideal for caesarean section
- Length of anaesthetic: a brief examination under anaesthesia may only require an injectable anaesthetic, whereas intubation and maintenance on inhalant anaesthetic are preferred for longer procedures

Injectable anaesthetics

Injectable anaesthetics may be used in a variety of ways:
- Induction of general anaesthesia prior to maintenance by **volatile agent** (or to top up volatile anaesthesia during a procedure)
- Sole general anaesthetic agent, whether as a single injection for brief procedures, or by repeated injections, or constant infusion. Some agents (such as propofol) are ideal as constant-infusion anaesthetics, being very short-acting and rapidly metabolised or distributed. Others, such as thiopental, are redistributed or metabolised slowly and constant infusion results in cumulative overdosage
- Treatment for **status epilepticus**, or toxin-induced seizures (for example, metaldehyde poisoning)
- Long-term sedation, for example, in critical care units

Individual agents will be considered in the next section. In general, the advantages of injectable anaesthetics are:
- They are simple to use, requiring little specialist equipment
- They are rapid- and either short- or ultrashort-acting
- They are not irritating to airways

Disadvantages are that:
- With the exception of ketamine, they require IV access, which may be difficult for aggressive animals
- Some agents (such as thiopental) are extremely irritant if administered perivascularly

- Once administered, they cannot be withdrawn
- Any adverse effects or overdosage must be controlled until the agent is metabolised or redistributed
- Most injectable anaesthetics result in temporary hypotension, or respiratory depression

The following is a summary of the more commonly used injectable anaesthetics.

Barbiturates

Barbiturate anaesthetics include phenobarbital, pentobarbitone, thiopental and methohexitone. Only thiopental and methohexitone are routinely used for general anaesthesia in small animals, although pentobarbitone is occasionally used in the treatment of **status epilepticus** and strychnine poisoning.

Barbiturates have little or no analgesic effect.

Thiopental (Thiovet, Novartis Animal Health UK)
- One of the older injectable anaesthetics, thiopental is still very popular due to its low cost and the small volume required to induce anaesthetic in large dogs
- Thiopental is highly lipid-soluble, resulting in quick transfer across the blood–brain barrier and hence quick-acting
- It is strongly alkaline (pH 14). This makes it highly irritant and results in pain and local tissue damage if injected perivascularly. It should only be administered via an IV catheter and should be used at the low concentration (1.25%)
- Thiopental crosses the placenta well, and may result in stupor and respiratory depression of the fetus. As a result it is not recommended for caesarean section
- It causes respiratory depression (especially in cats), hypotension and **apnoea** and reduces cardiac output. Metabolism (by the liver) is fairly slow and so recovery depends on redistribution to other tissues. As mentioned before, it is therefore unsuitable as a constant-infusion anaesthetic. Since greyhounds have very little

body fat, recovery in this and related breeds can be very slow
- Dose: 20 mg/kg dogs; not recommended for cats. Dose to effect

Methohexitone (Brietal, Eli Lilly – discontinued)
- Methohexitone is strongly alkaline, but less irritant than thiopental; perivascular administration does not result in tissue damage
- It is ultra-short-acting. Less 'hangover' effect is seen than with thiopental as redistribution and metabolism occur more rapidly. Animals with hepatic insufficiency will have prolonged recovery times and methohexitone is not recommended in these patients
- Greyhounds have a 2–3 times faster recovery than with thiopental
- Dose: cat: 5.7 mg/kg; dogs: <14 kg, 7.3 mg/kg; <14 kg, 5.5 mg/kg

Steroid anaesthetics

Alphaxalone/alphadolone (Saffan, Schering-Plough Animal Health)
- Two progesterone derivatives, alphaxalone and alphadolone, are combined together with a castor oil-derivative Cremophor to increase solubility
- The Cremophor component can cause acute anaphylaxis in dogs, and so Saffan should not be used in this species
- At the time of writing, Saffan is no longer being produced, but stores of the drug remain and so it is still in use
- It is used in cats, birds and small furry animals, but it has been widely superseded by newer **volatile agents** and propofol
- Saffan has a fairly wide safety margin, making it popular since a 'standard cat dose' can be given!
- It is metabolised rapidly by liver, so it is fairly short-acting (5–20 min), meaning that it can be topped-up or used as a total IV anaesthesia
- It provides good muscle relaxation
- It is not irritant to tissues
- A mild anaphylaxis is seen in some cats, resulting in oedema of paws and ears. In some cases

this can be marked, requiring treatment with IV corticosteroids
- Saffan provides moderate **analgesia**
- Although general anaesthesia is best achieved by IV administration; intramuscular (IM) injection results in reasonably deep sedation for 5–10 min, so that minor procedures such as radiography can be carried out
- Dose: cats: 9 mg/kg, 2.5–3.5 ml/cat

Ketamine (Ketaset, Fort Dodge Animal Health)
- Already discussed in Chapter 3 as a dissociative premedicant/sedative, ketamine provides a good level of anaesthesia
- Ketamine is effective by most routes, even oral
- Although not irritant to tissues, IM injection appears to be painful to many cats
- It is rapidly metabolised in the liver, with a very variable duration of action, ranging from 15 to 60 min after IM injection
- Ketamine has good analgesic properties and maintains cardiac output
- It can cause hypertension in certain instances
- It causes excessive salivation in cats; patients may benefit from premedication with atropine
- Postanaesthesia delirium can appear alarming
- Use as a sole agent results in plasticity of the patient, with hypertonicity of muscles. These effects are reduced when used in combination with other agents such as acepromazine (ACP), benzodiazepines, **opioids**, barbiturates and α_2-agonists
- Dose: cats: 11–33 mg/kg IM, IV, subcutaneously (SC). Dogs: 11–22 mg/kg. Not recommended as the sole agent for dogs due to postanaesthetic hyperactivity and delirium

Propofol (Rapinovet, Schering-Plough Animal Health)
- Propofol is a phenol-type chemical, presented as a white emulsion
- It has become one of the most popular injectable anaesthetics due to its properties and ease of use in many species

- It is ultra-fast-acting and cleared rapidly from the body, presumably by sites outside the liver, although the method of metabolism is still uncertain. Recovery is smooth
- Propofol is non-irritant to tissues, but has little or no effect unless given IV
- Rapid IV injection often causes temporary **apnoea**. As with most injectable anaesthetics, propofol causes a dose-related reduction in blood pressure and cardiac output
- As it is cleared so quickly, it is suitable as a maintenance anaesthetic and may be given by constant infusion over prolonged periods of time without apparent ill-effects. It is often used to treat **status epilepticus** for this reason
- Propofol is very mildly analgesic, but not clinically effective
- It is suitable for use in animals with liver failure
- The emulsion is protein-rich and can act as an effective bacterial culture medium. For this reason, propofol should be kept in the fridge when not in use and opened vials or bottles should be discarded within 24 h
- Dose: cats: unpremedicated 8 mg/kg, premedicated 6 mg/kg; dogs unpremedicated 6.5 mg/kg, premedicated 4 mg/kg, only IV

Inhalant (volatile) anaesthetics

Volatile or inhalant anaesthetics require sophisticated machinery to deliver a constant and precise concentration of agent as a percentage of carrier gas (usually oxygen (O_2)). They may be administered directly through an endotracheal (ET) tube, thus requiring prior induction by an injectable agent, or used to induce anaesthesia by 'masking down' or placing the patient in some form of anaesthetic chamber.

Although the newer **volatile agents** such as sevoflurane have less fragrant aromas, most inhalant anaesthetics smell unpleasant and are poorly tolerated by small animals when used to induce anaesthesia by masking down.

Solubility is an important factor in the uptake and distribution of volatile anaesthetics and distinguishes the agents from each other. The importance of solubility will be discussed later. The most soluble of these agents in blood is ether, then methoxyflurane, nitrous oxide (N_2O), halothane, then isoflurane, with sevoflurane and desflurane being least soluble of all. The lower the solubility, the quicker the induction and recovery.

The other important factor to take into account when considering volatile anaesthetics is the minimum alveolar concentration (MAC: Box 4.1). Generally, the lower the MAC, the more potent the **volatile agent**.

The most commonly used inhalant anaesthetics are briefly discussed below. Ether is rarely used these days due to its irritant action on mucous membranes and its highly flammable nature, but it is mentioned for comparison.

Ether (Ether, JM Loveridge)

- Ether was the first general anaesthetic agent to be used, in 1842
- It is a colourless, highly volatile liquid that is highly flammable
- It is very low cost
- Ether is safe for operating-room personnel (no long-term adverse reactions have been reported)
- It has a very wide safety margin and high level of **analgesia** (although it is irritant to mucous membranes)
- Induction and recovery by ether are fairly slow
- The flammable nature precludes its use with **cautery** instruments

Box 4.1

MAC: minimum alveolar concentration = the lowest concentration of anaesthetic in the alveoli that is required to produce anaesthesia in 50% of patients. MAC differs between species for different agents.

Methoxyflurane (Metofane, C-Vet – discontinued)

- Methoxyflurane is a fairly soluble inhalant anaesthetic, resulting in slow induction and recovery, so it is not recommended for induction
- The high solubility also makes it difficult to adjust the level of anaesthesia accurately or quickly
- It has a very low MAC (0.23%, as opposed to 0.87% for halothane), so it is highly potent. Low concentrations are required to induce and maintain anaesthesia
- Methoxyflurane produces excellent **analgesia** and muscle relaxation
- It is not hepatotoxic, but nevertheless it is not recommended in animals with liver disease
- It can be difficult to monitor levels of anaesthesia as palpebral and pedal reflexes are abolished at an early stage

Halothane (Fluothane, Pitman-Moore)

- Halothane is a member of the group of volatile anaesthetics known as halogenated ethanes
- It is less soluble than ether or methoxyflurane; it is thus faster-acting and recovery is quicker, making it suitable for induction, although it is odd-smelling and tends to cause unpleasant inductions
- The MAC value is higher than methoxyflurane – 0.87% in dogs and 1.19% in cats
- Halothane is not a very good analgesic
- It can cause arrhythmias (it sensitises the myocardium to catecholamines), and has a marked dose-dependent cardiac-depressant activity
- It is not suitable for patients with cardiac disease
- Halothane is mildly toxic to liver; this toxicity increases with raised carbon dioxide (CO_2) levels (**hypercapnia**). The liver toxicity seems to be cumulative: this has led to concerns over operating-room personnel, and was partially responsible for the introduction of mandatory scavenging of anaesthetic gases

Isoflurane (Isocare, AnimalCare)

- Isoflurane is another halogenated ethane, which has become more popular than halothane in recent years
- It has a higher MAC than halothane (1.5% in dogs, 1.61% in cats), but is less soluble, so induction and recovery are faster than halothane, with almost no 'hangover'. It is thus suitable for induction
- Recovery from anaesthesia tends to be fairly smooth
- Isoflurane may be used to induce and maintain anaesthesia safely in many species other than dogs and cats, including reptiles, birds and small rodents
- The relative expense of isoflurane is offset by its wide range of applications, and speed of induction and recovery
- Isoflurane is not metabolised by the liver, so it is not believed to be hepatotoxic. Only time will prove or disprove its safety to operating-room personnel
- The degree of cardiac depression is similar to halothane, but isoflurane is not arrhythmogenic
- Good muscle relaxation is achieved, like halothane, but there is a similar lack of **analgesia**

Sevoflurane (Sevoflo, Abbott)

- The newest licensed volatile anaesthetic agent, sevoflurane is more expensive than other agents
- Its very low solubility means that induction and recovery are extremely rapid. Added to this, the smell does not seem to be as noxious to cats and dogs, making masking down smoother
- The MAC value in dogs is 2.36%, meaning that more is used than isoflurane
- Some **analgesia** is seen, although this is believed to be minimal
- The greater expense, coupled with the higher usage, means that, at present, it may only be economically viable to use sevoflurane in closed anaesthetic systems

Desflurane (Desflurane, Minrad)

- MAC in dogs is between 7 and 10%: the variation in MAC seems to be due to several factors, including the temperament of the animal
- Desflurane is even less soluble than sevoflurane, with a correspondingly quicker induction and recovery
- It causes less reduction in tissue perfusion than isoflurane
- It causes airway irritation in humans, although this does not seem to be the case with dogs and cats
- It boils at close to room temperature, so it cannot be used in conventional vaporisers: it requires electronically controlled vaporisers
- As with sevoflurane, the greater expense of desflurane limits its use to low-flow or closed circuits

Nitrous oxide (BOC Gases)

- Its high MAC value (around 200% in dogs and cats) makes it impossible to use as a sole anaesthetic agent: hypoxia occurs long before anaesthesia!
- However, at subanaesthetic doses, N_2O is a very good analgesic (provided it comprises at least 50% of inspired gas). Note that there is no ongoing **analgesia** with N_2O: as soon as the gas is switched off, so is the **analgesia**
- It is usually administered with other anaesthetic gases to increase **analgesia** and decrease the amount of volatile anaesthetic agent required to maintain anaesthesia (optimal ratio of O_2 to N_2O = two-thirds N_2O to one-third O_2)
- N_2O should not be used in patients with respiratory compromise
- Nor should N_2O be used in patients with **pneumothorax** or **pneumoperitoneum**. The reason for this is that N_2O diffuses more rapidly into pockets of air, causing an increase in trapped gas
- For the above reason, N_2O should be withheld from an anaesthetised patient for the last 5–10 min of anaesthesia

Summary

Unfortunately, there is no such thing as an ideal anaesthetic (injectable or volatile): certainly there is no anaesthetic combination that will suit all anaesthetic cases. Whereas with injectable agents it may be possible to stock a range within the practice, with volatile anaesthetics a specific vaporiser is required with each agent.

For most minor surgical procedures, an appropriate anaesthetic protocol would be induction of a premedicated patient with propofol and maintenance with isoflurane, with or without N_2O. However, many other combinations are possible and individual or team preference is most important.

INTUBATION

In all but the briefest of anaesthetics tracheal intubation is warranted. An ET tube:
- Maintains a patent airway at all times during an anaesthetic
- Reduces the risk of aspiration during anaesthesia (N.B.: during certain procedures, such as dentals, the ET tube can act as a conduit for fluids to gain access to the trachea. For this reason, the use of swabbing material to pack the larynx is recommended during oral surgery and dentistry)
- Allows for accurate measurement of inspired and expired gases, provided an adequate seal is formed
- Allows for anaesthetic gas scavenging and reduces the likelihood of expired gases being breathed by operating-room staff
- Allows for IPPV

Selecting an ET tube

ET tubes are made from either polyvinyl chloride (PVC) or rubber.
- PVC tubes have the advantage that they become more flexible when warmed and conform to the curve of the trachea
- Rubber tubes are slightly irritating to the tracheal mucosa and have cuffs that are spherical in contour: this can result in pressure necrosis of the mucosa. The cuffs on PVC tubes are square-contoured, spreading contact with the trachea
- Rubber ET tubes suffer more than PVC tubes from heat damage due to repeated autoclaving: they can become brittle and crack

ET tubes may be further divided into cuffed and non-cuffed, referring to the inflatable seal at the distal end of the tube. In general, cuffed tubes are recommended in dogs, to ensure an airtight seal and reduce the risk of aspiration. Cuffs on ET tubes can damage the sensitive feline tracheal mucosa, and so it is not recommended that cuffed tubes be used for cats. Another consideration is that the external diameter of a 3.5-mm cuffed ET tube is greater than that of a non-cuffed tube: most cats, even smallish ones, will accommodate a 4.0-mm non-cuffed tube. If a cuffed tube is used on cats, the cuff should not be inflated: if necessary the pharynx may be packed gently with moistened swabs to improve the air seal.

This leads on to tube sizes: tube diameter has a tremendous impact on the resistance to airflow: half the radius = $16 \times$ resistance.

If the diameter is too small, airway resistance will increase and this may cause alveolar collapse and hypoventilation.

The largest tube that will fit comfortably should be chosen for the patient. Although, in general, there is a rough correlation with weight of animal and size of ET tube, this cannot be used as any more than a guide as individuals and breeds differ markedly. For example, a 25-kg labrador may take a 12–14-mm tube, whereas a 25-kg British bulldog with a severely hypoplastic trachea may only just fit a 5–6-mm tube. Bearing this in mind, it is wise to select a range of sizes for each patient. The size chosen should be marked on the anaesthetic sheet and preferably in the patient records, to facilitate correct choice in the future.

The length of tube is important (Figure 4.1): an ET tube should extend from the thoracic inlet (level with the spine of the scapula) to the incisors. An overlong ET tube increases mechanical dead space: a foreshortened ET tube may become dislodged during anaesthesia.

ET tubes are a potential source of infection and should be sterilised between patients. The cuff may be damaged by repeated autoclaving and should thus be checked before each use. This may be done using a cuff inflator or a 10-ml syringe. The cuff stopper on rubber tubes is especially susceptible to heat damage through repeated autoclaving and may not seal correctly. A **'Heath-Robinson'** fix for this is to fold the cuff tube over and insert the folded end into the plastic case of a hypodermic needle.

Procedure for intubation

Having induced anaesthesia, the animal is laid in sternal recumbency. An assistant holds the patient's head (or muzzle in a dolicocephalic breed) and rocks the head slightly backwards (dorsally flexing the neck). The anaesthetist then visualises the larynx by carefully grasping the tongue and retracting it **rostral** and ventrally.

Use of a laryngoscope, though not always necessary, may help here. Certainly a laryngoscope should always be on hand in case of emergency.

- Desensitising the larynx with local anaesthetic facilitates intubation. Intubeaze spray (Arnolds Veterinary Products) may be used, although in the author's experience a drop (0.1 ml) of lidocaine administered via a 1-ml syringe directly to the larynx seems to work very well and may reduce reactive salivation
- Allow the local anaesthetic some time to work!
- 30 s of patience markedly improves the anaesthetic effect. This is especially important for cats, which may suffer injury easily from a carelessly inserted ET tube
- The ET tube should be gently aimed between the laryngeal folds and slowly passed into the trachea, following the natural curve of the ET tube. No attempt should ever be made to force the ET tube down. If the larynx is closed, then either insufficient time has been allowed for the local anaesthetic to take effect, or insufficient injectable agent has been used

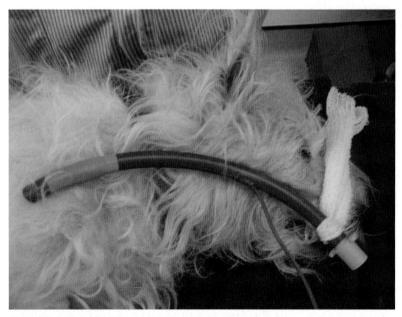

Figure 4.1 Selecting the correct length of endotracheal tube: the tube should extend from level with the spine of the scapula to the incisors.

- The application of a little lubricant (K-Y gel, Johnson & Johnson) may help the passage of the tube and reduce frictional damage to the tracheal mucosa
- It should be possible to visualise correct placement of the tube either directly or with the help of a laryngoscope. If the placement cannot be visualised, then listening for airflow may confirm placement, or else a small piece of cotton wool held over the end of the tube may be seen to move with respiration. Resist the temptation to pump air out of the patient by pressing on the chest: it is possible to be fooled by forcing air out of the stomach if the tube has been misplaced into the oesophagus
- The tube may then be secured with a bandage or tape around the muzzle in dogs or the back of the head in cats
- Once the tube is secured, the cuff is inflated using a cuff inflator or a 10-ml syringe, being careful not to overinflate, as this can cause collapse or narrowing of the tube. Inflating the cuff prior to securing may result in damage to the trachea if the tube moves

COMMON ANAESTHETIC BREATHING SYSTEMS

Various factors affect selection of a circuit for a particular patient:
- Size of patient: as with the ET tube, insufficiently sized anaesthetic circuit tubes will result in increased airway resistance and hypoventilation
- Controlled versus spontaneous ventilation: choosing a circuit that is inappropriate for IPPV will be of limited use for a thoracotomy
- Rebreathing or non-rebreathing: **rebreathing systems** have various advantages, such as reduced **volatile agents** and warmer air, but require more monitoring (for example, of CO_2 levels)
- Whether or not N_2O is to be used
- Mechanical dead space
- Circuit drag and valve position: is the circuit going to be 'clumsy' and difficult to prevent from twisting or falling off the table? Is the valve going to get in the way of oral or facial surgery?
- Ease of cleaning/sterilisation
- Ease of scavenging: for example, the risk of twisting the reservoir bag on a T-piece with added scavenging tube

Circuit factors

The tidal volume is the volume of air moved with each respiratory cycle and approximates to 10 ml/kg for cats, 15 ml/kg for dogs.

For ease of calculation, **minute volume** (Box 4.2) is usually taken to be:
- 200 ml/kg per min
- (800 ml/min for a 4-kg cat)
- (2 l/min for a 10-kg dog)

The **circuit factor** is the number of times higher than **minute volume** the fresh gas flow must be set to for a given circuit to ensure no expired air is rebreathed.

Non-rebreathing systems

Non-rebreathing systems have no CO_2 absorption and rely on high gas flow rates to flush expired CO_2 from the system. There are various circuits in common use: a brief summary follows and Table 4.1 suggests fresh gas flow rates for each system.

Magill (Figure 4.2)

- The flow rate must equal or exceed **minute volume** to prevent rebreathing (i.e. **circuit factor** = 1–1.5 × **minute volume**)
- The Magill works well for most animals up to 60 kg, but it does have a lot of expiratory resistance so it is not good for animals less than 5 kg

---

Box 4.2

Minute volume = tidal volume × respiratory rate

Table 4.1 Flow rates for various anaesthetic circuits

Weight of animal (kg)	Fresh gas flow rate (l/min)					
	Magill CF = 1–1.5	Bain CF = 1.5–2.5	T-piece CF = 2.5–3	Humphrey ADE CF varies	Lack CF = 1–1.5	Mini-Lack CF = 1–1.5
1	–	–	–	0.6	–	–
2	–	–	–	0.6	–	–
3	–	–	1.8	0.6	–	–
4	–	2	2.4	0.6	–	1.2
5	1.5	2.5	3	0.6	–	1.5
6	1.8	3	3	0.6	–	1.8
7	2.1	3.5	3.5	1	–	2.1
8	2.4	4	4	1	–	2.4
9	2.7	4.5	4.5	1	–	2.7
10	3	5	5	1	3	3
11	3.3	5	–	1	3.3	3.3
12	3.6	5.5	–	1	3.6	3.6
13	3.9	5.5	–	1	3.9	3.9
14	4.2	5.5	–	1	4.2	–
15	4.5	5.5	–	1	4.5	–
18	5.4	6	–	1	5.4	–
20	6	6	–	1	6	–
25	6	6	–	1	6	–
30	7	7	–	1	6	–
35	–	7	–	1	7	–
40	–	8	–	1	8	–
45	–	8	–	1	9	–
50	–	–	–	1	–	–
55	–	–	–	1	–	–
60	–	–	–	1	–	–

CF, circuit factor.
Below 20 kg, bag size should be 1 litre. Above 20 kg, bag size should be 2 litres.
N.B.: the above figures are calculated to allow a higher circuit factor for low body weights to prevent rebreathing and a lower circuit factor at high body weights to reduce wastage of fresh gas. They are provided as a guide: actual flow rates will vary according to individual patient tidal volume.

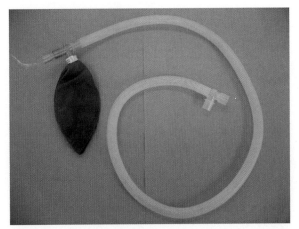

Figure 4.2 Magill circuit.

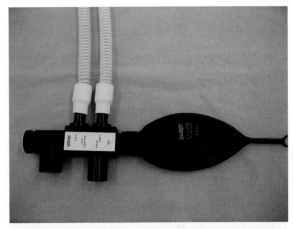

Figure 4.4 Mini-Lack circuit: close-up of valve to show connections.

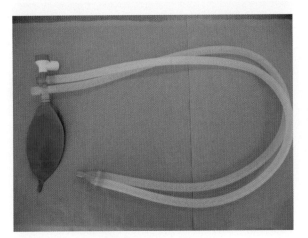

Figure 4.3 Lack circuit.

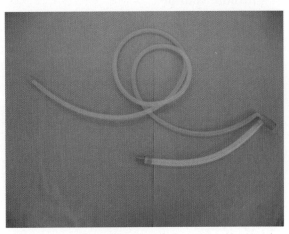

Figure 4.5 Ayre's T-piece circuit.

- IPPV causes rebreathing of alveolar gas and can cause **hypercapnia** unless high flow rates are used

Lack/parallel Lack (Figure 4.3)

- **Circuit factor = 1–1.5 × minute volume**
- The best advantage of this system is that it moves the valve away from the patient
- There are two forms: (1) the coaxial Lack has an inner and outer tube: the outer is inspiratory, and the inner expiratory; (2) the parallel Lack has separate inspiratory and expiratory tubes
- It is slightly more efficient than the Magill

- It has lower expiratory resistance so can be used in smaller animals
- It is suitable for IPPV

Mini-Lack (Figure 4.4)

- **Circuit factor = 1–1.5 × minute volume**
- The smaller design with smaller reservoir bag makes it suitable for smaller animals (4–13 kg)
- It is suitable for IPPV

Ayre's T-piece (Figure 4.5)

- High flow rates are needed (**circuit factor = 2–3 × minute volume**)

- There is minimal dead space and low resistance so it is good for small animals (<5 kg)
- It is suitable for animals up to 10 kg
- It is not suitable for IPPV

Jackson-Rees' modification (Figure 4.6)

- **Circuit factor** = 2.5–3 × **minute volume**
- It has an open-ended reservoir bag on its expiratory limb
- It can be used on animals less than 10 kg
- It is suitable for IPPV

Bain (Figure 4.7)

- **Circuit factor**: variable, between 1.5 and 2.5 × **minute volume**
- The Bain system comprises a coaxial T-piece, inner inspiratory tube and outer expiratory tube
- It warms inspiratory gases
- All configurations are suitable for IPPV
- There are three configurations: Mapleson D, E and F. E and F have no valves and have very small expiratory resistance: they can be used in cats and small dogs (4–10 kg). D is good for large dogs (10–50 kg)

Rebreathing systems

Rebreathing systems may be closed or semi-closed (low flow). Closed systems require more sophisticated monitoring of CO_2, O_2 and anaesthetic gas levels. There are two main types: circle system and to-and-fro.

Circle system (Figure 4.8)

- Gas flow is in one direction only
- The position of the reservoir bag between the expiratory valve and the absorber allows IPPV

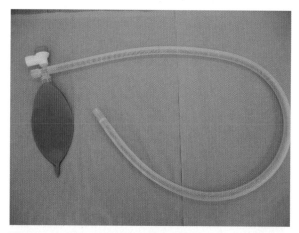

Figure 4.7 Bain circuit (Mapleson D configuration).

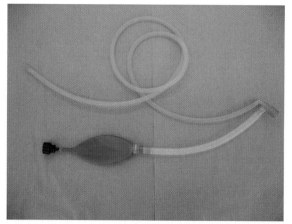

Figure 4.6 Jackson-Rees' modification of Ayre's T-piece circuit.

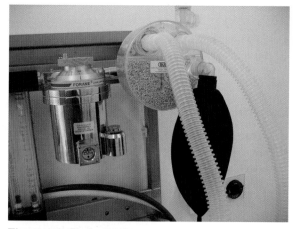

Figure 4.8 Circle circuit.

- The bag volume should be 3–6 times the animal's tidal volume
- Care should be taken to ensure that the soda lime canister is correctly filled as too much will increase resistance and too little will not allow for absorption of CO_2
- The older-style human-use circle circuits are suitable for dogs weighing 15 kg or more, but newer disposable paediatric systems may be used on patients weighing 8 kg or less

To-and-fro (Figure 4.9)

- Gas passes backwards and forwards over a horizontally placed soda lime canister
- This arrangement makes it possible for CO_2 to escape absorption if the canister is not completely full
- It is difficult to use this system for IPPV as the soda lime canister is between the reservoir bag and the patient. It is also possible for soda lime powder to be forced into the patient's airway
- This system is not suitable for animals weighing less than 15 kg

Humphrey ADE system (Figure 4.10)

- The Humphrey ADE system offers the advantages of **rebreathing systems** (low flow rates, warmed inspiratory gases, reduced volatile anaesthetic use) with the added advantage that it may be used on all but the smallest patients (3 kg, or smaller)
- As the reservoir bag is on the inspiratory limb, IPPV can be carried out
- The system is extremely efficient, allowing very low flow rates (70–100 ml/kg per min, although it is usually operated at a minimum of 300 ml/min)
- A patented four-stage valve system reduces wastage of clean air and allows release of alveolar air
- The circuit is operated semi-closed for animals below 10 kg. A soda lime canister is attached in parallel for larger animals. The recommended flow rates are 30 ml/kg per min for induction, reducing to 10 ml/kg per min for maintenance
- The same circuit can be used for animals between 3 and 100 kg in size, reducing the need for multiple circuits

MONITORING ANAESTHESIA

It is a legal requirement that monitoring of anaesthesia be continuous. There are various aids to monitoring, detailed below, but nothing beats human monitoring. It is frustrating (and frightening) to see a patient turning a deep shade

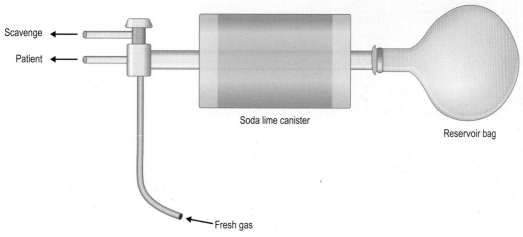

Figure 4.9 To-and-fro circuit.

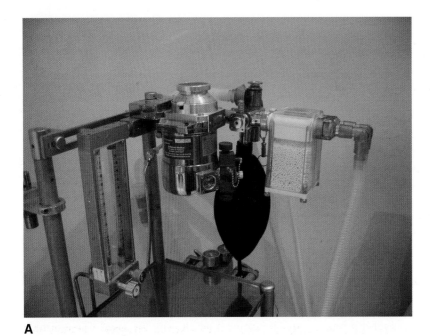

A

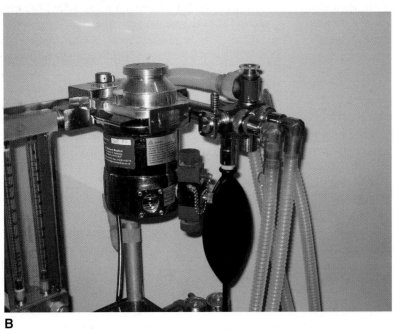

B

Figure 4.10 Humphrey ADE system (A) with soda lime canister for patients over 10 kg; (B) without soda lime canister for patients under 10 kg.

of blue on the operating table whilst the pulse oximeter is fiddled with to obtain a better reading! As mentioned in Chapter 1, it is not appropriate under any circumstances for a nurse to monitor the anaesthetic for a patient on whom she or he is performing surgery.

Continuous monitoring should result in instant alert should the patient's condition change suddenly: **apnoea**, for example. However, it is not easy to see trends or changes over time by simple monitoring. Use of a properly maintained anaesthetic record is important for several reasons:

- It shows trends in the patient's vital signs which allow the anaesthetic to be adjusted
- It can highlight problems with anaesthetic regimes or teams
- It improves the standard of monitoring by concentrating the mind
- It is strongly recommended for legal reasons

Figure 4.11 provides an example of a basic anaesthetic monitoring sheet.

Anaesthetic monitoring aids

Oesophageal stethoscopes

These are cheap and useful, allowing auscultation without having to risk disturbing drapes. Placement is easy: the oesophageal stethoscope should extend from the **caudal** border of the mandible to the manubrium.

Thermometers

If the patient becomes hypothermic then metabolism and rate of recovery from anaesthesia slow down. Shivering causes increased O_2 demand, which is not desirable postanaesthetic. Electronic probes are ideal for monitoring, but attention should be paid to positioning. For example, rectal temperature may not be accurate in prolonged abdominal surgery. In this case, nasopharyngeal temperature may be better: the probe may be placed into the ventral nasal meatus and positioned by the medial canthus of the eye. Measuring the core and surface temperature over a period of time may give an indication of peripheral perfusion and hence cardiac output.

Electrocardiogram (ECG)

The ECG trace can give us valuable information other than heart rate and rhythm, as it will alter characteristically with states such as **hypercapnia**, hyperkalaemia, hypercalcaemia and hypoxia. It is not necessary to place the leads perfectly: the trace may not be diagnostic for heart problems but will be satisfactory for monitoring. It is reassuring to see a beautiful QRS wave sweeping across the screen, but it is possible to get a normal ECG trace with no cardiac output, and so visual (nurse) monitoring is vital!

Pulse oximeter

This calculates relative concentrations of oxygenated and deoxygenated haemoglobin by measuring the relative transmission of red and infrared light. The value given is arterial haemoglobin saturation (SpO_2) as a percentage. Most healthy patients will have SpO_2 of more than 95%. Cyanosis becomes apparent when SpO_2 falls below 70%. As an aside, it is interesting to note that many British bulldogs have SpO_2 of less then 80% at rest: these dogs benefit from rapid intubation under anaesthesia! Pulse oximeters also give the pulse rate, and usually have alarms for low pulse rate or SpO_2. It is worth getting a vet-only machine rather than a converted human machine as the veterinary probes are much easier to place and the heart rate may be too high for human machines.

Pulse oximeters are extremely useful monitoring aids, but have several potential problems (Box 4.3):

- Lack of perfusion can lead to reduced or absent signal. The pressure of the probe itself can cause hypoperfusion, so it is a good idea to move it every 10–15 min
- Pigment or fur can reduce the signal
- Movement can dislodge the probe or cause a poor signal. You can use a bandage to hold the probe in place, but this can reduce perfusion
- Pretreatment with Oxyglobin can cause misreading
- A change in packed cell volume will not change SpO_2, so special attention must be given if SpO_2 falls in anaemic patients

The PetScan Clinic

Veterinary Surgery
1 Halstead Street
Lembert
Surrey

Record of Anaesthesia

Date: 19th April 2005

Client: Mr Smith   Animal: Alfie   Species: Canine   Breed: Labrador   Age: 8yrs 5 mths   Sex: male

Weight: 25kg   Surgeon: Ivor Scalpel   Anaesthetist: Hal O'thane

Operation proposed: Lumpectomy

Pre-anaesthetic blood sample: Pre-GA   GHP   Haem   PCV   Other tests _____

Physical examination: General physic good   temp 38.1°C   hrt 86   resp 20   CRT 2 sec

Other information: is on Rimadyl 50mg BID   sore hips

Risk category: G F P VP   fluids: route of administration: IV cephalic   type: Hartmanns   rate: 3 x maintenance

Pre-operative medication: none given

Premedication: ACP   dose: 0.3mls   route: IM   time given: 9am
                  Vetergesic   dose: 1.8mls   route: IM   time given: 9am
                  Rimadyl   dose: 1.8mls   route: IV   time given: 9.30am

Induction agent: Rapinovet   dose: 10mls   intubated: Y/N   tube size: 12   cuffed/uncuffed

Quality of induction: Good

Anaesthetic circuit: ADE/circle   posture: R lateral

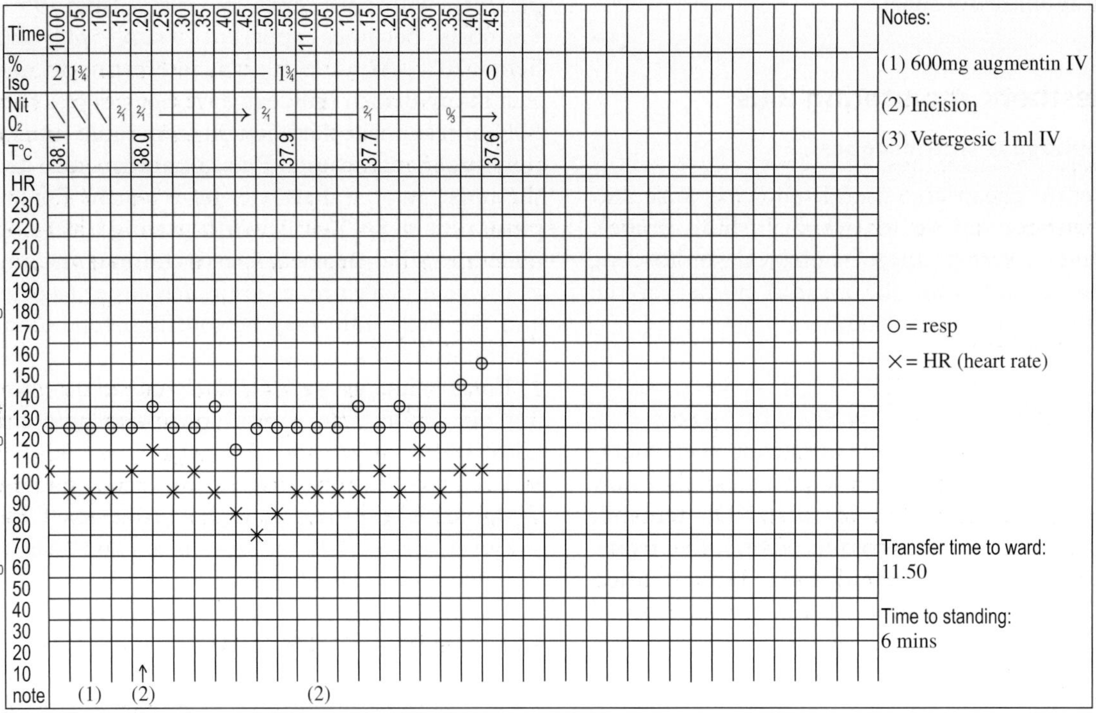

Notes:
(1) 600mg augmentin IV
(2) Incision
(3) Vetergesic 1ml IV

O = resp
X = HR (heart rate)

Transfer time to ward: 11.50

Time to standing: 6 mins

Figure 4.11 Example of an anaesthetic record sheet.

Box 4.3 Potential sites for placement of pulse oximeter probes

Tongue (as far back as possible)
Mandibular symphysis (cats)
Gastrocnemius tendon
Digit
Oesophagus
Rectum
Prepuce
Vulva
Scrotum
Pinna

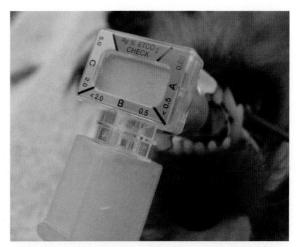

Figure 4.12 A disposable carbon dioxide (CO_2) monitor (Woodley Equipment) in use during routine surgery on a Yorkshire terrier. The central portion changes colour during the respiratory cycle: the CO_2 concentration is determined by comparing the colour of the central portion with the outer colour scale.

Reduced SpO_2 may be due to breathing a hypoxic gas mix, too low flow rate, increased shunt fraction, reduced cardiac output and reduced alveolar diffusion. Any reduction represents an immediate threat to the patient and must be acted upon quickly.

Respiratory gas analysis

Various new machines and disposable kits can give us information about O_2, CO_2, N_2O and anaesthetic gas levels in inspired and expired gas.

Carbon dioxide

The concentration of CO_2 is a sensitive indicator of rebreathing, whereas its absence suggests that there is no respiratory exchange. End-tidal CO_2 is a good measure of arterial CO_2 tension and gives a good indication of hyper-/hypoventilation. Inexpensive, disposable CO_2 readers are available (Figure 4.12), which may be connected to the ET tube and allow 2 h of measurement.

Oxygen

This is especially useful for rebreathing circuits as it demonstrates whether the patient is breathing a hypoxic mix. It can be used in combination with a pulse oximeter to look for changes in pulmonary function during surgery.

Nitrous oxide

Together with O_2 measurement this can be used to combine N_2O safely in a rebreathing circuit. N_2O measurement is also useful at the end of surgery when the patient is breathing pure O_2, allowing the anaesthetist to tell when N_2O concentration has reduced to low enough levels to remove the patient from the circuit safely.

Anaesthetic gas

This is probably less useful than measurement of the other gases; it can give an indication of the effectiveness of **analgesia**. Again, it may be useful in rebreathing circuits to ensure **volatile agent** concentration does not increase too much.

Arterial blood pressure

This is a very useful measure of cardiovascular function, and it is becoming easier to perform as better instrumentation becomes available. When blood pressure falls too far there is the risk of long- and short-term damage to organs such as the kidneys (through hypoxia and ischaemic damage). Trends and changes in blood pressure can also give us information about overzealous IV fluid administration, haemorrhage (hypovolaemia) and **analgesia**.

There are two ways of measuring arterial blood pressure: direct and indirect.

Direct measurement

Direct measurement requires placement of a cannula into a peripheral artery, most commonly the dorsal metatarsal artery in dogs. The cannula is then connected to a pressure-reader (**manometer**) via a heparinised saline tube. Depending on the **manometer** type, either mean arterial pressure or systolic and diastolic blood pressure can be measured. Cannulation of the artery can be tricky initially, but becomes easier with practice. Clotting can be a problem. Generally, direct measurement is probably inappropriate for anaesthetics for minor procedures.

Indirect measurement

A cuff tourniquet is placed on a distal limb or tail. This is used to occlude the blood flow and a measuring device is used to detect this. This can either be manual, using a **sphygmomanometer**, or electronic. Systems measure either systolic, or systolic and diastolic blood pressure. Although generally very reliable, problems with cuff placement or an inappropriate cuff width can affect the reading.

Central venous pressure (CVP)

Measurement of CVP requires placement of a jugular cannula so that the tip lies beyond the thoracic inlet. As with direct arterial blood pressure measurement, a heparinised saline tube is connected to this and thence to a pressure transducer. CVP is the first cardiovascular parameter to change in fluid balance so it gives a good indication of hydration status and integrity of the cardiovascular system. It is difficult to standardise CVP precisely, as placement can affect the reading tremendously, so trends are more important than individual readings.

Blood-gas analysis

Measurement of pH, O_2 and CO_2 tension, plasma bicarbonate, haemoglobin saturation and base excess gives us a lot of information about the health status of an anaesthetised patient. Although the most accurate machines require that samples be taken anaerobically and analysed immediately, machines such as the i-STAT (Woodley Equipment) give much of this information and are more readily available. Arterial samples give most information about oxygenation and acid–base status.

EXTUBATION

Once the procedure has been completed, the **volatile agent** is switched off, the system is purged and the animal is allowed to wake up. If N_2O gas has been administered during the surgery, then the **volatile agent** is continued for 5–10 min following withdrawal of nitrous to allow the N_2O to leave the body. At this stage, the cuff of the ET tube may be deflated and any tie holding the tube in place is loosened.

Dogs

The ET tube is left in place until a swallowing attempt is noted, or movement of the tongue is seen. The tie is taken off and the tube is smoothly drawn out of the trachea and mouth in a single fluid movement, following the curve of the tube.

Cats

The same procedure is followed, except that, due to the sensitive nature of the feline larynx, the tube is removed as soon as jaw tone has returned.

ANAESTHETIC EMERGENCIES AND RESUSCITATION (APPENDIX 2)

In the event of any problem under anaesthetic, a veterinary surgeon must be summoned immediately.

Problems and emergencies can occur at any time during an anaesthetic, but the most common time for anaesthetic disasters to occur is after extubation, when the patient has been returned to ward and the level of monitoring decreases. Closure of the larynx by dependence of the tongue causes suffocation in a patient not quite *compos mentis* enough to adjust its position. This can happen very quickly and so it is vital that monitoring is constant until the patient is in sternal recumbency and can lift its head.

The following information is just an overview of the treatment of anaesthetic emergencies. The interested reader is urged to read any of the excellent emergency trauma textbooks available.

Overdosage of injectable agent

This is most likely to result in **apnoea**. If this occurs, intubate the patient and perform IPPV until the animal starts breathing again. Unless a gross overdose has occurred, reversal agents or **antagonists** should not be necessary. However, in the event of gross overdosage, Table 4.2 lists available **antagonists** and doses. Unfortunately, for most agents, specific **antagonists** do not exist. Doxapram (Dopram-V, Fort Dodge Animal Health) is a respiratory stimulant that may be used to reverse the **apnoea** caused by anaesthetic overdosage. Although IV administration is recommended, the drug is also active if injected

Table 4.2 Antagonists and their doses			
Anaesthetic/sedative	**Antagonist**	**Dose**	
		Dog (10 kg)	**Cat (4 kg)**
Acepromazine	4-aminopyridine, 0.5 mg/kg (experimental)	(5 mg)	(2 mg)
	Doxapram[a] (Dopram-V, Fort Dodge Animal Health) 5.5 mg/kg	1–2.5 ml IV Puppies 2–10 drops sublingually	0.4–1 ml IV Kittens 2–4 drops sublingually
	Dopram-V drops		
Alphaxalone/alphadolone	Doxapram, 5.5 mg/kg Antihistamines, steroids to counter Cremophor reactions	As above	As above
Barbiturates	Doxapram, 5.5 mg/kg	As above	As above
Diazepam, midazolam	Flumazenil (Romazicon, Roche) 0.02–0.12 mg/kg IV	2–12 ml IV	0.2–4.8 ml IV
Ketamine	4-aminopyridine, 0.5 mg/kg (experimental)	(5 mg)	(2 mg)
Medetomidine	Atipamezole (Antisedan, Pfizer)	Same volume as Domitor IM	Half Domitor volume IM
Morphine, pethidine, fentanyl	Naloxone (Narcan, DuPont) 0.015–0.04 mg/kg IV, IM, IT, SC	0.37–1 ml IV	0.15–0.4 ml IV
Propofol	Doxapram	As above	As above

[a]Whilst doxapram is not a true antagonist to any of these agents, it has been included as a respiratory stimulant (thus antagonising apnoea).
Doses may differ if different concentrations of drugs are used: the suggested doses relate to the standard drug concentration.
IV, intravenously; IM, intramuscularly; IT, intratracheally; SC, subcutaneously.

(or dripped) sublingually. Another method of administration in an emergency is intratracheally (IT). To perform an IT injection, palpate below the cricoid cartilage and inject between cartilage rings.

Overdosage of volatile agent

As with injectable overdosage, this is most likely to cause **apnoea**. The **volatile agent** (and nitrous) is switched off and IPPV with O_2 is performed until voluntary breathing occurs.

Tips for IPPV

- IPPV is a very useful tool for anaesthesia and anaesthetic emergencies
- Although certain anaesthetic circuits are considered inappropriate for prolonged IPPV during procedures such as thoracotomy (e.g. Magill), all circuits can be used for IPPV in an emergency by increasing the fresh gas flow rate sufficiently to prevent rebreathing
- Aim for a rate of around 20–30 bag compressions per minute. A recommended way of timing is to have an inspiratory-to-expiratory ratio of 1:3
- With small animals care must be taken not to overinflate the lungs. With large dogs, it is easy to underinflate if the release valve is left open. To counter this, more vigorous or forceful compression of the bag should allow for inflation of the lungs, or else the valve may be partially closed
- Aim for a normal amount of chest movement for the size of patient

It is unusual for breathing not to recommence after IPPV. If this should occur, then administration of respiratory stimulants such as doxapram may be attempted.

It is also rare for breathing to stop in the middle of an anaesthetic during a minor surgical procedure. If this happens, IPPV should be immediately commenced. If the cause cannot be found immediately (**volatile agent** overdosage, obstructed ET tube and chest compression being

the usual culprits) then the procedure should be rapidly brought to a close and the **volatile agent**, and nitrous, withdrawn.

Circulatory arrest

Careful monitoring and rapid response to changes in patients' vital signs should reduce the risk of circulatory arrest. Particular attention should be given to:
- Reduction in pulse rate and quality
- Reduction in blood pressure
- Prolongation of the capillary refill time
- Pallor of the mucous membranes
- Any change in the ECG trace

Circulatory arrest is most often caused by a reduction in circulating blood volume, usually following haemorrhage. Other causes include sepsis, hypothermia, cardiac tamponade and myocardial injury. Excessive haemorrhage is unlikely to occur in minor surgery and may indicate underlying **coagulopathy**.

Impending circulatory collapse may be countered by increasing the fluid rate, or by adding colloids.

In case of circulatory arrest, then the procedures listed in Appendix 2 may be performed.

Cardiac massage

Cardiac massage may be performed externally or internally. With cats or small dogs, it may be possible to achieve adequate compression with external cardiac massage, but internal or direct cardiac massage is much more effective in larger dogs. Aim for a compression rate of 80–100 per minute. If resuscitation is not successful after 3 min, then internal cardiac massage should be started. A very brief surgical clip and prep should be performed over the incision area: from the **caudal** edge of the scapula to 5 cm from the sternum between the fourth and fifth ribs. Re-establishment of circulation is the most important thing here: infection can be controlled later. The heart is directly compressed between the thumb and first two fingers at between 80 and 100 times per minute.

IPPV should be maintained during cardiac compression, aiming for three ventilations every 20 compressions.

Emergency drugs

Although a variety of drugs are used during and after cardiopulmonary resuscitation, the three most commonly used emergency drugs are adrenaline (epinephrine), atropine and lidocaine, with dopamine or dobutamine used once cardiac arrest has been reversed (Box 4.4).

Adrenaline is considered to be the adrenergic agent of choice to increase arterial blood pressure by causing vasoconstriction. The emergency anaesthetic box should contain adrenaline vials and also syringes containing measured amounts of adrenaline. These should be diluted to 1:10000 (i.e. 1 ml adrenaline 1:1000 and 9 ml normal saline) for use in cats and small dogs and should be clearly labelled 'Cats' or 'Dogs'. The syringes should be discarded and fresh ones made every 2 weeks, or if they become discoloured.

Atropine is a **parasympatholytic** (anticholinergic) used to treat certain bradyarrhythmias,

such as those caused by **opioids**. In the absence of response to atropine, repeated doses should not be used as this can precipitate ventricular arrhythmias.

Lidocaine is very effective in treating ventricular arrhythmias and may be administered by bolus dose (see above) or by constant IV infusion at 60 µg/kg per min. If no response is seen to lidocaine administration, potassium levels should be checked to ensure hypokalaemia is not present.

Dobutamine and dopamine are catecholamines, which increase cardiac contractility through β-agonism. Both drugs have the potential to cause fatal ventricular arrhythmias and fibrillation in overdosage and must be administered by slow IV infusion, preferably with a controlled injection device. Dose rates are as follows:

Dobutamine: Dogs 5–20 µg/kg per min, cats 2–5 µg/kg per min

Dopamine: Dogs 2–10 µg/kg per min, cats 1–5 µg/kg per min

High-dependency anaesthetic patients

High-dependency anaesthetic patients include geriatric patients, pregnant patients and those patients with chronic illness or disease such as epilepsy or diabetes mellitus. Anaesthesia in these patients carries greater risk and precautions must be taken to ensure safety.

Geriatric patients

In the absence of specific diseases, the greatest risks to geriatric patients are dehydration, anorexia and recumbency for prolonged periods. In addition, geriatric patients may have less functional organ reserve and thus be prone to organ failure (liver, kidney, heart). Similarly, the respiratory system will have decreased function. Geriatric patients are frequently in a state of catabolism and being kept from food from the evening before anaesthesia until the evening after can prove to be quite a strain on their

---

Box 4.4

Adrenaline (epinephrine) may be given IV, IM, IT, IC at 0.1 mg/kg

Cats (4 kg): 0.75 ml (1:10 000)

Dogs (10 kg): 0.2 ml (1:1000)

Atropine should be administered IV at a dose rate of 0.04 mg/kg

Cats (4 kg): 0.2 ml

Dogs (10 kg): 0.7 ml

Lidocaine IV: cats 1 mg/kg, dogs 4 mg/kg (2% solution used)

Cats (4 kg): 0.2 ml

Dogs (10 kg): 2 ml

IV, intravenously; IM, intramuscularly; IT, intratracheally; IC, intracardiac.

metabolism. Anaesthetics with a long 'hangover' period can exacerbate arthritic pain if patients are left in a cage or kennel for long periods of time before and after surgery.

To minimise risk and improve comfort in these patients:

- A thorough physical examination (including blood biochemistry and urine tests) should be performed prior to anaesthesia
- Food should only be withheld for 3–4h before anaesthesia, and water for only 1h
- Wherever possible, theatre time for these patients should be arranged for early in the day, to reduce time spent in a cage prior to surgery
- Anaesthetic and premedication combinations should be very short-acting, to allow the patient to stand as soon as possible
- ACP should be used at the lowest dose, if at all
- α_2-agonists should be used with great caution, if at all
- A good premedication for these patients is diazepam (or midazolam) and ketamine (for doses, see Chapter 3), followed by induction with propofol and maintenance with isoflurane
- Patients should be preoxygenated for 2–3 min prior to induction to prevent hypoxaemia
- IV crystalloids should be maintained during anaesthesia and afterwards until the patient is eating
- Extra care should be taken to reduce heat loss, as geriatric patients are prone to hypothermia

Pregnancy

Wherever possible, anaesthesia should be avoided in pregnant dogs and cats: most minor surgery in the patients may be carried out under local anaesthesia. Where general anaesthesia is required, either due to the nature of the surgery, or to the temperament of the animal, the dose of all drugs should be reduced. It is an old adage to say that what the bitch gets, the puppies also get, but this is, by and large, true. **Opioids** will exert a sedative effect on puppies if given prior to cae-

sarean section, and there are few data to suggest that their use at other stages of pregnancy is safe.

Short- or ultrashort-acting injectable anaesthetics (such as propofol) should be used, or the animal can be masked down, provided its temperament allows. Administration of antiemetics such as metoclopramide (0.2 mg/kg) may help, as pregnant animals are prone to vomiting during or after anaesthesia.

Epilepsy

Assuming the epilepsy is well controlled and there have been no (or infrequent) seizures, epileptic patients may be at no significantly higher risk of anaesthesia than other patients, provided some precautions are taken:

- The premedication should include diazepam (0.25 mg/kg)
- Antiepileptic medication should be given as normal on the morning of surgery, preferably 3–4h before anaesthesia
- Certain drugs should be avoided due to the increased risk of seizures (ACP/ketamine should *not* be used)
- **Opioids** will have an increased **soporific** effect in dogs and cats being treated with phenobarbital and so should be used at the low end of the dose range
- Non-steroidal anti-inflammatory drugs should be used with caution in long-term epileptic patients: liver function should be investigated first
- Recovery should occur in as quiet an environment as possible, preferably with the lighting dimmed

Diabetes mellitus

Patients with diabetes mellitus are at greater risk with general anaesthesia because decompensation can occur due to the stress of anaesthesia and surgery.

- The diabetes mellitus should be controlled prior to anaesthesia
- Pre- and postoperative blood glucose levels should be measured: intraoperative blood

glucose should be measured if the surgery is prolonged
- Anaesthesia should be scheduled for as early in the morning as practice protocol will allow and the patient should be given half its normal dose of insulin
- IV crystalloids containing 5% dextrose should be administered during the procedure
- Short- or ultrashort-acting anaesthetics should be used

- A reasonable choice would be diazepam/buprenorphine premedication, followed by propofol induction and maintenance with isoflurane

As previously mentioned, care should be taken over any animal receiving medical treatment to make sure there are no known drug interactions or contraindications.

5 Wound dressings and bandages

TYPES OF DRESSING AND THEIR INDICATIONS

The terms 'dressing' and 'bandage' are often used interchangeably. In fact, the term 'dressing' refers more correctly to the primary layer in contact with the wound. A wound dressing must always be **sterile**. A bandage comprises the primary layer, or dressing; the secondary layer, which helps absorb exudates and provides support to varying degrees; and the tertiary layer, which helps protect the bandage and aids support.

Roles of dressings in minor surgery

Dressings are used in minor surgery to protect or cover traumatic wounds prior to closure, to protect the surgical wound after repair and to provide ongoing wound management for open wounds (see Chapter 6).

Dressings can perform several functions:

- Provide physical support to a wound
- Provide pain relief
- Help debride (remove necrotic or **contaminated** tissue from) the wound
- Deliver medication
- Absorb exudates, without allowing excessive fluid loss
- Aid **haemostasis**

Types of wound dressing

Dressings may be either adherent or non-adherent, and are subdivided into occlusive or non-occlusive, depending on whether or not they allow exchange of gases or water. Adherent dressings are generally used early on in wound management, when **debridement** of the wound is needed. Once wound-healing is under way, non-adherent dressings are chosen so as to minimise further damage to the wound when changing the dressing.

Adherent dressings

These may be gauze pads (swabs), or specialised adherent dressing. **Sterile** gauze pads may be used dry on wounds, or may be soaked with **sterile** saline. These applications are known as 'dry-to-dry' or 'wet-to-dry', and the function is to help debride the wound and remove necrotic tissue and loose debris.

Dry-to-dry dressings are best used on wounds that are moderately inflamed with obvious debris and pale, translucent-appearing necrotic tissue. Such wounds usually have watery exudates.

Wet-to-dry dressings may be applied to similar wounds when the exudates are sticky. The addition of **sterile** Hartmann's solution to the wound dilutes the exudate, allowing absorption and improving **debridement** of the wound. To reduce the risk of bacteria growing in the soaked dressing, it is possible to add 0.05% chlorhexidine to the Hartmann's solution.

Dry-to-dry and wet-to-dry dressings are covered by a bandage with an absorbent secondary layer (cotton wool or Soffban (Smith & Nephew)) and are removed once the primary layer has had a chance to dry, usually after 12–24 h. Removing the dressing removes the outermost surface of the wound, taking with it much of the exudate, foreign material and necrotic tissue.

OpSite (Smith & Nephew) is a transparent adhesive film dressing that may be used to cover granulating wounds that are highly exudative (Figure 5.1). This dressing allows water vapour through, but not water, thus reducing fluid loss from the wound site. It is also occlusive to bacteria, thus preventing secondary infection of the wound. It is usually not covered by a secondary layer. The dressing is usually left in place for several days, or longer, depending on the amount of fluid produced by the wound. An obvious advantage to this type of wound dressing is that the wound may be visualised without the need to remove the dressing. A disadvantage is that it can be difficult to get the dressing to adhere in the first place: clipping the hair 5 cm around the wound and degreasing the skin with surgical scrub solution may help.

Compeed (Johnson & Johnson) is a liquid film dressing that may be applied to small granulating wounds to provide an impermeable cover to prevent the wound drying out and to protect it from external damage, such as urine scalding. It

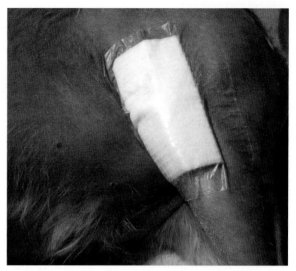

Figure 5.1 OpSite postoperative (Smith & Nephew) dressing used to cover a wound following removal of a small skin mass.

may be covered by a secondary layer, or left uncovered. This dressing is not removed but the application of further layers is required every 2–3 days.

Adherent dressings have several disadvantages:

- To work optimally, wet-to-dry dressings may need to be changed several times daily in very **contaminated** wounds
- Removal of an adherent dressing is often painful. The patient may require sedation or anaesthesia. Topical anaesthesia is often helpful
- Adherent dressings may adhere very strongly to a wound and prove difficult to remove without harming the underlying wound. Addition of a little warmed **sterile** saline can help soften the discharge
- Adherent dressings remove the surface of a wound and thus will slow the process of epithelialisation and wound contraction. They must only be used in the initial, inflammatory phase of wound-healing (see Chapter 6)

Wet-to-dry and dry-to-dry dressings are used less commonly now: the newer non-adherent dressings with highly absorptive hydrogels are much less traumatic to wounds, need to be changed less frequently and can be used later on in wound-healing, making them much more versatile.

Non-adherent dressings

These tend to disrupt the wound surface minimally and are recommended for wounds starting to granulate. Granulation tissue does not grow in the presence of infection and so its presence indicates that infection is controlled.

Non-adherent dressings prevent wound desiccation and allow moisture to be retained at the wound site, promoting healing. The degree to which they do this depends on whether they are occlusive or semi-occlusive.

Semi-occlusive non-adherent dressings include petrolatum-impregnated gauze pads (Jelonet, Smith & Nephew), calcium alginate pads (Kaltostat, ConvaTec) and polyester-covered absorptive cotton sheets (Melolin, Smith & Nephew). Occlusive non-adherent dressings include hydrocolloid sheets (Granuflex, ConvaTec), Hydrogels (Intrasite gel, Smith & Nephew) and foam dressings (Allevyn, Smith & Nephew).

Petrolatum-impregnated gauze is a tempting dressing to use as it rarely adheres to a wound and is usually very easy to remove, unless it has been in place for an extended period of time. Unfortunately, the petroleum jelly reduces oxygenation of the wound and is inhibitory to epithelialisation. This limits the use of these dressings to very early on in granulation. Newer dressings have rendered this rather obsolete.

Calcium alginate is an extremely useful dressing, as it has a tremendous absorptive capacity and a stimulatory effect on fibroblasts, as well as being haemostatic. The mesh pads rapidly form a gel in the presence of sodium ions and may be used in highly exudative wounds. In such wounds, an Allevyn pad may be placed over the alginate dressing to help absorption. In less exudative wounds, a Melolin pad may be used to cover the alginate. Calcium alginate dressings are low-maintenance, requiring changing only every 2–3 days.

Polyester-covered absorptive cotton sheets are used very commonly in wound management, but are a little disappointing. Frequently, they do stick to wounds, despite the plastic coating. Also, it is not uncommon to see local dehydration of a wound upon removal of the sheet, or else insufficient absorption of exudates from a wound. They are probably best used to protect an almost-healed wound from damage.

Hydrogels and other hydroactive dressings (Box 5.1) are very useful in early wound repair and are highly effective at debriding necrotic wounds. The gel readily conforms to the wound site and absorbs and retains water. This allows **autolysis** to occur: the dissolved necrotic material is then carried away from the wound edge into the gel. There is good evidence that hydrogels are inhibitory to bacteria. Hydrogels require a secondary dressing to cover them and hold them in place: they should be changed every 24–48 h. Most of the gel is removed by removing the overlying bandage: any remaining gel may be rinsed off with **sterile** Hartmann's solution or fresh gel placed over it.

Hydrocolloids are available in sheet, paste and powder form. The sheet form comprises a colloid matrix, usually carboxymethylcellulose covered by polyurethane sheets. Although not suitable for highly exudative wounds, hydrocolloids are very effective at keeping wounds moist but not excessively damp. Like hydrogels, there appears to be some antibacterial action. The retention of moisture at the wound site helps the ongoing process of wound **debridement** and speeds epithelialisation. The dressing may be left in place for 2–3 days.

Foam dressings are highly absorptive, multi-layered dressings, capable of absorbing large amounts of exudate even when compressed within a fairly snug bandage. In addition, they are excellent secondary coverings for hydrogels in moderately exudative wounds. They must be

---

Box 5.1

Hydroactive dressings are much easier to remove than other wound dressings, due to the gel nature. They are rarely painful and can usually be changed with no need for sedation.

used the right way round, as the backing layer is water-resistant, but when used correctly they will allow for rapid epithelialisation of a wound. Generally, they should be changed every 2 days.

Summary

Chapter 6 details wound care more thoroughly, but to make the choice of dressings easier one may use the following rough guide:

- Postsurgery (clean wounds) – non-adherent plastic-covered dressings (Melolin; use Allevyn or Kaltostat if there is any oozing from the wound)
- **Contaminated** and exuding wounds – use non-adherent dressings such as Intrasite gel or Allevyn for moderately exudative wounds, Granuflex for less exudative wounds

SECONDARY AND TERTIARY LAYERS OF THE BANDAGE

Roles of bandages

Other than helping to hold a wound dressing in place, bandages:

- Provide support (for an injured limb or a wound)
- Help to keep a dressing clean
- Help absorb exudates
- Protect the wound from self-mutilation
- Improve the environment of the wound site to improve healing
- Reduce swelling and haemorrhage
- Provide pain relief
- Restrict movement of the wound edges
- Keep intravenous cannulae in place

The secondary layer of a bandage provides most of these functions, with the tertiary layer providing protection from the environment and holding all the other layers in place.

Secondary layer

Essentially, the secondary layer is either cotton wool or a synthetic material such as Soffban (Smith & Nephew). These materials are both comfortable and absorptive.

Soffban is not as absorptive or soft as cotton wool, but it has the advantage that it is easier to apply, coming in suitably sized rolls (5 cm for cats, 7.5 cm for dogs, 10 cm for very large dogs). Soffban is also available with added triclosan to reduce bacterial growth, but it is questionable how much benefit this provides to the dressing as a whole. The padding layer must be thick enough to absorb any excess exudates and to provide padding for the wound and other parts of the patient covered by the bandage. In addition, the secondary layer provides most of the splinting effect of a bandage, preventing disruption of the wound. On the other hand, the secondary layer should not be too thick, or else the bandage will be unstable, susceptible to becoming dislodged and may also prove clumsy and annoying to the patient. A rough guideline is 2–3 layers of Soffban or 1–2 layers of cotton wool.

Tertiary layer

This is usually two layers and comprises a conforming layer and an outer protective layer.

The conforming layer should contour well to the area being bandaged: it compresses and holds the padding layer in place. Stretchy gauze bandages such as K-band (Parema) are ideal for this.

The outer layer should be relatively impervious to water, allowing water vapour and moisture out, but not allowing water in. It should also be fairly hard-wearing, especially if the bandage is to be placed on a limb. Self-adhesive bandaging tape such as Vetrap (3M) is ideal, but care must be taken when applying this as the tape tightens slightly after application and so it is easy to make the bandage too tight.

Plastic bags, rubber boots and such like can all help to protect the bandage from wear and tear, but should only cover the end of a limb bandage and should be removed when not required as this may otherwise cause the bandage to become unacceptably wet, through retention of moisture vapour.

APPLICATION TECHNIQUES AND MANAGEMENT OF BANDAGES

Most bandages relevant to minor veterinary surgery will be fairly simple bandages on the paws, limbs, ears, eyes, tail or trunk. These are covered here. Although not strictly relevant to minor surgery, Robert-Jones bandages, Ehmer and Velpeau slings are described for completeness.

Paws (Figure 5.2)

- Wounds may be ventral or dorsal, or may be on or between the digits
- If the nails are overlong, it may be wise to clip them before applying the bandage – this increases comfort
- The dressing is placed over the wound. It can be tricky to avoid the dressing slipping and to ensure it conforms to the wound: in the author's experience, applying a little Intrasite gel (Smith & Nephew) really helps at this stage. The dressing can be cut to fit, or wrapped round the paw. If it is wrapped, make sure that there are no creases that can cause pressure sores
- Small pads of cotton wool should be placed between the digits to reduce rubbing and moisture scalding. This is easier in some breeds than others. In stubby-toed breeds such as Staffordshire-bull terriers, it may be helpful to use very long strips of cotton wool that can be flattened over the paw or held in place by an assistant
- A padding layer (Soffban or cotton wool) is then wrapped around the paw, starting near the carpus or tarsus and folding round the paw back to the carpus or tarsus on the other side
- This is repeated once and then the bandage is wrapped spirally around the paw, neatly enclosing all digits and finishing 4–5 cm proximal to the tarsus or carpus
- The process is repeated with a conforming layer (e.g. K-band, Parema) and again with a tertiary layer (e.g. PetFlex, Andover; Vetrap, 3M), making sure that the bandage overlies itself by about one-third to two-thirds
- When completed, the bandage should look tidy and resist attempts to pull it off. There is

little point in being reluctant to try to pull the bandage off – it is likely that the patient will try!

Limbs (minor wounds)

- In most cases, the entire limb should be bandaged: in all but large, easy-going dogs a small bandage is likely to get in the way of movement or slip. Taping bandages in place is not recommended due to the risk of placing the tape too tightly. In the author's experience, stretchy sticking tape, such as Elastoplast (Smith & Nephew), either fails to stick or sticks so firmly that removal is difficult and painful to the patient
- Proximal limb wounds are especially difficult to bandage. In some cases, the bandage itself can cause movement of the wound edges. In these cases, either a combination of limb and trunk bandage may be used or else the wound should be covered by an adherent wound dressing such as OpSite (Smith & Nephew) or a non-adherent dressing with adherent edges such as Primapore (Smith & Nephew)
- Elizabethan collars may be helpful in these cases to prevent self-trauma to the wound. Otherwise, the dressing may be covered by a body-stockingette or a T-shirt
- If a full-length limb bandage is to be placed, the middle two digits should be left exposed, in order to monitor for discomfort, or any sign of reduced circulation
- In either case, the primary dressing should be applied and held in place by an assistant while the secondary layer is applied, again being careful to let successive layers overlap by one-third to two-thirds
- To reduce the chance of the bandage slipping, tape stirrups may be placed on either side of the limb, extending from twice the distance from mid-limb to toe. Elastoplast (Smith & Nephew) may be used, but the author's preference is to use white surgical tape (Micropore, 3M, or Durapore, 3M). The distal ends may be stuck together temporarily to keep them out of the way while the rest of the bandage is placed

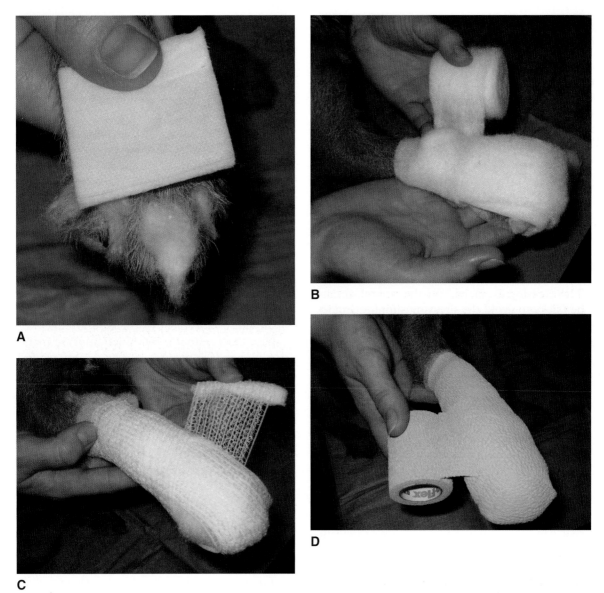

Figure 5.2 Application of a paw bandage. (A) A gauze swab is used to cover the wound: cotton pads have been placed between the digits. (B) A padding layer is applied. (C) Next, a conforming layer is applied. (D) A tertiary, water-repellent layer completes the dressing.

- Ensure adequate padding over the joints and contact points and take great care that no creases occur over the dorsal medial elbow or the dorsal tarsus – it is preferable to reduce the motion of these joints slightly rather than risk pressure sores

Pressure bandage

- If the function of the limb bandage is to minimise postoperative swelling and haemorrhage or to reduce dead space then a pressure bandage can be placed
- This is performed in the same way as a normal limb bandage, but great care must be taken not to reduce the blood supply to the limb by applying too much pressure
- In this case, it is preferable to leave the middle two digits out of the bandage. These should be checked 3–4 times daily for signs of poor blood flow (clamminess, swelling, cold or lack of capillary refill in white or clear claws)
- Any slipping or creasing of intermediate/ padding layer in this bandage must be corrected: a small crease under pressure can cause a point-pressure which may occlude blood supply
- These dressings should only be left in place for 12–24h and should be removed if the patient tries to mutilate them as this can be a sign of incipient problems

Ears (Figure 5.3)

- Ears may either be bandaged hanging down, or flapped back over the head, according to preference. It is important to make a note – ideally on the outermost bandage layer – of the ear position to avoid accidental pinnectomy when removing the bandage!
- A little surgical tape (Micropore, 3M) or zinc oxide tape may be used to hold a dressing in place, or else long strips of tape may be placed on the ventral and dorsal surfaces of the pinna, near the **rostral** and **caudal** edges directed from the head to the tip of the pinna. If the ventral tapes are made longer than the dorsal tapes, then the pinna may be flapped back over

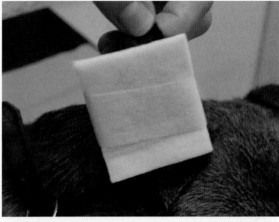

A

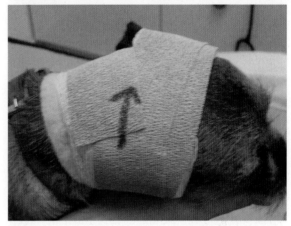

B

Figure 5.3 Application of an ear bandage. (A) A little surgical tape is used to hold a dressing in place. (B) It is a good idea to mark the orientation of the ear to avoid accidents when removing the bandage.

the head and the tapes used to help hold the ear in place on the head
- A dressing is applied to the wound and a conforming layer (e.g. PetFlex, Vetrap) is wrapped around the head. The contralateral pinna is not enclosed in the bandage
- There is usually no need for an intermediate layer of cotton wool or other padding: indeed, this increases the likelihood of slippage of the bandage
- Care must be taken to ensure the bandage does not restrict breathing. The bandage should not extend further forward than the

ramus of the mandible as this may interfere with breathing

Eyes

- Eye bandages are rarely warranted in minor surgery: postoperative swelling to the conjunctivae and palpebrae is usually fairly short-lasting and there are obvious advantages to being able to visualise the eye
- In most cases, an Elizabethan collar should be sufficient to prevent the patient from interfering with the wound
- If swelling is anticipated, or if a bandage is desired for comfort, then a non-adherent dressing should be applied to the wound (Melolin, Smith & Nephew, is usually appropriate) and cotton wool is used to pad out the area between the dressing and the outer bandage layer to ensure contact and a little pressure on the dressing
- A conforming layer (e.g. PetFlex, Vetrap) is then carefully wrapped around the head: the bandage should pass behind the ear on the opposite side to the affected eye, but the bandage may be wrapped both in front and behind the ear on the affected side to help maintain the position of the bandage
- As with the ear bandage, care must be taken not to restrict breathing

Tail (Figure 5.4)

- Tail bandages may be required for mid or distal tail wounds. Proximal tail wounds, near the perineum, do not normally lend themselves to bandaging
- Tail tip wounds can either be dressed with non-adherent dressings cut into strips and held in place by sticking tape under a bandage, or else covered by a plastic syringe case, with the end cut off to provide ventilation
- Padding, if provided, should not be more than one layer thick
- The tertiary layers should be snug but not tight to prevent a tourniquet effect
- It is often helpful to trap some hair in the proximal part of the bandage to reduce slip-

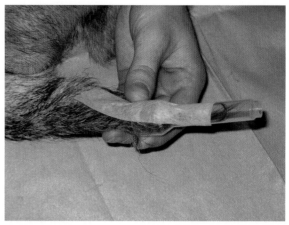

A

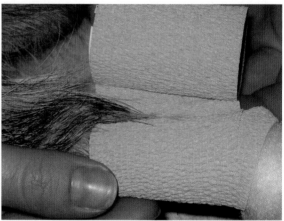

B

Figure 5.4 Application of a tail bandage. (A) A plastic syringe case can be held in place by surgical tape. (B) Trapping hair between bandage layers helps reduce the likelihood of the bandage slipping off.

page. It is also possible to wrap some surgical sticking tape loosely around the end of the bandage, trapping hair within this; care must be taken, however, to ensure the tape is not wrapped too tightly

Chest

- A variety of body-stockingettes (Monarch Textiles) are available for dogs and cats, or else tube bandage (Tubigauze, Millpledge) may be used to hold a dressing in place

- Otherwise, cotton wool or Soffban may be wrapped around the chest, followed by a conforming layer (e.g. PetFlex, Vetrap), being careful not to restrict breathing if around the chest, or to restrict venous return if around the abdomen
- The bandage should start at the withers and progress round the front of the right shoulder to the left axilla, back up to the withers and down to the right axilla, round the front of the left shoulder and so on, in a figure-of-eight style until sufficient coverage is obtained
- Minor wounds near the forelimbs may be covered with a T-shirt
- Small surgical wounds may be covered by a self-adhesive dressing (e.g. Primapore), or similar

Abdomen (Figure 5.5)

- Bandages around the abdomen can be very difficult to keep in place: they have a tendency to slip or concertina up
- Having placed the dressing, the bandage (use a fairly wide size) is built up in a simple spiralling pattern around the body: padding layer (Soffban) and then conforming layer(s) (K-

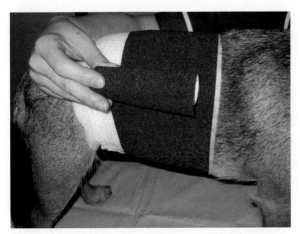

Figure 5.5 Application of an abdominal bandage. Wide tape is used to spread pressure evenly over the bandaged area.

band and/or Co-flex), being careful not to apply the bandage too tightly
- A strip of adhesive tape, such as Elastoplast or wide zinc oxide, may be used to anchor the bandage down – do not wrap the adhesive tape around the whole body as this can severely restrict breathing: usually a strip either side of the body will suffice
- Alternatively, a stockingette placed over the dressing may suffice – holes may be cut to allow placement over the fore or hind limbs, making sure the dressing will not be soiled during urination

Robert-Jones bandage (Figure 5.6)

- This is a development of a pressure bandage that has the added advantage of effectively immobilising the distal limb, making it suitable for management of some fractures and sprains
- Any appropriate dressings are applied
- Tape stirrups may be placed to reduce the risk of slippage
- Cotton-wool pads are placed between the toes and a padding layer (Soffban) is wrapped around the limb
- Cotton wool is neatly wrapped around the limb, being careful to avoid creases or areas of poor padding
- Stretchy gauze bandage (K-band, Parema) is wrapped around the limb, to help conform the cotton wool. Make sure the proximal bandage does not end at the elbow or stifle joint, but as high up the limb as possible. Do not apply much tension at this stage, and rewrap any areas that bulge. The middle toes are left visible
- A second layer of cotton wool is wrapped around the limb, again making sure that the coverage is even and that there are no poorly padded areas
- A second layer of K-band is wrapped around the limb. The bandage at this stage should be slightly 'squishy' to the touch
- The stirrups can be folded back at this stage to adhere to the K-band
- If necessary, a third layer of cotton wool may be added

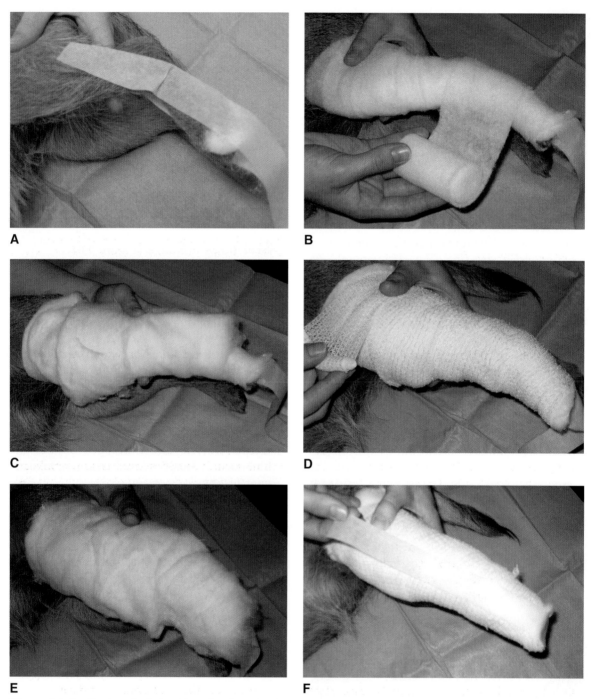

Figure 5.6 Application of a Robert-Jones bandage. (A) Cotton pads are placed between the toes and stirrups (if desired) are attached to the limb. (B) An initial layer of padding is wrapped around the limb. (C) A single layer of cotton wool is wrapped around the limb. (D) A conforming bandage is used to provide a small amount of pressure and to even out the cotton wool layer. (E) A second layer of cotton wool is wrapped around the limb. (F) A second conforming layer is placed, applying a little more tension this time and ensuring there are no wrinkles or creases in the bandage. The stirrups are folded back and stuck to the conforming layer. (G) A final, water-resistant layer is applied. The bandage should be firm and smooth, with no visible creases.

(cont'd)

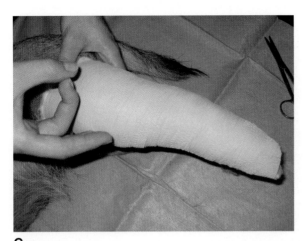

G

Figure 5.6 (Continued).

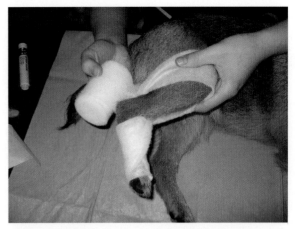

Figure 5.7 Application of an Ehmer sling. Only the padding layer has been applied to illustrate the direction of travel of the bandage.

- Starting from the distal end of the limb, wrap 1–2 layers of conforming bandage (e.g. PetFlex, Vetrap) around the limb, using enough tension to smooth out the dimples in the surface of the bandage
- The resulting bandage, when flicked, should make a satisfying noise of which a good greengrocer would be proud! The bandage should not deform under fingertip pressure
- The toes should be checked several times daily, as with the lighter pressure bandage. Any slippage should be monitored closely: slipping of a Robert-Jones may cause uneven pressure on part of the limb and occlude blood supply
- Provided no slippage is seen, the toes appear healthy and the animal is comfortable, and provided the bandage remains tidy and dry, a Robert-Jones may be left in place for up to 2 weeks

Ehmer sling (Figure 5.7)

- This type of bandage is used to prevent weight-bearing of a hind limb and may be used after reduction of hip luxation
- It is often poorly tolerated by the patient and can cause severe pressure sores if placed incorrectly or inadequately monitored
- Consideration should be given to the animal's other hind limb: elderly or arthritic patients may find it difficult to cope with one less limb
- A thin layer of Soffban or cotton wool is placed over the metatarsals (around the foot)
- A conforming bandage (e.g. K-band) is wrapped several times around the foot in a clockwise direction (looking from the patient's front) in the right hind and in an anticlockwise direction in the left hind
- The stifle is then flexed as far as possible and the K-band is passed medially (i.e. between the limb and the body) and out over the quadriceps muscle (if possible, a wad of cotton wool is placed over the quadriceps as padding at this stage)
- The bandage is kept under tension as it passes round the back of the tibia to wrap around the metatarsals from medial to lateral. This should look like a figure-of-eight from the front of the patient
- The process is repeated 3–4 times
- Finally, a layer of cohesive bandage is applied in the same manner to provide further support and protect the conforming bandage

Velpeau sling (Figure 5.8)

- This is used to prevent weight-bearing of a fore limb, for example after scapular fracture or shoulder dislocation

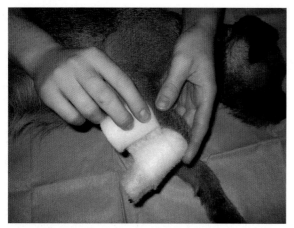

A

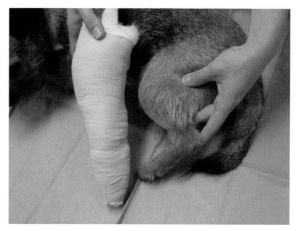

Figure 5.9 Incorrect application led to this bandage slipping off immediately. Stirrups may have helped, although a correctly tensioned bandage should not require stirrups to keep it in place.

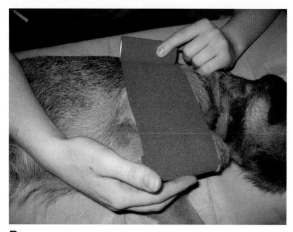

B

Figure 5.8 Application of a Velpeau sling. (A) A padding layer is applied to the carpus and paw. (B) A tertiary layer is wrapped over the completed bandage to improve support.

- As with the Ehmer sling, care should be taken, particularly in older dogs, that the other limbs are able to cope with the extra load
- The carpus and paw are padded with cotton wool
- The forelimb is flexed as close to the trunk as possible and a conforming bandage (e.g. K-band) is wrapped around the carpus and brought up over the lateral carpus, elbow and shoulder
- The bandage is continued round the body, passing behind the opposite elbow to wrap several times around the body, spreading

tension evenly over the whole of the bandaged limb
- A cohesive layer (e.g. Vetrap, PetFlex) may then be applied to improve support

COMPLICATIONS FROM DRESSINGS

Unfortunately, as useful as dressings and bandages are, they are subject to various complications: ranging from inconvenient to disastrous. The most common complication is slippage, or falling off entirely (Figure 5.9). Any slippage should be treated seriously, as it could cause a crease in the bandage to exert undue pressure on part of the animal, leading to discomfort or trauma.

It can be very embarrassing waving a client out of the consultation room, only to receive a call 20 min later to say that the bandage has come off! Practice is the only way to avoid this (and using stirrups on limb bandages) as you will get a feel for the tension required to keep a bandage in place.

Using too much padding in the secondary layer may make a bandage susceptible to loosen, as after only a few minutes, the padding begins to pack down and lose volume. However, this should not be seen as an excuse to reduce the padding: too little padding may not confer enough absorption to the bandage, as well as reducing comfort and protection against the bandage rubbing.

If a bandage is found to have slipped, resist the temptation to push it back into place: it is unlikely to remain there a second time and you may cause damage to the underlying wound or move the primary dressing.

Other complications include pressure sores, infection and hypoxic damage due to bandages being too tight:

- Always make sure the client returns for a bandage check at the appropriate time: any cancellations should be followed up by phone call to make sure a bandage is not allowed to remain unchanged for too long
- Clients should be shown how to monitor their pet's bandage: checking for slippage and feeling any exposed digits for cold, pain or swelling. Any obvious signs of discomfort should be reported: if in doubt, change the dressing earlier than planned
- When changing a dressing, it may be advisable to take into account the client's temperament: remember, clients are often unused to seeing wounds on their pet. It may be considerate to ask them to wait outside while performing a dressing change, or to admit the patient
- There may often be a faint musty smell associated with a bandage, especially if the outer layers of the dressing have been allowed to become wet. This need not be any cause for concern, although a damp dressing needs to be changed, or it will increase the risk of 'strikethrough' of infection. However, very unpleasant smells are often indicators of infection
- Hydrogel and hydrocolloid dressings collect fluid and become quite viscous – there is frequently obviously necrotic tissue within the fluid, which is extremely pus-like. If the client is present, this should be pointed out to avoid concern. It should be fairly easy to distinguish between pus and hydrogel: the lack of odour with hydrogel compares to the foul smell of anaerobic infection. Examination of the wound will usually confirm healing: a smooth, salmon-pink granulation tissue is extremely unlikely to have formed in the presence of infection

- If there are any signs of infection (smell, pain, lack of granulation tissue, gaping of the wound) then various steps should be taken:
  - A swab should be taken for culture and sensitivity, and broad-spectrum antibiotics should be commenced
  - The wound should be washed copiously with **sterile** Hartmann's solution. Any substantial wound breakdown should be treated as appropriate (see Chapter 6), removing any sutures not holding tissue as these may be sites for bacterial persistence
  - The wound should be re-bandaged, preferably using a hydroactive dressing. Depending on the degree of infection or of necrotic tissue, this dressing may need to be changed daily
- Any sign of rubbing or pressure sore should be treated by dressing the sore if it is open, or re-bandaging with more padding over the area if it is very mild. Even very mild pressure sores will progress to partial- or full-thickness sores if unattended
- Particular attention should be paid to projections of bone (the lateral malleolus of the tibia is commonly affected in hind-limb bandages). If concerned about rubbing, then a pressure-relieving pad may be placed over the area of concern: this may be as simple as a length of cotton wool rolled into a tube and curled into a doughnut-shape. Placing this around the sore point will take pressure off; however, care must be taken to ensure that the pad does not slip, or this will exacerbate the injury
- Over-tightening of dressings can cause disastrous complications: the lore of veterinary practice abounds with stories of cats' hind limbs coming away with the dressing. Fortunately these disasters are rare and they should be avoidable by meticulous bandage care and good client communication

It cannot be overstated that dressings need to be checked several times daily and any sign of discomfort (particularly in a patient that was previously comfortable) should be reported as soon as possible. Printed bandage care sheets are an

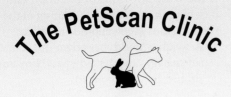

The PetScan Clinic

Veterinary Surgery
1 Halstead Street
Lembert
Surrey

_____Alfie_____ has required a dressing and some care is needed to ensure that it provides both comfort and protection.

The dressing should not be allowed to become wet or dirty.

If the bandage has been applied to a foot then this must be covered by the plastic bag provided and secured with tape whilst the animal is outside. The nurse will demonstrate this for you.

The cover must not be left on for long periods as animals sweat through their pads and this will cause the bandage to become soggy and uncomfortable. It may also cause damage to the wound.

Please contact the surgery immediately should any of the following occur:

- Any unusual odour or discharge from the bandage
- Swelling or redness around the bandage
- Excessive discomfort is noticed

Aggravation (biting, gnawing, etc.) of the bandage by _____Alfie_____ should be discouraged. A special collar (called an 'Elizabethan collar') can be obtained from the surgery as necessary.

An appointment will be made for you for the removal or replacement of the bandage.

Figure 5.10 Example of a bandage care client information sheet.

excellent idea and should be encouraged (Figure 5.10).

It is not uncommon for our patients to try to remove dressings themselves. Whilst some animals may be difficult and attempt to remove any dressing placed on them, alarm bells should ring if an animal which has had a bandage on for several days starts to mutilate it. This is often a sign of pain and needs to be investigated.

Elizabethan collars, bitter apple spray or bandaging paws are all ways of reducing mutilation of dressings: in many cases these can be avoided by judicious use of **analgesia**.

Part 2:
Minor surgical techniques

Wound management

WOUND CLASSIFICATION

Wounds are classified according to the type of injury sustained and the contamination/sanitary status of the wound. The type of injury may be:

- Incisional
- Abrasions/grazes
- Degloving/shearing/avulsion
- Puncture
- Burns
- Firearm
- **Iatrogenic** (bandage wounds)
- Miscellaneous (bite or sting from e.g. snake, arthropod, jellyfish)

The sanitary status of a wound may be:

- Clean: there is no inflammation present and no sign of contamination (surgical wounds)
- Clean **contaminated**: there is no inflammation present but some superficial contamination. Flushing the wound will generally remove contamination and revert the wound to a clean wound
- **Contaminated**: there is little or no inflammation present, but contamination is fairly heavy and may involve high bacterial numbers. If left unattended, infection will occur
- Dirty: inflammation is present and there is a purulent discharge. Necrosis of the wound is evident and debris may be substantially present

Incisional wounds

- These types of wound usually arise from a sharp instrument or object being drawn along the skin surface (Figure 6.1)
- They are characterised by gaping of the wound with a sharply defined wound edge and minimal damage to surrounding tissues
- Generally, contamination is not usually a problem

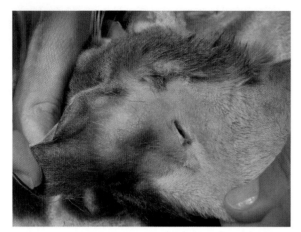

Figure 6.1 Incisional wound to cat's head: this wound occurred due to the patient mistaking a broken windowpane for a cat flap!

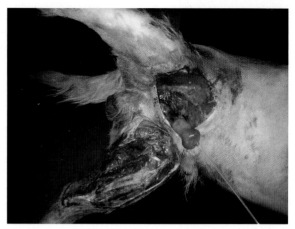

Figure 6.2 This dog has received shearing and avulsion injuries following an RTA.

- These types of wound are generally amenable to primary closure

Abrasions/grazes

- These wounds are usually seen following road traffic injuries and are caused by frictional damage to the skin
- Grazes typically only involve the more superficial layers of the dermis, although wounds rarely fall into discrete classifications; thus deeper layers may be affected
- Due to the nature of the injury, debris, along with bacteria, has usually been pressed deep into the wound. Such injuries are thus classed as **contaminated** wounds
- These types of wound are rarely amenable to primary closure and often require prolonged wound management

Degloving/shearing/avulsion

- Degloving is usually the result of a road traffic accident (RTA) and involves the tearing away of skin from a limb (Figure 6.2)
- It may be immediate, or progress over several days. In the latter case, the degloving is due to damage to blood vessels supplying the area of skin

- Avulsion injuries are frequently seen following encounters between dogs and badgers. Areas of skin, often around the mandible, may be torn off
- Shearing injuries are a combination of abrasional injury and degloving and usually result from an RTA. Distal limbs are most commonly involved and there may be substantial damage to underlying tissues
- Degloving or avulsion injuries generally have minimal contamination, whereas contamination of shearing injuries is likely to be substantial
- All of these types of wound require extensive and prolonged wound management, often including skin grafting or reconstructive surgery after management of infection. Shearing wounds may also require extensive orthopaedic repair

Puncture wounds

- Puncture wounds are usually caused by bites (Figure 6.3), but may also be caused by staking injuries
- The skin wound is usually rather small, whereas the deeper tissues sustain extensive crushing and tearing damage: body cavities may be involved; including abdominal visceral rupture or **pneumothorax**

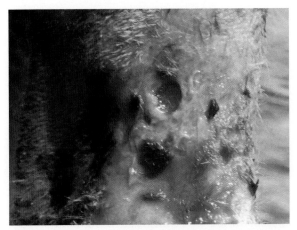

Figure 6.3 Puncture wound on cat forelimb. The wound is approximately 24h old and was caused by a cat bite. Fur has been clipped from the area prior to **debridement**.

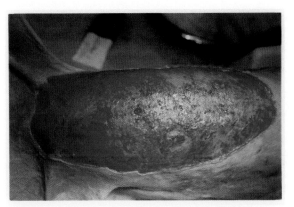

Figure 6.4 This greyhound received extensive full-thickness burns to the ventrum after lying on an uncovered electric blanket.

- Contamination by bacteria is generally quite marked: in addition, hair and dirt may be driven deep into the wound. Stake injuries in particular may be very heavily **contaminated**, with fragments of stick and dirt deep in the wound
- Management of these wounds may be fairly complicated and prolonged: infection and damage to underlying organs are the main determinants of treatment

Burns

- Extreme heat or cold, various chemicals, electricity or radiation may all cause burn injuries (Figure 6.4)
- Burn injuries, regardless of their aetiology, often result in loss of skin several days after the injury: indeed, it can be impossible to predict the severity of a burn immediately
- As the extent of the burn becomes apparent, there is often a clear distinction between devitalised tissue and healthy tissue
- Contamination is rarely a problem initially, although bacterial contamination rapidly ensues as the wound progresses
- Management of burns will depend on the size of the wound, but usually consists of early sharp excision of affected tissue

Firearm wounds

- Firearm wounds differ depending on the calibre and velocity of the weapon, ranging from small puncture wounds to massively destructive wounds with large exit sites
- Generally, tissue damage through the shockwave effect is more of a problem than contamination, although this tissue damage often leads to massive infection potential

Iatrogenic (bandage wounds)

As mentioned in Chapter 5, bandages may cause damage through rubbing or, more usually, through restriction of blood supply due to over-tight bandages
- Injuries may be severe, involving the loss of digits or large areas of skin
- Contamination is usually not the major problem in these wounds, although in very severe cases gangrene may set in
- Management usually consists of prolonged wound management

Miscellaneous (bite or sting from e.g. snake or spider)

- These wounds are frequently small and superficial, with the main complications arising from local damage due to necrotising toxins, or more widespread damage due to venoms

- Although spider bites and scorpion stings are not classed as **contaminated** wounds, snake bites are often associated with high numbers of bacteria
- Jellyfish stings can cause quite widespread chemical burns, resulting in necrosis and sloughing of skin
- Management of these wounds usually consists of prolonged wound management and specific antitoxins where appropriate

REVIEW OF WOUND-HEALING

Wound-healing is often divided into three or four phases, although the phases overlap considerably:

- Inflammation/debridement phase: injury to blood vessels in the skin triggers the haemostatic pathways that result in coagulation and clot formation. Other chemicals, such as **cytokine** and growth factors, are released and these draw inflammatory cells into the area. The blood clot helps to stabilise the wound edges and limits ingress of bacteria. As inflammation progresses, the inflammatory cells (macrophages and neutrophils) aid in **debridement** by phagocytosis of bacteria and debris, release of collagenases and formation of purulent exudates. This phase starts within minutes of injury and becomes maximal at 2–3 days after injury
- Proliferation phase: growth factors and **cytokines** released by macrophages stimulate the migration and reproduction of fibroblasts. The fibroblasts produce collagen and other components of fibrous tissue. **Angiogenesis** is also stimulated by macrophages, directing growth of capillaries into the area. It is this mix of fibroblasts, collagen and new blood vessels that comprises granulation tissue, which usually becomes apparent 3–5 days after injury. Once granulation tissue has developed, epithelialisation begins, although this process occurs much earlier (within 24–48 h) with sutured wounds. Epithelial cells migrate over the surface of the wound to cover it completely. Once this has happened, further cell

division occurs and stratified epithelium begins to be produced. Specialised cells, called myofibroblasts, help wound contraction at this time, reducing the size of the wound

- Maturation phase: the number of collagen fibres deposited by the fibroblasts usually reaches its peak 2–3 weeks after injury. After this time, the apparently random deposition of collagen fibres reorganises to increase wound strength. Fibroblasts and capillaries decrease in number, causing the scar to become paler and flatter. The process of maturation is ongoing, but scars rarely attain more than 80% of the skin's original strength

FIRST AID FOR SIMPLE AND COMPLEX WOUNDS

First aid for wounds simply means preventing the wound (and the patient) from worsening in any way: in other words, first aid does not involve wound-suturing. The aims of wound first aid are:

- To reduce or stop further haemorrhage
- To provide **analgesia** (either in the form of drugs, or by applying a dressing)
- To reduce contamination of a wound
- To minimise further damage to surrounding tissues or to tissues deeper within the wound (by preventing drying of tissues or damage by wound movement)
- To begin the process of wound **debridement** by suitable selection of dressings
- To stabilise the patient until wound management proper can be carried out

In some cases, definitive wound repair can be carried out immediately; in most cases, some delay is necessary until time or circumstances allow for wound repair. For example, relevant personnel may not be available, or the patient may have injuries that require more urgent attention.

Triage/emergency assessment

Wounds may present to the practice as simple cut pads on a sprightly young pointer, or as extensive

debridement injuries following a RTA on a cat. Regardless of the cause or type of wound, following a standard protocol should facilitate the best treatment in every case.

The ABC is familiar to most people as the basic first-aid mnemonic: D stands for danger and refers in this case to danger of injury to the first-aid provider (Box 6.1).

- Danger: wounded animals are likely to be in pain and may behave abnormally: the most placid of pets could well become aggressive if frightened or in pain, or may simply snap or strike out if a painful area is touched. Precautions must be taken to ensure that neither the staff nor the clients are at any risk of injury. It is reasonable to ask the owner whether a pet normally resents being handled. Wherever possible, a nurse or trained member of staff should assist in restraining the patient so that your full attention can be given to assessing the wounds. Muzzles may be a sensible precaution
- ABC: certainly any wound obtained as a result of an RTA or other traumatic incident may have caused other injury to the patient. Alternatively, animals may have concurrent illness or be otherwise debilitated (e.g. geriatric patients). Checking for an adequate airway, signs of respiratory distress and assessment of the cardiovascular system should be carried out rapidly and accurately:
  - A brief history of the trauma should be obtained
  - If the patient is presented in a container then take the animal out and examine it: it is useful to examine any blankets briefly to assess the amount of blood loss
  - The respiratory rate and effort should be assessed: any open-mouthed breathing in cats should be viewed with concern as it may indicate underlying pulmonary dysfunction rather than simple stress. It may be worth considering oxygen supplementation for these patients, or, if no life-threatening injuries are detected, allowing them to calm down in an oxygen cage or tent for several minutes before examining them further
  - The mucous membrane colour and capillary refill time (CRT) should be assessed, together with heart rate and pulse quality. Rapid or slow pulse, together with decreased CRT and pale mucous membranes, should alert the observer to the possibility of shock or at least circulatory compromise and measures should be taken to counter this
  - A brief assessment should be made of the nervous system: the patient's level of awareness should be fairly obvious and may give an indication as to whether or not cranial damage has occurred

Once any life-threatening complications have been ruled out, the animal should be examined more closely and a (mental) list made of any obvious or possible trauma. Nails/claws should be examined for scuffing or tearing that may indicate RTA: these patients should always have chest radiographs to rule out diaphragmatic rupture. However, in more stable patients some attempt at wound first aid should be carried out first.

Fractures or severe soft-tissue injures may underlie fairly innocent-appearing wounds. These may not be life-threatening, but an accurate assessment of them early on may allow for a more appropriate bandage to be placed as a first-aid procedure.

Burns may often appear relatively superficial, but are often associated with appreciable fluid losses, which, if not corrected, can lead to shock and death.

Bite injuries are often 'traumatic icebergs', especially bites inflicted by large dogs on small dogs or cats: these wounds often have substantial underlying damage, even penetration into the abdominal or the thoracic cavity, and must all be properly explored and debrided.

Box 6.1

- **D**anger
- **A**irway
- **B**reathing
- **C**irculation

First aid

Any haemorrhage should be controlled first.

- Placing **sterile** swabs or bandage over the wound and applying pressure for 4–5 min may often be enough to control minor haemorrhage
- Calcium alginate dressings may be applied to aid **haemostasis**
- In cases with more severe haemorrhage, direct pressure over the supplying artery may be considered (for example, in the groin to exclude the femoral artery, or over the biceps to reduce bleeding in the distal fore limb: again, 4–5 min of pressure may be sufficient to control haemorrhage)
- Tourniquets should be avoided unless absolutely necessary due to the risk of pressure damage to underlying nerves and blood vessels
- An alternative to tourniquets is to use a blood-pressure cuff on a limb proximal to the wound and inflate that to 20 cmH$_2$O above measured arterial pressure. Provided it remains inflated, this may be left in place for 2–3 h

For small lacerations, placing a simple bandage (non-adhesive contact layer and conforming bandage layer) may be a sufficient first-aid measure, until preparations can be made for wound **lavage**.

The first 6 h following injury represent the 'golden period' (Box 6.2). During this time, a wound may be considered **contaminated**, rather than infected. Wounds cleaned within this time are amenable to cleaning and primary closure. After this time, bacterial numbers in a wound will have risen to a level at which infection is inevitable and these wounds must be treated by secondary intention or delayed primary healing (see later).

Box 6.2

Wherever possible, wounds should be closed within the first 6 h to take advantage of the 'golden period'.

This should be borne in mind when dealing with wounds that are nearing the end of the golden period. These wounds should be covered with a **sterile** dressing (as with other wounds), but preparation should be made to deal with these wounds definitively as soon as possible.

Analgesia should be a priority of wound first aid. Several steps may be taken to ensure adequate pain relief:

- **Opioids** may be administered at analgesic doses: if the patient is stable for anaesthesia, a routine premed may be administered at this time
- Provided there is no concurrent hepatic or renal disease, and provided the fluid status of the patient is adequate, non-steroidal anti-inflammatories may be administered
- Dilute lidocaine (1 ml in 10 ml **sterile** water or saline) can be applied directly to the wound by syringe or spray bottle (a small plastic perfume spray bottle is useful for this). This may not provide appreciable **analgesia** if the wound is bleeding copiously, but the author has found it to be considerably analgesic for his own climbing injuries!
- The dressing, if snugly placed with padding extending some distance away from the wound, will provide some fair measure of pain relief
- Placing the patient in a cage, thus restricting movement, will aid **analgesia** and may increase the 'comfort factor' in patients that are stressed

Wound **lavage** should then be performed:

- Depending on the nature of the wound and the temperament of the patient, sedation or even general anaesthesia may be necessary to facilitate adequate wound **lavage**
- For smaller wounds and calmer patients, the **analgesia** described above may well be sufficient to enable a thorough inspection of the wound and **lavage**
- **Sterile** gloves should be worn – ideally full operating gear (mask, hat, gown). Although the wound is considered already **contaminated**, further contamination, especially by hospital bacteria, is to be avoided
- The hair around the wound should be carefully clipped: in order to avoid getting hair in

the wound, a covering of Intrasite gel (Smith & Nephew) or saline-soaked gauze swabs may be used

- Using a 20-ml syringe with a 19 G needle, the wound should be copiously flushed with **sterile** saline or Hartmann's solution. The syringe and fine needle increase the jet pressure and enable a much more effective flush to be carried out
- Enough fluid to clean the wound visibly should be used (500 ml is usually considered the minimum). The needle should be positioned just off the surface of the wound so as to avoid spreading contamination deep within the surrounding tissues
- A bacterial swab should be taken for culture. This will not provide a result for 2–3 days, but it will ultimately save time if bacterial resistance is demonstrated to the chosen antibiotic. It will also monitor for the presence of unusual pathogens or potentially very serious bacteria such as methicillin-resistant *Staphylococcus aureus* (MRSA: see Chapter 10)
- A suitable dressing and bandage should then be applied. This may only be left in place for a short while, until definitive closure or **debridement** is performed, but attention should be given to the quality of the bandage: irritation at pressure points at this stage could well lead to pressure sores and bandage disease later on

First aid for complex wounds

Burns, penetrating foreign bodies (sticks), gunshot wounds and compound fractures can all be managed appropriately by first aid, in the manner described above, but with the following precautions:

- Burns should be cooled by **lavage** and by cooled moistened swabs for at least 30 min. Clients should be instructed to do this prior to bringing the patient in, provided the animal is otherwise stable. Heat damage can progress for some time after the initial heat source has been removed and the true extent of burn damage can often not be fully assessed for 48–72 h. Particular attention should be paid

to fluid management of these patients: they are likely to be dehydrated, anaemic and hypoalbuminaemic. Early use of intravenous fluids such as Hartmann's solution and colloids (e.g. Haemaccel, Intervet UK) is necessary to stabilise these patients and protect renal function

- Sticks or other penetrating foreign bodies should not be removed without first taking radiographs to assess the extent of penetration, although it may make movement of the patient slightly easier if the object is cut short, say 2–3 cm from the body wall. The wound should be assessed from a first-aid point of view, gross contamination removed by **lavage** and a dressing placed over the wound and foreign body until the patient is ready for exploratory surgery. If possible, conscious radiographs should be taken to assess thoracic or other life-threatening damage. Securing the foreign body with a bandage should restrict further movement and thereby limit tissue damage
- Gunshot wounds and compound fractures can be treated in a similar way from a first-aid perspective. Severe soft-tissue injury is likely to have occurred in addition to fractures, so some form of splinting may be advisable: plastic gutter splints are light and may be cut to fit and are ideal for lower-limb trauma. The upper limb or trunk may be less amenable to splinting, but thick pads of cotton wool or disposable nappies may provide a good deal of support to a wound and limit further damage until definitive repair can take place

OPEN MANAGEMENT AND MINOR SURGICAL DEBRIDEMENT

By observing the golden period and performing adequate **lavage**, simple incisional wounds can be closed primarily (see Chapter 8). These wounds will have fresh edges and no visible sign of contamination (Figure 6.5). Wound-healing should proceed without complication in these types of injury.

Where the 'magical' 6 h have elapsed, or considerable contamination has occurred, which

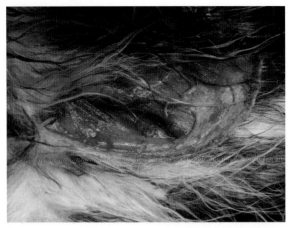

A

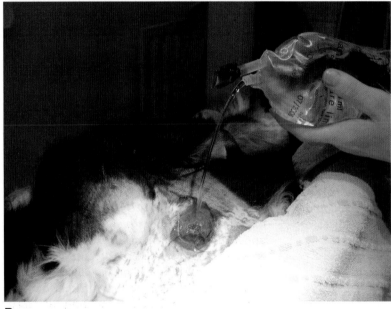

B

Figure 6.5 (A) Stake injury. X rays are indicated to assess damage to internal organs. (B) Saline is used to remove gross contamination from the wound.

cannot be removed by **lavage**, the wound is not amenable to simple primary closure and will require some form of **debridement** (Box 6.3).

In almost every case, this will require general anaesthesia, or at least sedation. Attention should be given to the level of **analgesia**. As discussed in Chapter 3, it is far more effective to utilise several types of analgesic than to increase the dose of a single agent (sequential **analgesia**).

Box 6.3

Debridement is the removal of contaminated, infected, necrotic or otherwise non-viable tissue and debris from a wound.

Wounds with appreciable contamination may be treated in a number of ways:

- By minor **debridement** of the wound edges and immediate closure of the wound (primary)
- By regular dressing changes and antibiosis until infection is controlled, then **debridement** and closure (delayed primary)
- Allowing a granulation bed to form and then closing by grafting techniques (secondary closure)
- Allowing the wound to heal by granulation and re-epithelialisation (secondary-intention healing)

Primary closure following debridement

In order to be amenable to **debridement** and primary closure, a wound must fulfil certain criteria:

- The wound must be in an area where there is sufficient skin to enable primary closure following **debridement**. For limbs, wounds that can be easily closed are limited to lacerations, tears and small puncture wounds. On the torso, where skin is more elastic, relatively large wounds can be debrided and closed in a primary fashion
- Damage must be limited to more superficial tissues. An exception to this is where the wound is still within the 6-h grace period and minimal **debridement** of deeper tissues is required; especially where ligament or tendon injury has occurred, it is best to try to repair these structures as soon as possible. If in doubt, the skin may be left open or a surgical drain placed; however, a drain should not be used as an alternative to meticulous **debridement** and **lavage**
- There must be no sign of infection. It may be easy to spot infection: there may be purulent discharge or inflammation around the wound. However, in some cases it may be difficult to assess whether a wound is infected or merely **contaminated**. If there is any doubt, the wound should be left open and treated by delayed primary or secondary closure

Debridement

- Hair should be clipped around the wound (if not already done)
- The skin surrounding the wound should be prepped as for surgery, using povidone-iodine or chlorhexidine. The wound itself should be lavaged again with **sterile** saline: detergents should be avoided as they damage tissues and will delay healing. However, dilute chlorhexidine (0.05%) and povidone-iodine (0.01%) may be used if desired
- The wound should be considered a **sterile** surgical site: **sterile** drapes should be used and mask, hat, gloves and gown worn
- The wound should then be re-examined; any remaining debris should be removed using forceps or swabs (being careful not to force debris deeper into the wound)
- Any obviously necrotic tissue should be removed by dissection: sharp dissection using a scalpel is preferred to scissors, as the latter tend to cause crushing injury to tissues. A large blade (no. 10 scalpel blade) may be used to scrape the deeper wound to remove crusting contamination. Necrotic muscle tissue may be cut away, but care should be taken to avoid nerves and blood vessels. Ligaments and tendons should be minimally debrided (as this will lead to problems of foreshortening)
- The skin edges should be 'freshened up' by sharp dissection, using a no. 11 scalpel blade perpendicular to the skin. Practice is needed here to create straight cuts: holding the 'dead' line of skin with a forceps and applying a little tension helps to direct the line of the cut. Aim to remove 2–3-mm strips around the wound edges. The aim is to see bleeding at the cut edge: if no blood is seen then a further strip should be removed. Burn wounds often require fairly brusque **debridement** as the damaged tissue (**eschar**) is often more extensive than it first appears
- Gentle **lavage** during the **debridement** process aids in removing dissected debris. Surgical suction, if available, is most useful
- Haemorrhage should be controlled with care (see Chapter 7), as blood is an excellent culture

medium for bacteria. On the other hand, blood vessels should not be needlessly crushed or ligated as they are ultimately the providers of growth and repair factors for the wound

- En bloc **debridement** is a useful technique for speedy **debridement** of a moderately deep **contaminated** wound (Figure 6.6). The wound is lavaged and closed using a simple continuous suture pattern (see Chapter 7) or else tissue glue may be used. The closed-off wound is then treated as a 'lump' and excised, being careful not to penetrate the wound cavity. The excised wound is thus kept isolated from the surgical site, providing a **sterile debridement** and reducing the chance of wound infection
- Once **debridement** of the wound is complete, **lavage** with **sterile** saline is repeated
- At this stage, a swab may be taken from the deep part of the wound and sent for culture and sensitivity
- The wound may now be closed (see Chapter 8)

Delayed primary closure

In some cases, it may be difficult to **lavage** a wound adequately to the degree of readying it for primary closure. In these situations, application of an adherent dressing (see Chapter 5) such as **sterile** gauze soaked in saline (wet-to-dry) will aid **debridement** of the wound.

- The dressing should be changed daily. In some cases, with heavily **contaminated** wounds, the frequency of dressing change may be increased to twice daily
- Each dressing change should be performed under aseptic conditions, with hat, mask, gown and gloves
- Removing an adherent dressing is often painful and the patient may require sedation or even general anaesthetic for each dressing change. Lidocaine 2% dripped or sprayed on to the dressing may provide some **analgesia**
- It is usual to see some greenish discharge for the first 2–3 days. Provided the animal is non-pyrexic and there is minimal inflammation, this should not cause too much concern. There

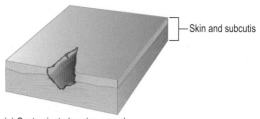

(a) Contaminated gaping wound

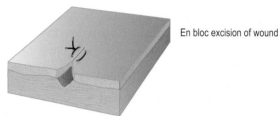

(b) Wound closed with one or more horizontal mattress sutures

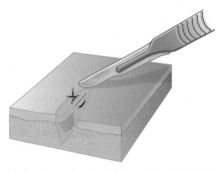

(c) Closed wound excised with a small margin of excision

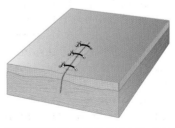

(d) Simple interrupted sutures used to close new (clean) wound

Figure 6.6 En bloc **debridement** of a **contaminated** wound.

should not be frank pus when the wound is palpated

- After 3–5 days, the dressing should come away from the wound bloody, but not covered with discharge. At this stage the wound is ready for delayed primary closure
- Sharp dissection is carried out to provide fresh skin and wound edges and the wound is closed (see Chapter 8)

Secondary closure

Avulsion injuries, shearing injuries, burns and other wounds that result in skin deficits may require closure by reconstructive skin closure techniques or by grafting. In all cases, it is necessary to have a recipient bed of granulation tissue over the wound. This recipient bed provides support, nutrition and growth and repair factors to the overlying repair.

- Initially, the wound should be cleaned by **lavage** and gross contamination removed (as above). Sharp **debridement** should be used to remove as much necrotic tissue as possible
- An adherent dressing (**sterile** saline-soaked cotton gauze: wet-to-dry) should be applied to the wound and the dressing changed daily or twice daily until granulation tissue can be seen to be forming in the wound (usually 3–5 days)
- Strict aseptic technique (hat, mask, gown, gloves and drapes) should be used at each dressing change
- Once granulation tissue has appeared, a non-adherent dressing should be used. A hydro-colloid gel (e.g. Intrasite, Smith & Nephew) is ideal at this stage and will aid in micro-debridement of necrotic tissue. A non-adherent cotton pad (e.g. Melolin, Smith & Nephew) is placed over a layer of Intrasite gel and a bandage applied
- The dressing should be changed daily until the granulation tissue has formed a smooth bed. There should be no sign of necrotic areas and the granulation bed should have an even texture and colour
- Presence of a mature granulation bed implies absence of infection and at this stage an

attempt may be made to close the skin over the bed by a variety of reconstructive techniques

Second-intention healing

Where skin closure is not considered advisable or achievable (for example, when the wound overlies a fracture with a fixator in place, or in the distal limb where less spare skin is available), the wound may be left to heal by second-intention healing (Figure 6.7). Since this takes longer and may result in a less cosmetic appearance than primary or delayed primary or secondary closure, it is often avoided. However, careful attention to dressing construction early on in management of the wound will accelerate wound-healing and lead to a much better end-result.

- The wound is cleaned by **lavage** and sharp **debridement** of necrotic tissue as above
- Steps are followed as above to induce a bed of granulation tissue
- Once a uniform granulation bed has been achieved, a hydrofoam dressing such as Allevyn (Smith & Nephew) is used to maintain a good environment for wound-healing. The dressing may be changed every 3–5 days at this stage (strict asepsis should be maintained)
- Re-epithelialisation and wound contracture (**cicatrisation**) will result in wound-healing after 4–6 weeks, depending on the size of the wound
- Dressings are required until an epithelial layer covers the entire wound

Antibiotics

In deciding whether to use antibiotics in wound management, and which antibiotics to use, there are several guidelines to follow:

- Uncomplicated wounds which are treated within the 6-h golden period should not require antibiotics
- For more complicated or long-standing wounds, start with a broad-spectrum antibiotic (an amoxicillin/clavulanate, e.g. Synulox, Pfizer, 12.5–25 mg/kg PO BID)

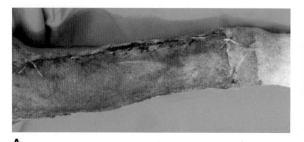

A

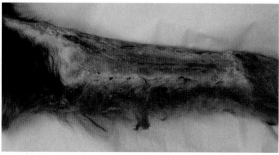

C

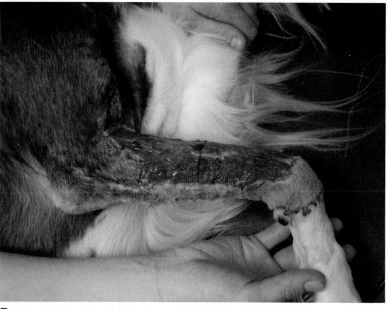

B

Figure 6.7 Second-intention healing. (A) An axial pedicle flap was used to repair a skin deficit following removal of a **tumour** from the forelimb of this border collie. Five days after surgery, the distal pedicle began to dehisce. At first the flap became darkened and oedematous; over the next 3 days the entire distal flap lifted off the wound. (B) The wound was debrided over several days using a combination of Intrasite gel and Allevyn (Smith & Nephew). Twelve days after surgery, a layer of granulation tissue covers the deficit. A small patch of necrotic tissue remains (central wound). The dressings and limb were supported by a Robert-Jones bandage and changed daily until day 14, then every 2 days for a further week. Sedation was not required for the dressing changes, but buprenorphine was administered 45 min before each dressing change. (C) By 8 weeks following surgery, epithelialisation and wound contraction have reduced the size of the wound by over 70%. The newly epithelialised skin is relatively fragile at this stage. A non-adherent dressing (Melolin, Smith & Nephew) is used to protect the wound. The dressing is changed every 5 days.

- This course should then be continued for 5–7 days and re-evaluated once the results of the culture and sensitivity are back
- In the case of severe wounds (for example, burns, degloving injuries or any wound necessitating intensive medical or nursing care)

intravenous broad-spectrum antibiotics (e.g. a second-generation cephalosporin, such as cefuroxime (Zinacef, Glaxo, 20–50 mg/kg IV) should be commenced immediately
- When dealing with heavily **contaminated** wounds, topical antibiotic therapy can also be

used: soaking the primary dressing in gentamicin or lincomycin may aid in reduction of bacterial numbers

If infection persists despite antibiotic usage:
- Reappraise the dressing regime to ensure an appropriate dressing is being used
- Check for any breakdown in aseptic technique when changing dressings
- Repeat bacterial swabs (aerobic and anaerobic culture) to check for appropriate antibiotic selection
- Consider radiographs to look for signs of underlying osteomyelitis or remaining foreign bodies
- Monitor the patient's haematology for evidence of immune suppression or problems due to chronic infection (**lymphopenia**, anaemia)

MANAGEMENT OF COMPLICATED WOUNDS

Most wounds are amenable to treatment following the guidelines above. However, some wounds require slightly different management. Situations of note are: shearing wounds associated with compound fractures; **perineal** wounds; slow-healing wounds and **ulcers**; and management of wound breakdown following surgery.

Wounds associated with compound fractures

- A compound fracture is one where the bone has exited the skin at some time during the fracture genesis. Such fractures may present in any one of a number of ways: a fragment may still be protruding from the wound; there may be extensive skin and tissue loss overlying the fracture; or else the only indication of a compound fracture may be a small puncture wound at the affected area
- In any case, the bone must be considered **contaminated**. In the case of a small overlying puncture wound, if the wound is treated well, observing strict aseptic precautions, there are usually few complications. In more extensive injuries, the prognosis depends on the degree of contamination and damage to other tissues
- These wounds must be managed with some haste: early wound **lavage** under general anaesthesia, application of a dressing (with the addition of a topical antibiotic such as gentamicin) and stabilisation with a gutter splint or a good Robert-Jones bandage will all help to improve the prognosis
- A swab should be taken for bacterial culture and intravenous antibiotics commenced
- Internal/external fixators are the treatment of choice for these fractures, as there are no implants at the **contaminated** fracture site and the wound is disturbed as little as possible for implant placement
- The wound may then be managed open, by application of dressings as above, either until a delayed primary closure may be performed, or, more usually, to allow healing by second intention

Perineal wounds

These present various problems in management, mainly due to the fact that they are in an area that is considered heavily **contaminated** and also because they are difficult to apply dressings to. Due to their painful nature, animals are prone to self-mutilating **perineal** wounds, thus worsening them; patients may also become aggressive and difficult to handle when examining the wounds.

In most cases, it is necessary to sedate or anaesthetise the patient to deal with these wounds. As with all other wounds, the basic principles of **lavage** and **debridement** of necrotic tissue, observing aseptic technique (hats, masks, gowns, drapes) stand true here. Simple wounds may be amenable to primary closure: more complex, long-standing or infected wounds will have to be dealt with by secondary closure or second-intention healing. Dressings are usually impossible to apply, so it may be necessary to perform **lavage** on a sedated or anaesthetised patient daily (applying Intrasite gel to the wound can often speed up healing). Elizabethan collars may be used to prevent self-trauma, and the use of a tail bandage may reduce recontamination of the wound.

The perineum is gifted with a very good blood supply and repair is usually rapid and uneventful in this area. An exception is seen in German shepherds with anal furunculosis – a disease of controversial origin. Anal furunculosis should be considered a medical problem and treated with a combination of drugs and diet; surgical management is aimed at performing delayed primary closure on persisting furuncles towards the end of medical management.

Slow-healing wounds and ulcers

An **ulcer** is defined as a wound involving loss of a basal epidermis. Such wounds are uncommon in animals, but may be seen following radiation treatment for cutaneous **tumours**, chemical injuries (for example, perivascular administration of irritant drugs, including vincristine and thiopental) and in diabetic patients. In addition, **ulcers** arising from inadequately padded or monitored bandages or from recumbent patients (pressure sores or decubitus **ulcers**) are seen.

- Repair entails **lavage** and **debridement** of the wound under aseptic conditions, application of suitable and appropriate dressings and regular dressing changes
- In addition, the underlying cause should be identified and dealt with: recumbent patients should be placed on padded beds and moved at least every 2 h

Slow-healing wounds to the axilla

These are commonly seen in cats, following entrapment of the affected limb in a collar. These wounds often fail to heal due to the constant movement of the wound edges. **Debridement** and dressing changes are usually ineffectual at healing these wounds and they are best treated by reconstructive surgery techniques utilising advancement or rotational flaps. Omentalisation of the wound (drawing a flap of greater omentum into the wound from a separate **laparotomy** site) often aids healing.

Wound breakdown following surgery

It would be lovely if all wounds treated within a veterinary practice healed without event and produced minimal scarring. However, for various reasons wounds can and do break down.

- The wound management may have been inappropriate (due to incorrect assessment of viability of tissues, level of contamination or lack of aseptic technique)
- The repair may have been performed badly, or without consideration of other factors (for example, a repair under tension or over a moving joint)
- Foreign material may be present in the wound or in the deeper tissues (sticks, grit, swabs!)
- The patient may have self-mutilated the wound
- The owner may have failed to notice a slipped or soiled dressing or may not have been well-informed as to correct bandage care
- The patient may have concurrent illness that delays wound-healing (e.g. diabetes mellitus, hyperadrenocorticism, feline leukaemia virus (FeLV) or feline immunodeficiency virus (FIV) in cats), or there may be underlying **neoplasia** at the wound site
- There may have been a reaction to the suture materials used
- There is an inherent wound breakdown rate of any surgical repair, which is highest in skin grafts, but still present in simple repairs

It can be very depressing to encounter wound **dehiscence**, both from a personal perspective and also for the sake of the patient and the owner's expectations. However, wound breakdowns should be seen as a learning opportunity and a chance to improve client communication. This does not mean that one should be dismissive of failures, but merely that one should approach them as interesting challenges. If more wounds break down than heal well, then, of course, there is a problem with technique or management that needs to be addressed.

When presented with a wound that has regressed in its healing, several factors must be ascertained:

- Why has the wound broken down?
- How much of the wound is still progressing well?
- Is the remaining wound at risk?
- How can the breakdown process be halted?
- Is the patient otherwise well?

This demonstrates one of the values of taking a bacterial swab for culture at the time of initial wound management. Not only can one then be a step ahead in terms of antibiotic selection, but, importantly, it is useful to be able to differentiate between a pre-existing infection and a **nosocomial** infection (one acquired in hospital).

It is usually unrewarding to resuture wound breakdowns unless the patient has very recently ripped the sutures out. If attempts are made to repeat suturing, then this should be performed under aseptic conditions and the wound thoroughly lavaged and the wound edges freshened.

- In most cases, the wound is best treated by open wound management, by performing **lavage**, repeating bacterial swabs and dressing the wound with an appropriate contact layer. If the wound has become very **contaminated,** this may require **debridement** under general anaesthesia, application of wet-to-dry dressings and a progression through hydrogel dressings to non-adhesive dressings. These wounds may then be allowed to progress to healing by second intention, or else a delayed primary closure may be performed
- Small wounds may be closed by en bloc **debridement**, although this must be performed with meticulous care, as if wound breakdown recurs, then the wound will be considerably larger
- Very minor breakdowns (single sutures becoming loosened in very shallow incisions) may just be monitored for complications
- It may be worth considering biopsy of the wound edges to rule out **neoplasia**
- Any loosened sutures, especially subcutaneous sutures, are best removed as they may act as reposits for bacteria. It may be worth removing all sutures, debriding the wound edges and replacing with surgical staples

- Antibiotics should be chosen according to the results of culture and sensitivity (if no results are available, then a broad-spectrum antibiotic such as a second-generation cephalosporin or potentiated amoxicillin may be used)
- Consideration should be given to **analgesia**
- Any wound breakdown caused by self-trauma must be countered by appropriate measures (such as Elizabethan collars, body stockings and bitter apple spray)

PREPARATION OF SKIN FOR GRAFTS

Wounds with large skin deficits are amenable to closure by various reconstructive techniques, including second-intention healing, skin flaps of varying complexity and skin grafting.

We are fortunate with our animal patients that they have very elastic skin. This means that it is possible to close almost any trunk wound utilising some form of flap or skin movement procedure. However, the limbs, in particular the distal limbs, are not so readily covered by these methods.

Leaving these wounds to heal by second intention often works well, but can have several disadvantages:
- It can take 2–3 months for healing to progress to the stage where dressings are no longer required
- The end-result may be cosmetically unattractive – hairless, heavily scarred skin
- **Cicatrix** (scar) formation may result in a painful area, or, if over a joint, can result in reduction of movement
- Such scars are often considerably weaker than normal skin and may be prone to trauma

The use of skin grafts can reduce many of these disadvantages, when properly placed.

Skin grafts may be full- or partial-thickness, depending on whether epidermis and entire dermis or part of the dermis is included in the graft. They may be placed entire (sheet grafts), or meshed to allow greater coverage and conformation of a wound. Small islands of skin (pinch, punch or stamp grafts: Figure 6.8) may be placed on to a granulating wound to increase the rate of epithelialisation of the wound.

Skin grafting requires a donor skin (the graft) and a recipient bed.

- The recipient bed should be free of all necrotic tissue and contamination, containing only healthy, viable tissue
- Suitable recipient beds include healthy mature granulation tissue, fresh uncontaminated wounds and surgical wounds
- Other wounds should be managed as described above, by debriding under general anaesthesia, careful wound **lavage** and serial application of appropriate dressings until healthy granulation tissue is seen covering the entirety of the wound
- If chronic granulation tissue is present, this is unlikely to have sufficient surface vasculature to allow a graft to take. This should be converted to healthy granulation tissue by surgical **debridement** 24–48h before skin grafting and covered by a **sterile** saline-soaked gauze (wet-to-dry dressing)
- Immediately prior to application of the graft, the skin edges at the recipient bed should be debrided using a scalpel perpendicular to the wound plane, to 'freshen up' the edges, allowing repair between the edges of graft and the wound. If this is not done, the spreading epithelial cells underrun the graft, causing lifting of the edges and risking **dehiscence** of the entire graft

Sheet grafts

- Most sheet grafts used in small animals are full-thickness: that is, they comprise the epidermis and full dermis
- Partial-thickness grafts require the use of special instruments (dermatomes), are prone to failure and tend not to produce cosmetically acceptable results
- The selected skin should come from an area that is easily amenable to primary closure (the flank) and preferably on the same side as the affected limb, to reduce the need to reposition the patient

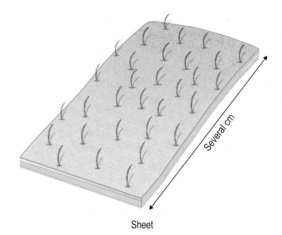

Sheet

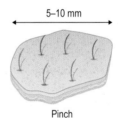

5–10 mm

Pinch

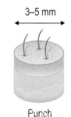

3–5 mm

Punch

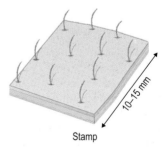

10–15 mm

Stamp

Figure 6.8 Sheet, pinch, punch and stamp grafts.

- The donor skin should be collected under aseptic conditions and the skin, once harvested, should be kept moist by covering or rolling in saline-soaked swabs until required (usually immediately, although it may be stored at 4°C for 2–3 days)
- All hypodermic tissue (fat, panniculus muscle) should be carefully removed from the graft, although direct handling of the graft should be kept to a minimum to avoid crushing damage to the tissue
- The sheet may then be grafted entire, or meshed as required, prior to suturing on to the wound

Pinch, stamp and punch grafts

- These must also be collected in a strict aseptic manner; they are usually harvested from the flank on the same side as the affected limb
- The easiest method of collection is to use a skin biopsy punch (3–5 mm diameter), otherwise pinches of skin may be removed
- The grafts may be stored in **sterile** glass dishes on saline-soaked swabs until required. The donor sites are closed by simple sutures or tissue glue
- Any hypodermic tissue should be snipped off and discarded, prior to placing into slots cut into the granulation bed. No sutures are used
- For a 10×5 cm wound, as many as 20 patches of graft tissue may be required, making the process very time-consuming

Care of the graft and complications

- Most grafts fail due to lack of take. The donor fails to adhere to the recipient bed or receives insufficient nourishment from the underlying tissue. Until new blood vessels begin to grow into the graft (from day 3 onwards, but not providing appreciable nutrition for some days after that), the graft obtains nutrition by a process called **plasmatic imbibition**. Essentially this is a diffusion process, aided by

a sponge-like uptake of fluids and nutrients by the graft
- The first few days are thus critical for graft survival. The most important factor is stability of the graft: any movement or slippage of the graft will drastically reduce the chances of success. Paramount to this is the application of a well-constructed bandage
- The primary (contact) layer must be non-adherent. A polythene-covered cotton pad (e.g. Melolin, Smith & Nephew) may be used, or else silicon non-adherent dressings are available. Petrolatum-soaked swabs should not be used as they inhibit epithelial cell growth
- A Robert-Jones or thick support bandage is ideal; a plastic gutter splint may be used to restrict movement for the first 5 days following surgery
- Wherever possible, the first dressing change should be delayed until 48 h postsurgery: great care must be taken to ensure no lifting of the graft occurs when the dressing is removed. This procedure is best carried out under sedation or general anaesthesia to ensure the patient does not move while the dressing is taken off. It is at this stage that most pinch or punch grafts are lost, as they simply pull off with the dressing
- Strict aseptic technique must be adhered to at each dressing change
- Subsequent dressing changes are carried out daily: due to the process of **plasmatic imbibition**, there is often considerable discharge. At this stage the graft commonly appears an unpleasant oedematous bluish colour. Any focal swelling may indicate fluid accumulation beneath the graft and may be removed using a syringe and 22 G needle
- It may be difficult to distinguish a failing graft from one that is progressing well: it is best to give it the benefit of the doubt and continue treatment as planned. Ultimately, graft failure results in thinning of the graft, pallor or blackening and a papery feel to the donor skin. Any necrotic tissue must be trimmed away to prevent bacterial colonisation
- Infection should not be a problem provided meticulous care in aseptic procedure has been maintained throughout. Any infection tends

to be disastrous to the graft and is best treated prophylactically by judicious use of systemic antibiotics

- The regular dressing changes should be continued for several weeks, reducing in frequency and level of support as dictated by the appearance of the wound. The graft will not reach full strength until at least 45 days, and will thus be prone to damage by even small knocks or bumps

WOUND-HEALING PRODUCTS

Most wounds are amenable to healing by following the basic premises of thorough wound **lavage**, **debridement** and selection of suitable dressings, coupled with appropriate antibiosis and strict adherence to aseptic technique. However, some wounds fail to heal adequately or else heal very slowly. The market worldwide for wound-healing products is massive, indicating the need for more rapid and more successful modes of treatment.

Wound-healing products fall into several main categories: peptide growth factors, larval 'dressings', apitherapy and engineered skin substitutes.

Peptide growth factors

- Including epithelial growth factor, insulin-like growth factor and transforming growth factor-β, these are small subprotein chemicals released from many tissues within the body
- Their role is variously to stimulate and coordinate wound repair, cell growth and chemotaxis
- Their addition topically to wounds has been found to be beneficial in speeding up wound repair, especially in slow-healing **ulcers**
- Although at the moment largely experimental, it is likely that their use will be more widespread as biotechnology brings down the price of production of these growth factors

Larval 'dressings'

- Now accepted as routine use in many hospitals as part of wound care programmes, the appli-

cation of larvae of the common greenbottle, *Lucilia sericata*, helps debride wounds prior to delayed primary closure or skin grafting

- **Sterile** larvae are placed into the wound and restricted by the use of cut-out dressings to the wound itself
- The maggots secrete collagenases and various other enzymes that break down necrotic tissues. There is a suggestion that maggot excretions are antimicrobial, and an alkaline environment is produced which aids wound disinfection
- Exudates are removed by covering the maggot 'cage' with absorptive dressings and the maggots are left in place for up to 3 days, after which time the wound is lavaged, further **debridement** carried out as necessary and definitive wound repair performed

Apitherapy

- The term refers to the use of honey as a wound dressing
- It is likely that much of the benefit of honey derives from the strong osmotic pressure produced by the high sugar content, although the presence of antioxidants, production of hydrogen peroxide and even natural antibiotics derived from plant pollens have all been suggested as having a role to play in the use of honey as a wound treatment
- Benefits include rapid resolution of inflammation around the wound and a reduction in wound malodour. Honey creates a moist environment that favours epithelialisation. Its use in chronic rabbit **abscesses** favours the production of a more watery exudate that drains from the **abscess** more readily

Engineered skin substitutes

- Examples include: VetBiosyst (Global Veterinary Products) porcine collagen, chemically treated and formed into sheets; Transcyte (Smith & Nephew), a polymer membrane comprising porcine dermal collagen; and human collagen derived from newborn human

fibroblasts. The cells are killed during freezing, leaving behind the tissue matrix and growth factors
- These are presented as sheets, which may be placed or sutured on to wounds such as burns or degloving/shearing injuries
- The sheets act as a framework for epithelial regrowth and may provide growth factors and essential nutrients

- Sheets are covered with dressing and regular dressing changes performed under aseptic conditions until either a suitable granulation bed has formed for delayed primary repair or grafting, or else, more usually, the wound is allowed to heal by second-intention healing

Principles of soft-tissue surgery

ASEPTIC TECHNIQUE: HAND-SCRUBBING, GOWNING AND GLOVING

Core to successful surgery is meticulous attention to aseptic technique. It is much easier to prevent infection than to treat it, and this will only become more valid as antibiotic resistance increases.

All possible precautions should be taken to avoid transfer of bacteria from your own body to the surgical site:

- The use of scrub suits and shoes or at least shoe covers is to be encouraged
- Hats and masks reduce contamination from personnel and should be worn at all times in theatre
- **Sterile** gowns present an aseptic barrier between the surgeon and the patient. This is necessary because the surgical scrub process reduces but does not eliminate microorganisms from the arms. It is therefore pointless wearing **sterile** short-sleeved gowns. These gowns are essentially long scrub suits and should be treated as such. If a **sterile** barrier is to be worn, then the gown should be long-sleeved, with the sleeves tucked into **sterile** gloves
- **Sterile** gloves must be used to cover scrubbed hands. They may not be used as an alternative to hand-scrubbing, as research has shown that gloves will develop small tears during surgery: these tears may allow transfer of bacteria from non-scrubbed hands to surgical site. Surgical scrubbing only reduces or suppresses bacteria and so it is vital that **sterile** gloves are worn

Hand-scrubbing

As already mentioned, surgical hand-scrubbing does not sterilise hands and forearms; it merely reduces the microbe count to a very low level and suppresses numbers for a short time. It is therefore important to choose an effective antimicrobial soap based on the effectiveness in terms of microbe kill and residual activity.

In addition, a hand-scrub solution should be fast-acting. Most hand-scrubbing protocols take 3–5 min to perform, but some parts of the hand or arm may only receive attention for a fraction of this time.

Finally, the soap should be non-irritant and preferably not cause chapping or drying of the skin.

Table 7.1 lists common hand and skin disinfectants.

There are two phases to hand- and arm-scrubbing: the first phase is to remove dirt and debris from the hands, arms, fingers and nails. The second phase is the disinfection phase, allowing contact time over each portion of the hand and forearm in a methodical manner.

- All jewellery (watches, rings, bracelets) is removed
- Taps are turned on and, if possible, water is mixed to a comfortable temperature (washing hands in very hot or very cold water may lead to short cuts being taken)
- The hands and forearms are wet thoroughly
- Using an electronic or elbow-operated dispenser, 2–3 pumps (10–15 ml) of surgical scrub solution are applied to the hands
- The hands are then rubbed against each other and the forearm to create a rich lather and to clean them fully

Table 7.1 Properties of common hand and skin disinfectants used in minor veterinary surgery

Disinfectant	Trade name and manufacturer	Properties and uses
Wet scrub soap Chlorhexidine	MediHex-4, MediChem Hibiscrub, Zeneca Hospiguard, Brosch direct	4% Chlorhexidine, surgical scrub and hand-scrub preparations. Lower incidence of allergies than iodine-based disinfectants
Povidone-iodine	MediDine, MediChem Betadine/Pevidine Perdue, Pharma	7.5–10% Povidone-iodine, surgical scrub and hand-wash preparations. Inactivated by pus; may discolour instruments and surfaces. Causes a high incidence of allergies
Triclosan	MediScrub, MediChem Dymapearl, Dyma	1% Triclosan. Surgical scrub. Residual activity, low incidence of allergies
Cetrimide	Hibicet, Zeneca	15% Cetrimide, 1.5% chlorhexidine. Surgical scrub. Low incidence of allergies, due to lower concentration of chlorhexidine
Waterless soap Chlorhexidine	MediHex-05, MediChem	0.5% Chlorhexidine in a foaming base. Rapid-acting
Alcohol (ethanol)	Trigel, MediChem Cutan, Deb	70% Ethanol in a gel base. Contains skin humectants to prevent skin drying from frequent use
Combined alcohol–chlorhexidine	Hibisol, Zeneca Hydrex hand rub, Adams	0.5% Chlorhexidine, 70% alcohol Hydrex contains glycerol to prevent drying of hands

- The nails are cleaned with a nail-cleaner and the hands and arms are rinsed fully
- A **sterile** nail brush is then taken and 2–3 pumps of scrub are applied to this and to the hands and arms

Beyond this stage, if anything other than the nail brush is touched (i.e. another part of the body, the sink or taps), the process must begin again.

- Starting with one hand, the palm is scrubbed gently, making sure that the skin overlying the carpal tunnel is not missed
- The heel of the hand is then scrubbed, followed by the back of the hand
- Each finger (and thumb) is then scrubbed carefully. It may help to consider each finger as having four sides and a top, to make sure no part is missed. The webbing between fingers and between thumb and first finger should be scrubbed well
- The process is repeated for the other hand. Scrubbing each hand should take at least 2 min
- Keeping the hands held higher then the arms, the brush should be used to scrub the forearms, to about three fingers-width above the elbows. This should take a further minute
- The hands and arms should be rinsed off, being careful at all times not to allow the hands to drop lower than the elbows. The hands should be rinsed carefully, starting with the fingers, so that the lather is rinsed down towards the elbows
- The hands are kept raised and away from the body whilst proceeding to the gloving and gowning area

Various adaptations can be made to the above procedure: one rather laborious method is the counted stroke hand-scrub, in which each part of the hand and arm is subjected to 20–30 strokes of the brush. Many surgeons no longer use a scrubbing brush to apply soap through fears that the brush may increase bacterial counts by disturbing bacteria firmly entrenched in crevices in the stratum corneum. Whatever method is used, care must be taken to ensure that no part of the hand or forearm is neglected.

Many companies now produce a waterless scrub solution, comprising alcohol with chlor-hexidine. This has been shown to have a faster action and is more effective than antimicrobial soaps without alcohol. Since it also saves money and time by negating the need for hand towels, it is likely that the waterless scrub alternative will increase in popularity.

Hand-drying

Sterile hand towels should be absorbent, free from lint (or loose bits of cotton) and large enough to be able to dry each hand and forearm on a fresh area of towel. Old drapes make particularly poor hand towels, being relatively non-absorbent, and may be mistakenly repacked as drapes. Fairly inexpensive hand or tea towels are far better suited to the task and are also less likely to be wrongly packaged.

Hand towels should be folded in a concertina fashion and either sterilised individually or in a sterilising drum together with the gown. A corner of the towel is grasped in one hand and the opposite hand and arm are dabbed dry, starting at the fingers and working down to the elbow. If the towel is of a sufficient size, the diagonally opposite corner can then be held in the dry hand and the other hand and arm dried.

Gowning

Gowns may be either single-use (disposable) or cotton reusable. Table 7.2 lists some advantages and disadvantages of each.

Gowns should be considered as having two sides: an inside and an outside. On no account should an ungloved hand touch the outside, and on no account should a gloved hand touch the inside. When taking a gown out of its packaging, it should be held by the inside front of the gown, just below the neck of the gown (Figure 7.1). As it is picked up, it should unfold so that the outside of the gown faces away. The free arm is then inserted through a sleeve, being careful not to touch the outside of the gown and also being very careful not to allow the arm to touch anything (when starting to learn how to gown, it is important to allow a good deal of clear space around

Table 7.2 Relative merits of disposable and reusable gowns

Disposable (single-use) gowns	Cotton (reusable) gowns
Advantages	**Advantages**
Guaranteed sterility (gamma-sterilised)	Better conforming material so increased comfort
Water-resistant material prevents strike-through	Better for the environment as less paper/material waste is produced
Time saving – no need to wash and resterilise	Less storage problem, as fewer gowns needed
Additional cost can be offset by reduced laundry bills and cost of autoclave packaging	
Disadvantages	**Disadvantages**
Relatively expensive (but cost can be offset by reduced laundry bills and less staff time and can be passed on to client)	Cuffs tend to fray over time, and elasticity is lost, making gloving difficult
Bulky waste, so increased disposal costs and increased environmental impact	Time-consuming to prepare (laundry, packaging, autoclaving)
Poorly conforming material so not very comfortable	Washing-machine effluent has a high environmental impact
Storage can be a problem as a new gown is required for each procedure	Fairly absorbent material, so risk of **strike-through**

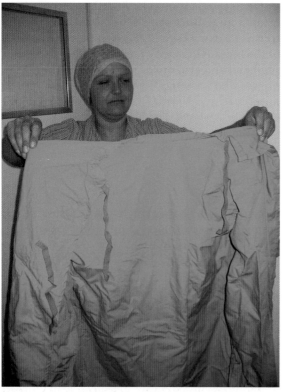

A

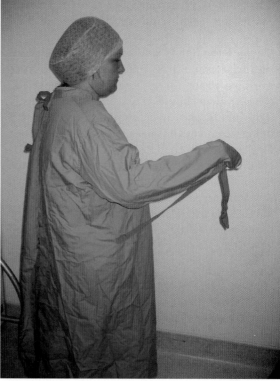

B

Figure 7.1 Gowning. (A) The inside of the gown is held near the collar and the gown is allowed to unfold. (B) The waist loop is handed to an assistant. Note that the hands are retained inside the sleeves. (C) The waist loop is tied around the back. Hands should be held in a praying position to avoid contact with non-sterile surfaces. (cont'd)

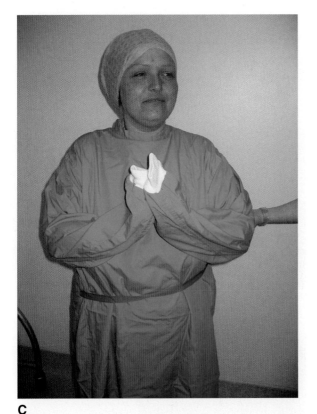

C

Figure 7.1 (Continued).

the gowning area). The other arm can then be slid into its sleeve. Keeping both arms up and shrugging a little helps this process. The hands should not be pushed out of the cuffs at this stage.

An assistant will then be required to secure the gown ties: some gowns require that the wearer ties the waist loop in front (**sterile**-backed gown), while others require that the assistant secures all ties from behind. If a **sterile**-backed gown is worn, the waist tie should not be secured until **sterile** gloves are worn, although an assistant may secure the neck tapes.

Gloving

Sterile gloves may be lubricated or non-lubricated. Non-lubricated gloves are very difficult to put on unless the hands are completely

dry and so lubricated gloves are preferred. Cornstarch, used as a lubricant in many gloves, is very irritating to tissues and should be rinsed off well with **sterile** saline (although this may not remove all traces of it). Ideally, gloves should be chosen which are only lubricated on one side.

There are three methods of applying **sterile** surgical gloves: closed gloving, open gloving and assisted (or plunge) gloving.

Closed gloving is the preferred method of gloving for **sterile** procedures, but requires a little practice to perfect (Figure 7.2):
- Keeping the hands inside the sleeves of the gown, the **sterile** inner pack of gloves is taken and placed on to a **sterile** surface
- Feeling through the gown, one glove is picked up by the cuff and laid over the sleeve, fingers pointing towards the body
- Whilst still pinching the cuff of the glove, the other hand is used to bring the cuff of the glove over the end of the gown cuff
- The folded-over section of glove cuff is then straightened out over the gown sleeve and the hand is wriggled out of the sleeve into the glove
- The process is repeated for the other hand and the gloves are adjusted to make them comfortable and eliminate floppy ends to the fingers

Open gloving is easier, but is not considered aseptic as there is a potential for microbe transfer from the hand to the outside of the gown's cuff:
- The fingers (but not the hands) are allowed to exit the gown cuffs
- The **sterile** inner pack of gloves is taken and placed on to a surface (this need not be **sterile**, but if not, care must be taken not to touch the surface – special care should be taken to ensure that the pack, once opened, does not fold over again, as the outer surface will be **contaminated**. Opening the packet on the edge of a table helps to avoid this)
- The right glove is held open at the inside cuff by the left hand and the right hand is inserted into the glove
- The right hand (in the glove) is then run down the left glove so that the fingers slide into the fold formed by the outside of the cuff (giving

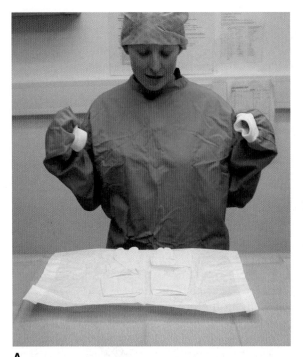

A

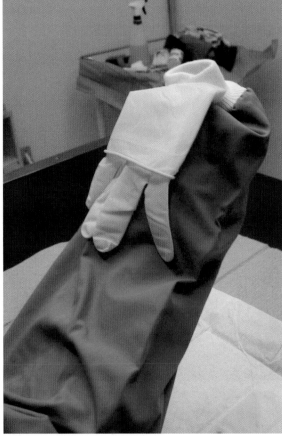

B

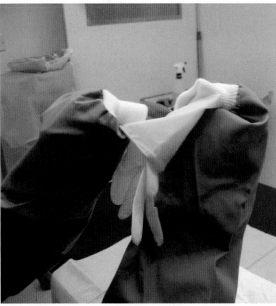

C

Figure 7.2 Closed gloving. (A) The **sterile** glove packet is opened on a **sterile** surface, with the glove fingers pointing towards the gown. (B) The right glove is picked up by the right hand. (C) The left hand pulls the cuff of the right glove over the right hand. (D) Once the glove is over the wrist, the fingers can be allowed out of the gown sleeve. The process is repeated for the other hand. (E) Any floppy ends are adjusted. (cont'd)

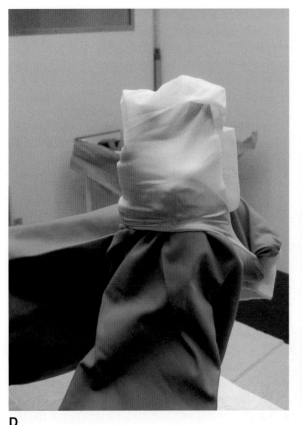
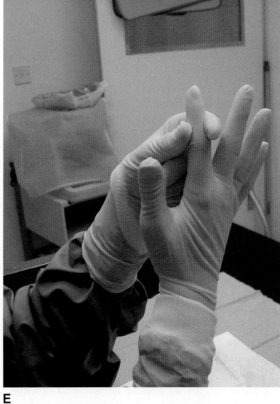

D   E

Figure 7.2 (Continued).

the glove a gentle tug on the end of the cuff with the left hand helps to open the fold here)
- The right hand can then lift the left glove and hold it steady while the left hand is placed inside
- The right hand then pulls the glove's cuff over the cuff of the sleeve. The same is done for the right glove
- The gloves can then be made comfortable

Plunge or assisted gloving requires that a member of the surgical team be already aseptically attired:
- The fingers (but not the hands) are allowed to exit the gown cuffs
- The **sterile**-gowned and gloved assistant holds a glove, fingers down, with the cuff stretched open. It is important that the glove is held by

the outside surface, so that the inner glove is presented
- The hand is firmly inserted into the glove and the assistant repeats the process with the other hand
- This is the technique that should be used if fresh gloves need to be put on during surgery

PREPARATION OF THE SURGICAL SITE

Preparation of the surgical site involves five stages:
1. Removing hair from the site
2. Performing a disinfectant scrub to remove contaminating bacteria
3. Moving the patient to the aseptic operating theatre
4. Positioning the patient for surgery
5. Draping the patient

Although several methods exist for hair removal from the patient (clipping, shaving, application of hair-removal cream), clipping remains the method of choice.

Shaving causes multiple small lacerations on the skin, which may predispose the site to infection. Depilatory creams are expensive to use and are often not very effective on coarse hair.

Before use, the clippers must be checked for blunt or broken teeth and lubricated as necessary. A no. 40 clipper blade is appropriate for most instances.

- The hair is clipped from around the surgical site, to provide a clear margin of between 10 and 20 cm
- If the margin is too small, the site may become **contaminated** by movement of the drapes during surgery
- It is good practice to clip a slightly larger area, to allow for enlargement of the wound should it be required
- The hair is clipped in two stages: firstly with the clippers travelling in the direction of the hair, and secondly, against the hair growth, to close-clip
- A vacuum cleaner should be used to remove clipped hair from the patient
- The paws can be very difficult to clip adequately: care should be taken to avoid cutting the interdigital webbing. Having an assistant spread the digits apart may make this easier
- Alternatively, if the paws are not included in the surgical area, they may be wrapped in conforming bandage or covered by a surgical glove
- It is not recommended to shave the surgical site on the day before surgery: although it may seem to be a good time-saving procedure, the small amount of skin trauma caused by shaving increases the bacteria numbers and can create tiny pockets of infection

Next, the surgical scrub is performed. Table 7.1 lists the commonly available skin disinfectants. The most common contaminants of surgical wounds are the regular skin commensals, *Staphylococcus aureus* and *Streptococcus* spp., and so disinfectants must be highly effective against these organisms. As with hand-scrubbing, surgical skin preparation does not render the skin **sterile**, but reduces the bacterial population to very low numbers and depresses the recolonisation of these organisms.

- Latex gloves should be worn during the scrub procedure: some texts recommend the use of **sterile** gloves and **sterile** swabs. This should not be strictly necessary, provided attention to aseptic technique is adhered to
- Disinfectant is applied to damp gauze swabs (or else dry swabs are dipped into a dish of diluted disinfectant). Warming the scrub solution helps reduce the incidence of hypothermia
- The site is gently scrubbed in a spiralling motion, working from the centre outwards
- Rough or harsh scrubbing should be avoided as this will irritate the skin and release bacteria from hair follicles
- Swabs should never be returned to the central area of the site once they have reached the outer area
- The process is continued until no dirt is seen on the discarded swabs
- Limbs and paws should be prepped in the same way, but in order to gain access to all surfaces a tie or rope may be used to raise the limb off the table. Intravenous (IV) stands or lights may be convenient tying-off points
- Next, a skin antiseptic (final prep) is applied to the site. This is usually 70% alcohol (ethanol) with or without povidone-iodine or chlorhexidine. The solution is applied from the centre outwards by swab, or else may be sprayed. The alcohol will increase the disinfectant effect and displace water from the surgical area, aiding drying

The patient is then transferred to the **sterile** theatre and positioned for surgery.

- To reduce patient heat loss during anaesthesia, some form of heating device should be used. Electric blankets, hot-water bottles, heated bean bags and warm water beds are all useful, but great care must be taken to avoid the risk of **iatrogenic** burns: blankets should be placed between the patient and the heating device

- Plastic troughs or conforming beds are tremendously useful positioning aids. Ties or ropes, if used, must not be allowed to place unnatural tension on a joint (especially in old or arthritic patients). Slipknots should not be used, as these may become tourniquets if the patient is repositioned during surgery!
- The hanging-limb technique may be used to prevent a scrubbed limb or paw becoming recontaminated prior to surgery (i.e. the limb is suspended from a suitable stand, such as an IV drip stand). Some form of quick-release knot should be used on the limb and the hanger so that the tie may be removed by an assistant very easily during draping without allowing contact between the surgeon and the rope or assistant
- Skin antiseptic should be applied to the surgical site, working outwards from the centre. If any contact with the surgical site has been made during movement of the patient, the entire surgical scrub is repeated

DRAPING THE PATIENT

Drapes provide a **sterile** barrier between the patient and the surgical process. They also reduce heat loss from the patient.

Drape material may either be disposable or reusable. Both have advantages and disadvantages:

Disposable drapes:
- Are water-repellent and resist wicking of fluids
- Do not require cleaning
- Are relatively expensive
- Are often less conforming to the surgical site

Reusable drapes:
- Conform better to the surgical site
- Are cheaper, since they are reused
- Require time-consuming cleaning and sterilisation
- Are moderately absorbent and allow wicking

A combination of disposable and reusable drapes may be used, to allow the advantages of both to be exploited.

Two layers of drapes are applied. The first layer usually consists of four reusable drapes; the second layer consists of one fenestrated drape.

Drapes are applied over the patient in an aseptic manner, being careful not to fan or shake the drapes, as this will cause disturbance of hair and debris and increase the risk of infection. Folding the corners of the drape over the gloved hand, each drape is positioned accurately inside the edge of the prepped site. Once placed, the drape should not be moved. Any drape that has been incorrectly placed should be gently removed from the patient, rolling away from the **sterile** site, and discarded.

Drapes are placed nearest first, then to either side and finally furthest away. If a **sterile** assistant is to be present during the surgery, the second drape may be placed furthest away to enable him/her to assist draping. **Sterile** Backhaus or bulldog towel clamps are used to secure the corners of the drapes. Once placed, the towel clamps may be tucked behind the edge of a drape: this not only keeps the operating field tidy, but also reduces tangling of suture material around the clamp, which can be very annoying. The tips of the towel clamps should now be considered **contaminated** and thus should not be removed and repositioned. Care should be exercised during the draping procedure not to allow contact between the gown and the table.

The second layer of drapes is now placed. This should be a single large sheet with a suitable-sized hole, or fenestra. The fenestra should cover the surgical site with room to spare should the wound need to be lengthened. The drape should cover the entire operating table to provide an uninterrupted **sterile** surgical field. Any area of drape hanging over the table or below waist level should be considered **contaminated** and not handled (Box 7.1).

> **Box 7.1**
> Once drapes have been placed, they should not be repositioned.

Draping a limb requires care and planning. Four **sterile** drapes are placed around the base of the limb while it is hanging. A **sterile** drape is then wrapped around the limb, the surgeon or **sterile** assistant holds the limb steady and the tie is removed. The **sterile** drape is then clipped to the limb by **sterile** towel clamps, or else a **sterile** bandage or stockingette is placed over the limb. A large fenestrated drape is placed over the limb and then opened out to cover the table.

This may seem a little excessive in terms of draping simply to remove a small skin tag. However, it is important not to cut corners in sterility. Any breakdown in aseptic technique may lead to infection, and with an increasing number of resistant, or multiply resistant, bacteria there is increased demand to follow protocol and to be seen to do the right thing.

REVIEW OF APPROPRIATE SURGICAL INSTRUMENTS, THEIR USE AND CARE

Figure 7.3 shows a selection of surgical instruments appropriate to minor veterinary surgery.

Scalpel holders and blades

- Blades should always be removed from and applied to a holder using needle holders, never by hand
- For most skin incisions, a no. 10 or 15 blade will be most useful. For sharp **debridement** of a wound edge, some users may find a no. 11 blade easier
- The scalpel may be held in several ways: for most minor surgery techniques, the pencil grip is best as it allows precise incisions (Figure 7.4). However, the scalpel handle may also be held by the fingertips (useful in longer incisions) or within the palm, using the thumb to press down on the blade. The latter hold is more suited to cutting very tough tissue and is not appropriate for most minor surgery

Blades should be discarded after use: it is never acceptable to resterilise them, due to risk of injury to personnel and also to the fact that they will not retain the edge sufficiently.

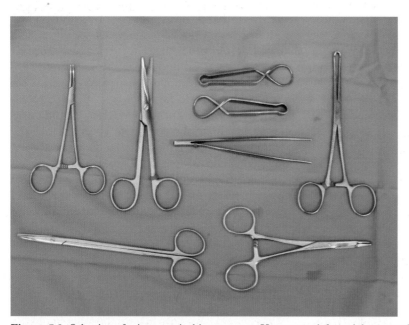

Figure 7.3 Selection of minor surgical instruments. Upper row, left to right: curved mosquito forceps, straight Mayo scissors, bulldog (Jones) towel clamps, rat-toothed (Semkin) thumb forceps, Allis tissue forceps. Lower row: Metzenbaum scissors, Olsen-Hegar needle holders.

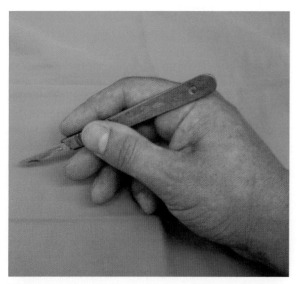

Figure 7.4 The pencil grip for the scalpel provides fine control over the blade.

Cutting tissue may be performed in several ways with a scalpel blade:

- One may use the tip of the blade to enter tissue (a stab incision). This is useful if lancing an **abscess**. It is difficult to control the depth of penetration of the blade, although placing a finger just back from the end of the blade may help to prevent the blade from going too deep
- Drawing the blade along the tissue in a finger grip (slide cutting) provides the easiest way of making skin incisions. Using the free hand to steady the skin and provide a little tension reduces the effort needed to incise and thus makes control of the wound more precise
- A no. 10 scalpel blade may be used to scrape tissue and may be useful for **debridement** of mildly **contaminated** wounds. Care must be taken that all **contaminated** tissue is removed this way and the blade does not push debris further into the wound
- The blade can be used in a sawing motion, pushing and pulling along the tissue. Although useful for thick hypodermic tissue, this technique is not recommended as it is difficult to control the depth of the cut adequately

Needle holders

These may be simple, or combined with scissors. They may be self-locking (ratcheted, e.g. Mayo-Hegar) or non-locking (e.g. Gillies).

- Needle holders without scissors are recommended, as it is possible inadvertently to cut the suture material with the scissors portion while trying to grasp the needle (a cause of some muttered oaths, usually)
- Another reason to choose simple needle holders (e.g. Mayo-Hegar needle holders) rather than those with cutting blades (e.g. Gillies or Olsen-Hegar) is that the former have boxed hinges that are longer-lasting (less prone to loosening)
- Needle holders with a ratchet lock are preferred over non-locking ones as they facilitate more accurate suture placement and are not so tiring for suturing large wounds
- Buying needle holders with tungsten-carbide inserts is worth the extra small expense, as they resist wear from the needles and last longer
- Needle holders should never be used for twisting orthopaedic wire: this causes misalignment of the ends and renders the holders useless

Thumb forceps

These are called thumb forceps to distinguish them from haemostatic forceps and tissue forceps; also they are generally held between the first finger and thumb.

- They are generally of two types: tissue forceps that have little projections (teeth) at their end to enable them to hold tissue, and dressing forceps, which have no such projections and are designed to hold gauze swabs without getting the swabs tangled. Dressing-thumb forceps should not be used on tissue as they are fairly damaging
- Tissue-thumb forceps may have a 'rat tooth' design (e.g. Semkin or Adson tissue forceps) or a complex toothed design (e.g. De Bakey tissue forceps) (Figure 7.5). The latter is very much recommended as the arrangement of

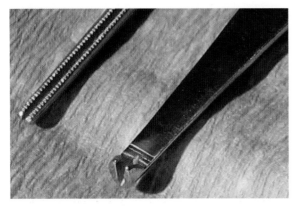

Figure 7.5 Close-up view of toothed end of De Bakey (left) and Semkin (right) thumb forceps. The fine interdigitation of the De Bakey forceps provides extremely atraumatic tissue-handling.

teeth is much less traumatic than other forceps

Tissue forceps

These are generally of a scissor style and ratcheted. Examples include Allis, Babcock and Doyen tissue forceps (Doyen tissue forceps are more usually called bowel clamps). Non-ratcheted tissue forceps include Noyes alligator forceps.

- Alligator forceps are used extensively as foreign-body extractors and are particularly useful in removing grass awns from ears or interdigital spaces
- Allis tissue forceps are highly traumatic and should not be used on any viable tissue. They are quite useful for holding necrotic wound edges during **debridement**
- Babcock tissue forceps are much less traumatic and may be used for intestinal surgery. They are of limited use for minor surgery

Towel clamps

The two commonest forms of towel clamp are the Backhaus (ratcheted) and Jones (bulldog-clip style).

- Backhaus towel clamps are much easier to place and less traumatic to skin and so are preferred

- They may also be used to secure cables or tubes (e.g. for electrocautery or suction) in place on the drapes
- Sharp towel clamps damage drapes, causing puncture marks and small tears. They also have the potential to cause real damage to the skin, or to other structures lying beneath the drapes. Great care must be exercised when draping the head or face not to damage the eye with towel clamps

Scissors

Scissors are classified according to their use (dissecting scissors, suture scissors, bandage scissors) and according to the configuration of the blades and whether the ends are sharp or blunt (straight, curved, blunt/blunt, blunt/sharp, sharp/sharp).

- Scissors should only be used for their intended purpose. For example, fine dissecting Metzenbaum scissors should not be used to cut skin or sutures – this will blunt the blades and loosen the hinge
- Dissecting scissors tend to have a blunt/blunt configuration to prevent inadvertent 'pranging' of vessels while advancing the scissors
- The most popular scissors for minor surgery are the Mayo and the Metzenbaum. Mayo scissors are somewhat sturdier than the fine, delicate Metzenbaum scissors and are more useful for cutting tougher tissue such as fascia
- Straight scissors have a stronger cutting ability than curved scissors, but curved scissors provide better visibility as the blade tip is not obscured by the hand while cutting
- Scissors crush tissues as they are cutting. They should thus not be used in the skin as the tissue damage delays healing and leads to a less satisfactory wound closure
- Scissors have handedness. In other words, some scissors are designed for right-handed people, others for left-handed people. Using the wrong hand makes the scissors slightly less comfortable to handle and over time will cause loosening of the hinge as undue shearing pressures are used

Scissors may be held in a number of ways:

- The usual way is to place the thumb and the third finger in the thumb holes and direct the scissors with the index finger (the tripod hold). This allows for a very precise cut and a high shearing force (Figure 7.6A)
- In the thenar eminence grip, the thumb replaces the index finger and the bulge at the base of the thumb (the thenar eminence) is used to support the thumb hole on the scissors (Figure 7.6B). This is a fairly difficult grip to master, but is a very stable grip when cutting fine tissues
- The backhand grip can be used to extend an incision in the opposite direction. A variation of the tripod grip can be used for this, or else the scissors can be held with the thumb and index finger with the blades passing along the palm to the heel of the hand
- Blunt dissection is a useful technique for dividing tissues and undermining skin.

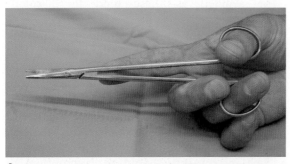

A

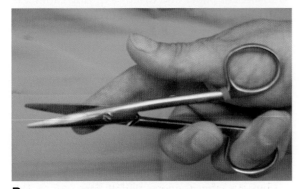

B

Figure 7.6 (A) The tripod hold for scissors. (B) The thenar eminence grip for scissors.

Repeatedly inserting scissors between tissues with the blades closed, opening the scissors and removing them reduce the risk of inadvertently cutting important structures. Fine Metzenbaum scissors are generally used

Haemostatic forceps

These are instruments designed to crush and hold blood vessels

- They vary in size, the smallest being the Halstead mosquito forceps, used to clamp small blood vessels (point bleeders); Kelly and Crile haemostats, for use on larger vessels or small pedicles; and Rochester-Carmalt haemostatic forceps for use on larger clumps of tissues containing blood vessels, such as ovarian pedicles
- They also vary in the orientation of the jaw serrations, with mosquito, Kelly and Crile forceps having transverse serrations and Rochester-Carmalt forceps having longitudinal serrations. Transverse serrations are generally more traumatic to tissue. To prevent slippage from a pedicle or blood vessel, Rochester-Carmalt haemostats have cross-hatched serrations at the tip of the jaws
- With use, the ratchet teeth may wear, causing the jaws to snap open during use. This is not good, and such instruments must be discarded
- Haemostats should be held in the tripod grip, being careful only to insert the very tips of the fingers through the rings, so that the fingers do not get caught

Retractors

Retractors are used to improve visibility within the surgical field and to improve access to tissues to enable precision of instrument placement or procedures:

- Retractors may be finger- or hand-held (Hohmann, Senn, Army-Navy, malleable: Figure 7.7), requiring that a **sterile** assistant holds the instrument, or else self-restraining (Gelpi, Travers, Weitlaner: Figure 7.8), which have some manner of ratchet-lock

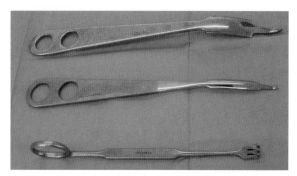

Figure 7.7 Hand-held retractors. From top to bottom: Hohmann, mini-Hohmann, Senn.

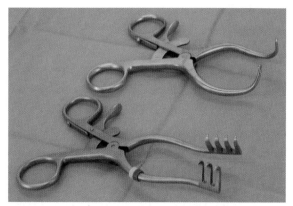

Figure 7.8 Self-retaining retractors: top: Gelpi, bottom: Weitlaner.

- Senn are finger-held retractors, and are very useful in minor veterinary procedures for retracting skin
- Hohmann retractors are more useful for orthopaedic procedures and can be used to lever muscles out of the way carefully or to provide retraction in joints
- Gelpi retractors are the most useful self-retaining retractors, causing less tissue damage than Weitlaner retractors. They provide a very good degree of retraction and are of particular help in exploratory surgery (**laparotomy**, arthrotomy). They are of some use in minor surgery, especially if greater visibility is required when dealing with **haemostasis**
- The ratchet-lock on self-retaining retractors is an ingenious contraption and can be a little difficult to master. Practice is advisable before using it on a patient

Cleaning and maintaining instruments

- To observe the regulations of the Control of Substances Hazardous to Health Act 1988, rubber gloves and aprons should be worn
- Instruments should be cleaned as soon as possible after surgery to prevent blood drying and fixing and to reduce the build-up of bacteria
- All sharps should be disposed of in an approved sharps container (suture needles should be carefully inspected and handled separately)
- Delicate surgical instruments (ophthalmic or other fine dissecting instruments) should be separated to reduce risk of damage
- Instruments should first be rinsed in cold water: rinsing in hot water tends to fix blood and makes it more difficult to remove from surfaces
- Debris should be removed by soaking in warm water containing (pH-neutral) detergent. Detergents containing ammonia should be avoided as these tend to discolour instruments
- The detergent and remaining gross soiling should be removed by gentle scrubbing and rinsing with clean water
- An ultrasonic cleaner should then be used to remove fine debris. Overloading of the cleaner is to be avoided as this may cause damage to instruments – it is better to run several loads. Ratcheted instruments should be left open
- The instruments should be laid out on to absorbent paper and dried (a drying cabinet is a tremendous time-saving purchase for a busy practice), prior to inspection (see below) and lubrication with a high-quality instrument lubricant
- Finally, the instruments are grouped together into kits and packaged according to appropriate sterilisation methods

Instruments should be carefully checked during cleaning:
- The ends of needle holders should be examined for sharp edges which may cause the suture material to tear
- Instrument clasps or ratchet locks should be tested to ensure correct closure and easy

release: with the teeth of the instruments closed, the clasp edges should just touch
- Scissors should be sent for sharpening regularly
- All instrument hinges should be checked and if loose sent for repair or discarded
- Forceps should be examined to make sure the bite is aligned
- Poor-quality or worn-out instruments are damaging to tissues and frustrating to use, resulting in longer operating times. It is far more economical in the long run to invest in good-quality surgical tools

Markers for instruments (tapes or coloured bands) are useful as they simplify separation of instruments into different kits during cleaning. However, frayed ends of tape and the underside of tight bands can act as deposits of bacteria and potential sources of contamination. Also, adhesive from tapes can spread along the instrument and make cleaning difficult. When fitted, coloured bands or tapes should not interfere with closure of instruments and should not be placed so as to cause rubbing or chafing of the surgeon's fingers.

REVIEW OF SUTURE MATERIALS AND THEIR APPLICATIONS

Suture material is required for apposing tissues or ligating vessels.

The correct choice of suture material will depend on the biophysical properties of the tissue and of the suture material and will vary according to the state or condition of the wound (whether or not infection is present) and the rate of healing of the tissue.

There are several criteria that make for the ideal suture material (Box 7.2):

- It should be easy to handle with instruments and hands
- The security of the knots should be excellent on a minimum number of throws (ideally 2–3)
- It should not induce or cause any tissue reaction (inflammation or allergy)
- It should resist capillary action (wicking)
- It should be stable in tissue, resisting shrinking or swelling which may impinge on the wound edges or loosen knots
- There should be no long-term reactions or carcinogenesis with permanent suture material
- It should last as long as it is required, and at the tensile strength it is required, until wound-healing is complete. It should then disintegrate as quickly as possible, leaving no residue

Suture materials are classified in several ways (Box 7.3):
- Absorbable, e.g. catgut, polyglycolic acid, polyglactin 910, polydioxanone, polyglyconate, poliglecaprone 25, glycomer 631, polyglytone 6211, lactomer 9-1. All lose most of their strength within 60 days and are eventually removed by phagocytosis or hydrolysis
- Non-absorbable, e.g. silk, nylon (polyamide), polyester, polypropylene, polybutester, polymerised caprolactum, stainless steel. These are not degraded during the healing process and generally cause little tissue reaction

Box 7.2

Although advances in suture material are rapidly being made, there is no one material that fulfils all these criteria for every wound.

Box 7.3 Recommended suture materials and sizes for minor surgery

Skin: synthetic non-absorbable suture material (e.g. nylon: Monosof, Vetoquinol or Ethilon, Ethicon).

Subcutaneous or subcuticular layers: a synthetic absorbable suture material should be used (e.g. polyglactin 910 (Vicryl, Ethicon) or lactomer 9-1 (Polysorb, Vetoquinol)).

3/0 (2 metric) or 4/0 (1.5 metric) is suitable for dogs and cats.

- Monofilament, e.g. polydioxanone, polyglyconate, poliglecaprone 25, glycomer 631, polyglytone 6211, polybutester, nylon (polyamide), polypropylene. These tend to have little capillarity and reduce wicking
- Multifilament, e.g. nylon (polyamide), silk, polyglactin 910, lactomer 9-1, catgut, polyglycolic acid. These are more likely to cause wicking by capillary action
- Synthetic, e.g. polyglycolic acid, polyglactin 910, polydioxanone, polyglyconate, poliglecaprone 25, lactomer 9-1, glycomer 631, polyglytone 6211, polymerised caprolactum. These generally cause little tissue reaction (although multifilament synthetic suture material causes more tissue reaction than monofilament)
- Non-synthetic (natural), e.g. catgut, silk. These tend to cause considerable tissue reaction. Because of this and because of poor latent knot security (loosening after several hours within tissues), catgut is no longer recommended. In any case, fear of contamination by transmissible spongiform encephalopathies has led to halts in manufacture of this material.

Table 7.3 lists common suture materials used in veterinary practice.

Table 7.3 Commonly available suture materials and their properties

Suture material	Trade name	Properties	Manufacturer
Non-synthetic			
Catgut (chromic catgut)	–	Absorbable (gone by 60 days), multifilament. Loses one-third tensile strength within 7 days. Made from sheep/cow intestinal submucosa. 90% collagen	Ethicon
Silk	Mersilk	Non-absorbable, multifilament. Loses one-third tensile strength within 14 days	Ethicon
Synthetic			
Glycomer 631	Biosyn	Absorbable, monofilament. Loses two-thirds tensile strength within 21 days (but initially 30% stronger than PDS). Very strong, but low memory, so easy to handle. Extremely good knot security	Vetoquinol
Lactomer 9-1	Polysorb	Absorbable, multifilament. Loses two-thirds tensile strength within 21 days. Completely absorbed by 56–70 days. Excellent knot security, very good handling characteristics	Vetoquinol
Poliglecaprone 25	Monocryl	Absorbable, monofilament. Loses one-half tensile strength within 7 days. Excellent handling, reasonable knot security	Ethicon
Polydioxanone	PDS II	Absorbable, monofilament. Only loses one-eighth tensile strength within 14 days, lasts at least 180 days. Quite springy and high memory so can be difficult to handle. Good knot security, provided care is taken when tying	Ethicon

(cont'd)

Table 7.3 (Continued)

Suture material	Trade name	Properties	Manufacturer
Polyglactin 910	Vicryl	Absorbable, multifilament. Loses one-third tensile strength within 14 days; complete absorption by 60 days	Ethicon
	Vicryl rapide	Very quick hydrolysis, complete absorption by 42 days	Ethicon
Polyglycolic acid	Dexon	Absorbable, multifilament. Loses one-third tensile strength within 14 days. A coated form is available, which lasts longer and reduces wicking	Davis & Geck
Polyglyconate	Maxon	Absorbable, monofilament. Loses one-third tensile strength within 14 days	Davis & Geck
Polyglytone 6211	Caprosyn	Absorbable, monofilament. Loses all tensile strength by 21 days; completely absorbed by 56 days. Excellent handling and knot security. Ideal for oral cavity	Vetoquinol
Polyamide	Monosof Ethilon, Surgilon	Non-absorbable, mono- or multifilament. Relatively poor knot security and poor handling (quite springy, but Monosof is better). Little or no tissue reaction	Vetoquinol Ethicon, Davis & Geck
Polybutester	Novafil	Non-absorbable, monofilament. Good handling, secure knots	Davis & Geck
Polyester	Mersiline, Dacron	Non-absorbable, multifilament. Poor handling and poor knot characteristics. Fairly tissue-reactive	Ethicon, Davis & Geck
Polypropylene	Prolene, Fluorofil	Non-absorbable, monofilament. Very good handling and knot characteristics	Ethicon, Malinckrodt Veterinary
Stainless steel	Flexon	Non-absorbable multi- or monofilament. Very strong. Excellent knot security, but prone to metal fatigue. Poor handling characteristics	Davis & Geck

Other wound closure methods

Tissue adhesives

- These are cyanoacrylate adhesives (e.g. Vetbond, 3M), similar to domestic strong rapid adhesives
- They may be used to **appose** skin, and are especially useful in rodent surgery or for small wounds. They are especially useful in closing small biopsy wounds

- The use of cyanoacrylate adhesives to provide **haemostasis** in abdominal surgery can result in granuloma formation and so care should be taken to avoid overuse
- A **sterile** 23 G or 25 G hypodermic needle can be placed on to the tip of the dispensing bottle to improve accuracy and precision of placement
- Although wounds to the cornea can be successfully **appose**d with tissue glue, the potentially disastrous consequences associated with

accidental misapplication mean that this procedure should only be performed by experienced surgeons

Surgical staples

- There are various surgical stapling machines, designed either for internal use (TA (thoracoabdominal), GIA/ILA (gastrointestinal anastomosis stapler), Vetoquinol, LDS (ligating and dividing system stapler), Vetoquinol) or for external use (Royal or Appose skin stapler, Vetoquinol)
- Surgical staples cause little or no tissue reaction and provide excellent apposition and **haemostasis** when used correctly
- Stapling equipment and staples are relatively expensive (although some companies will lease the equipment), but this can be offset by the dramatic reduction in surgical time
- The choice of staple size can be bewildering, and some degree of experience is required until the technique can be mastered
- Removal is simple, but a dedicated staple removal device is required

SELECTION OF NEEDLE TYPE

Suture needles are chosen on the basis of the type of tissue to be sutured, the size of wound, suture pattern and choice of suture material. They may either be separate from the suture material (eyed needles) or else fused to the suture material (swaged needles). They also differ in shape (straight, half-curved and part-circle) and type of point (non-cutting, taper point, cutting, reverse cutting, spatula-point: Figure 7.9).

- Swaged needles benefit from being sharper and quicker to use, since no threading is necessary. Suturing is generally easier with swaged needles as there is no tissue drag at the junction between needle and suture material
- The advantages of eyed needles are that suture material is usually cheaper when supplied without a swaged needle and the length of suture material can be chosen more readily (swaged needles often come with either far too little suture material, so that several packs must be opened, or else too much, increasing tissue-drag and the likelihood of tangling)

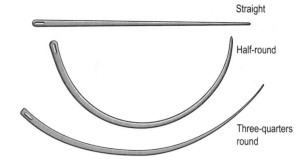

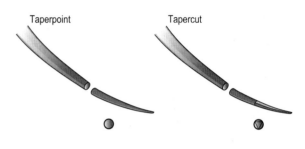

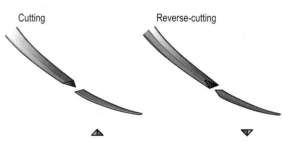

Figure 7.9 Suture needle shapes.

- The curve of the needle determines its path through tissue. Thus a curved (3/8th or half-circular) needle will follow a circular path through tissue and is easier to place skin sutures with than a straight needle, which would require that the skin be manipulated more to pass the needle through (Box 7.4)
- The shape of the point is important when deciding which tissue requires suturing. For example, a round-bodied (non-cutting) needle would require considerable effort to pass through skin: a cutting needle is more suitable for this. However, a blunt-point round-bodied needle would easily pass though softer liver

Box 7.4 Recommended choices of needles

Subcutaneous tissue, subcutis or muscle
3/8th or half-circular reverse-cutting (or tapercut)

For skin
3/8th curved or half-curved cutting or reverse-cutting

tissue and is less likely to cause tearing or inadvertent cutting of blood vessels than a cutting needle. Reverse-cutting needles have the advantage that they are less likely to create cuts along the tension plane of the suture. Spatula-point (side-cutting) needles are used in ophthalmic surgery to suture the cornea without allowing the suture material to cut out of the tissue

- The needle should make a hole the same diameter as the suture material (the exception to this is swaged vascular sutures, in which the suture material is wider than the needle to facilitate a watertight seal)

Needles should be held with needle holders approximately one-third of the way along the needle (from the eye or suture end).

HALSTEAD'S PRINCIPLES OF TISSUE-HANDLING

It is thanks to William S. Halstead, late of Johns Hopkins University, that we have many of our basic aseptic precautions. He introduced the use of thin rubber gloves for surgery in the 1890s and gave his name to a list of precautions or surgical principles. Now over 100 years old, these principles still remain as important today:

- Tissues should be handled gently, so as to minimise damage to vital tissues (using atraumatic instruments wherever possible)
- **Haemostasis** should be performed as accurately as possible, to avoid damage to surrounding tissues (ligatures should be placed over vessels rather than clumps of tissue)

- Every effort must be made to preserve the local blood supply (consideration should be given to the blood supply to an area prior to surgery, and vasculature should be handled with care during surgery)
- Strict aseptic technique must be maintained at all times
- Wound closures should be tension-free (see Avoiding skin tension, below)
- Wounds should be reconstructed accurately, paying attention to careful approximation of tissues
- All dead space should be eliminated from wounds (by careful wound closure and the use of drains where necessary)

The above principles, when followed, maximise the chances of a rapid and acceptable wound repair. Tissues tend to repair despite certain breakdowns in attention to the above principles, but it is not good practice to hope that will be the case. Attention to detail, and, above all, pride in your work, is the best way of ensuring rapid and uneventful wound-healing.

PRACTICAL SUTURE PATTERNS FOR MINOR SURGERY

Although a wide variety of suture patterns exist, not all are appropriate to minor surgery and some are of historical interest only.

It is far better to know and be competent at a small number of useful suture patterns than to dither over a large choice.

Tension-relieving sutures are covered later; appropriate to this text are skin suture patterns, which may be categorised thus:

- Subcutaneous or subcuticular sutures
- Skin sutures:
  - Interrupted (simple, horizontal mattress or cruciate)
  - Continuous (simple continuous, Ford interlocking)

Instruments (needle holders and tissue forceps) should be used to place skin sutures: it is much easier to control tension using instruments and allows for more accurate suture placement.

Subcutaneous or subcuticular sutures

Simple interrupted sutures may be placed deep within a wound, away from the skin edges to close down dead space. They may also be used to reduce skin tension at the wound edge. When placing subcutaneous sutures:

- Care must be taken not to produce unwanted ligature effects by entrapping blood vessels or nerves within the suture
- A 3–5-mm bite of suture may be placed through underlying muscle or fascia and through dermis as hypodermic fat has no holding power for sutures and will pull through
- Absorbable suture material should be used
- Using a swaged-on needle will cause less tissue damage and create less drag, making suturing easier
- Avoid a surgeon's knot (with an initial double throw) and restrict yourself to three throws as knots provide the greatest source for bacterial persistence within a wound
- Similarly, do not place too many sutures – there is a fine trade-off between necessary sutures and unwanted foreign material within a wound. This can be difficult to assess, but proper planning of wound reconstruction makes it easier to reduce dead space with fewer sutures

When a long wound is to be closed and there is a need to close subcutaneous dead space, a continuous suture pattern is recommended. This has several advantages:

- It is quicker to perform than simple interrupted sutures
- There are fewer knots (and so less likelihood of bacterial sequestration)
- Tension within the wound is more evenly distributed

The needle is passed perpendicular to the wound from left to right (for left-handed surgeons) and a knot is tied. The needle is then advanced along the wound about 10 mm and again passed through the skin across the wound from left to right. This is repeated along the wound so that the suture travels along the wound on the surface and per-

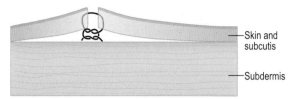

Figure 7.10 Subcuticular suture: if the suture is passed from deep to shallow then the knot is buried.

pendicular to the wound edges subcutaneously (providing good apposition). Tying a knot between the free end and the last loop completes the suture.

A disadvantage of continuous subcutaneous sutures is that, if the knot fails, the entire wound reopens. Also, should it become necessary to provide drainage to the wound, one or two simple interrupted sutures may be removed.

Subcuticular sutures may be used instead of skin sutures for reasons of surgeon's preference, or a difficult patient. In addition, they reduce skin scarring (Figure 7.10).

Care must be exercised when placing subcuticular sutures that the sutures are not placed too deeply, or they will enter the weaker dermis or hypodermis (leading to wound-gaping). Nor should they be placed too superficially, as this may lead to suture material bursting out through the skin.

Skin sutures

Skin sutures may be interrupted (a series of individual sutures: Figure 7.11) or continuous (one long suture: Figure 7.12). Continuous sutures have the advantage that they are quicker to perform and distribute tension more evenly: they also improve tissue apposition. As with subcutaneous continuous suture patterns, they have the disadvantage that if one suture fails (or the patient removes it) the whole wound is liable to open. In practice, this is rarely a problem.

To reduce scarring, skin sutures should be placed 2–3 mm away from the skin edges, there should be no tension on the sutures and fine suture material should be used (3/0 (1 metric) or 4/0 (1.5 metric) in dogs, 4/0 (1.5 metric) in cats).

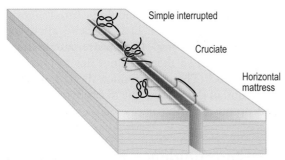

Figure 7.11 Interrupted skin sutures.

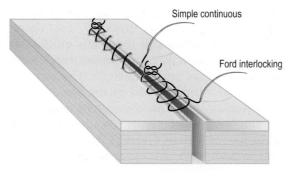

Figure 7.12 Continuous skin suture patterns.

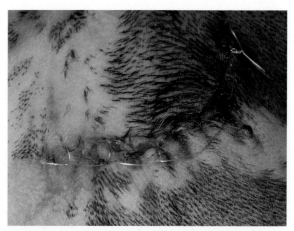

Figure 7.13 The stake injury from Chapter 6 (Figure 6.5A) has been repaired using a Ford interlocking suture pattern.

Needle holders and thumb forceps should be used to place the sutures and hold the skin steady, respectively. This allows for more accurate suture placement and reduces skin trauma.

Simple interrupted

These are very easy sutures to place, but care must be taken not to place them too tightly, as this may cause inversion of the wound edges. The needle should enter the skin about 2–3 mm away from the wound edge on the side closest to the surgeon's hand (left side for left-handed surgeons, right side for right-handed ones).

Cruciate

Although it initially appears complicated, this is a very easy suture to perform. It covers a greater length of wound than the simple interrupted and is thus speedier: it also tends to improve apposition. Its greatest disadvantage is that it is easy to

make the suture too tight, which not only places undue tension on the skin, but also causes the suture to cut into the skin, making removal difficult. To avoid this, it may help to pull tight on the second throw of the knot, rather than the first, to bed it down.

Horizontal mattress

Although they are quick to apply, if over-tightened these can cause wound eversion and reduce blood supply to the wound edge. Eversion of the wound edge can be reduced by not allowing the needle to go much deeper than the dermis. Horizontal mattress sutures placed some way away from the wound edges are useful in reducing skin tension (see later).

Simple continuous

This suture pattern may be used in the skin, but it is difficult to tension correctly to avoid puckering of the skin edges.

Ford interlocking suture

This is the author's preferred suture pattern for long wounds. With practice, it is very quick to perform and provides excellent apposition (Figure 7.13). However, it can be difficult to avoid over-tightening (which causes the sutures to dig into a wound). Although the pattern works best on straight wounds, it can also be used adequately on slightly curving wounds.

For right-handed surgeons, the needle is first passed from the right side of the wound to the left and a knot tied. The needle is then moved along the wound 8–10 mm and a second pass is made from right to left (as for a simple continuous suture). However, as the needle exits the skin, it catches the previous loop in a lock. To finish the suture, the needle is reversed and the free end is knotted against the last loop.

Hand ties

Knowing how to tie a ligature by hand is useful in deep wounds or areas with difficult access. Although a simple reef or square knot can be tied in just the same way as on a parcel, a more useful and rapid technique is the one-handed tie. Although both hands are used for this tie, only one hand places the throws: the other hand just brings the suture into position. The sequence of photographs in Figure 7.14 best explains this technique. It may take a little while to master, but allows for extremely rapid knot-tying when perfected.

Knots

The knot is the weakest part of any suture and consequently care must be taken to ensure it is well tied. Although several knot patterns exist, the recommended one is the square or reef knot (Figure 7.15). The surgeon's knot is a variation of the square knot in which a double twist is used on the first throw to increase friction and avoid the knot opening. Although it can be very frustrating to see the first throw loosen as you begin to lay the second throw, the surgeon's knot is no longer recommended as the extra twist dramatically increases the bacterial load within the suture material. In order to make it easier to tie the knot under tension, either a sliding knot may be used or else an assistant can **appose** the wound edges. An extra throw over a square knot should provide good knot security.

Once the knot is tied, it should be lifted slightly to make sure there is a little slack to allow for postoperative swelling. The suture should then be repositioned so that the knot lies to one side of the wound. This is to reduce the risk of contamination of the wound due to exudate or debris build-up on the knot.

Practising suturing

Suturing a skin wound once the surgeon has finished the surgery can improve practice efficiency by freeing the surgeon to make clinical notes, arrange medication or speak to the client. However, in practice, it is frequently quicker for the surgeon to complete the skin suturing than it is for the less experienced nurse to. The suturing may be neater if performed by the more experienced worker. This creates a catch-22 situation wherein, with more experience the nurse can suture just as well and just as quickly, but the nurse cannot gain the experience in the first place.

There may certainly be opportunities to practise suturing real tissue: for example, after a postmortem investigation has been performed. However, this is unlikely to provide enough experience to make one competent at suturing. Attending suture courses (wet lab courses) or using a suture dummy may help. An excellent and inexpensive suture dummy may be made from a sheet of adhesive Allevyn dressing (Smith & Nephew) simply stuck on to a surface. The texture and feel of this material are extremely lifelike, and there is good resistance to pulling through of suture material (the author is grateful to Duncan Henderson for this suggestion).

Pursestring sutures

Although used more commonly in gastrointestinal surgery or vascular surgery to secure tubes entering hollow viscera or blood vessels, pursestring sutures are very useful when performing **perineal** surgery. To avoid risk of faecal contamination when suturing a **perineal** wound, for example, or removing anal sacs, it is convenient

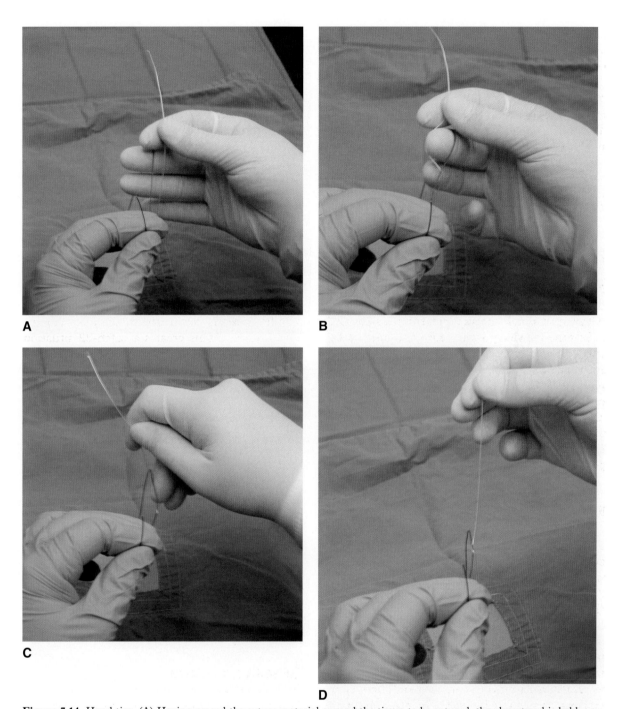

Figure 7.14 Hand ties. (A) Having passed the suture material around the tissue to be sutured, the closest end is held between finger and thumb. The far end is laid next to this and held in the other hand. (B) The middle finger is used to hook the close strand round and over the far strand. (C) The middle and fourth fingers are used to hold the close strand and it is pulled around the near strand. (D) The close strand is then pulled away to form the first throw. (E) The first throw is settled on to the suture site. The close strand has become the far strand. (F) The two strands are laid over the index finger, next to each other. (G) The index finger is used to hook the far strand over the near strand (H) to form a loop. (I) The far strand is pulled through the loop, and towards the surgeon. (J) The knot can now be tightened. (K) The finished square knot. More throws may be added by following the sequence through from (A) again.   (cont'd)

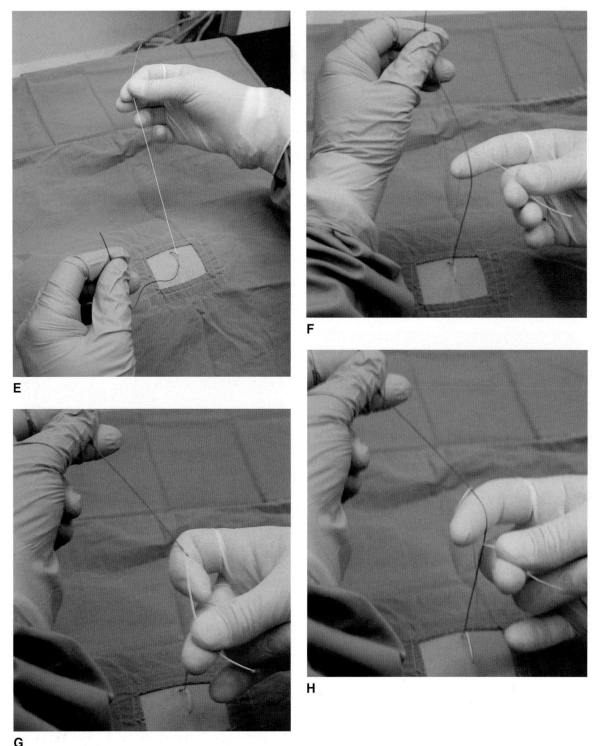

E

F

G

H

Figure 7.14 (Continued).

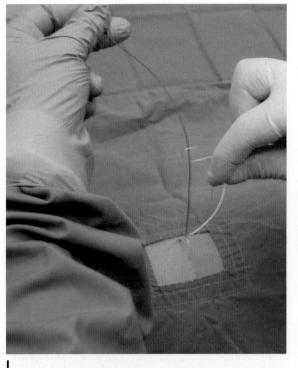

I

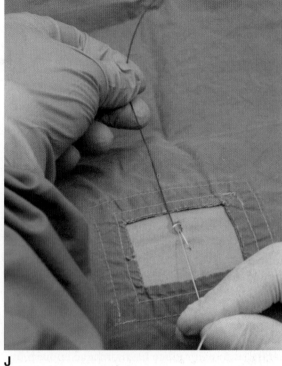

J

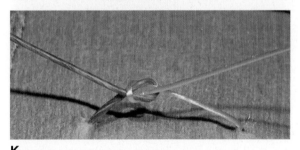

K

Figure 7.14 (Continued).

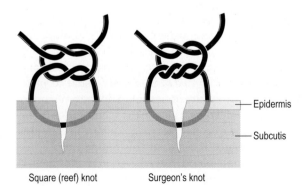

Square (reef) knot   Surgeon's knot

Figure 7.15 Surgical knots.

to place a circumferential suture around the anus temporarily.

A brief surgical prep of the perineum is performed and some cotton wadding is inserted into the rectum. A round-bodied curved needle is used to introduce 2/0 or 3/0 suture material (synthetic non-absorbent or monofilament absorbent) into the mucocutaneous junction at the ventral anus. The needle is passed just subcutaneously to one side of the anus and allowed to exit dorsal to the anal ring. The needle is then reintroduced through the exit hole and passed ventrally on the other side of the anus. The two ends are tensioned to reduce the diameter of the anus small enough to prevent exit of the cotton wadding and a knot is tied. This may be left in place for the duration of surgery, *but must be removed before the patient regains consciousness*! It may be prudent to secure an instrument or gauze swab to the pursestring suture to act as a reminder.

This technique usually works very well, but the suture should be untied immediately if the patient begins to strain against it.

HAEMOSTASIS – DEALING WITH BLEEDING

Depending on the level of bleeding and the nature of the wound, bleeding may be controlled in a number of ways. Regardless of the method used, keeping a calm head and methodically searching for the bleeding vessels will accomplish resolution quicker than blundering into a wound and clamping everything in sight. Direct pressure on a supplying artery or in the wound itself with a **sterile** swab will reduce haemorrhage enough in almost all instances to allow time for definitive **haemostasis** (Box 7.5).

Swabbing

The application of **sterile** gauze swabs to areas of bleeding is the standard method of dealing with bleeding in most wounds. Swabs should be used in a dabbing or blotting manner, as wiping will tend to wipe off a forming clot as well as any blood. Applying pressure to a small blood vessel for 3–5 min should cause thrombus formation. The swab should be removed carefully, to avoid removing the thrombus.

Swabs should be counted before, during and after surgery, and a record of these counts entered into the anaesthetic form. This is done for two reasons. The first is that it reduces the risk of

Box 7.5 Golden rule
The golden rule of haemostasis is: 'Don't panic'.

leaving swabs in wounds. The second reason is that examination of the swabs can give an idea of the amount of blood loss from a wound. Swabs can be weighed to give an accurate estimate of blood loss, but as a rough rule of thumb a blood-soaked 10×10 cm cotton gauze swab will contain 15 ml of blood.

Haemostatic forceps

As mentioned above, haemostats should ideally be placed over isolated blood vessels or small vasculature pedicles, rather than used to crush blindly large areas of tissue. In order to visualise the bleeder more clearly, the area should be blotted with a **sterile** cotton-gauze swab. If the degree of haemorrhage is such that blood returns too quickly to be able to spot the bleeding vessel, then the following methods may help:
- The swab should be reapplied and then slowly rolled off the area, ideally against the direction of blood flow. This may allow the end of the blood vessel to be seen while hand pressure occludes the proximal portion of the vessel
- A **sterile** assistant can apply pressure on the surrounding tissue in the hope of reducing blood flow to the haemorrhaging vessel

Haemostats should be left in place for 5–10 min to allow thrombus formation. The area should be monitored closely during removal and if haemorrhage recurs then the haemostats should be replaced and left for longer or a ligature placed.

Ligatures

Once a bleeding vessel has been identified and a pair of haemostats used to control the bleeding, the vessel may be tied off with a ligature.

Although metal ligature clips are available and are very quick to place, it is more usual to place a ligature of suture material. Slippage of incorrectly placed ligatures is the most common reason for postoperative haemorrhage. There are various ways to reduce the risk of this happening:
- Individual blood vessels should be ligated wherever possible, rather than large clumps of

tissue. This will allow for a greater ligature pressure and reduce the likelihood of other tissue pulling out of the ligature. Excess tissue caught up in the haemostats should be carefully bluntly dissected away or the haemostats removed and replaced more accurately

- If it is not possible to reduce the amount of tissue needing to be ligated, then suture material may be passed through rather than around the tissue (a round-bodied needle is ideal for this purpose). In this way, the pedicle can be tied off in a series of overlapping ligatures, each one more effectively tying off a smaller amount of tissue. This technique is known dramatically as 'divide and conquer'
- A transfixion ligature can be used. This involves passing the needle through a section of the blood vessel, tying a single throw (to secure the suture material in place) and then passing the suture material around the vessel to ligate (Figure 7.16)
- The ligature should be applied at least 0.5 cm from the end of the vessel
- The finer the suture material, the more stable the knot. 3/0 (2 metric) or 4/0 (1.5 metric) suture material should be suitable for most subcutaneous ligatures
- Hand-tying ligatures uses more suture material, but makes it easier to tie ligatures in deep wounds
- The choice of suture material affects the success of the ligature. In the author's experience, polydioxanone (PDS II, Ethicon) or glycomer 631 (Biosyn, Vetoquinol) produces satisfactory ligatures

Cautery

If available, **cautery** may be used. Various **cautery** machines are available, from a simple heat **cautery** device resembling a soldering iron, to complex electrocautery (or, more correctly, electrocoagulation) machines. Bipolar or unipolar **cautery** may be used. In the former, a charge is applied across a gap between two metal points (conveniently styled as thumb forceps). In unipolar **cautery**, a charge is applied between a

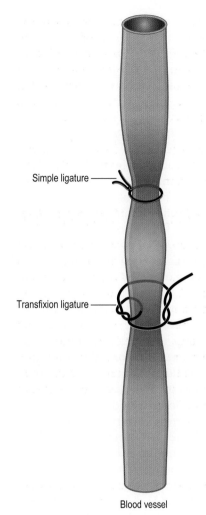

Figure 7.16 Ligatures.

probe and a base plate, placed under the patient. If electrocoagulation machines are to be used, care must be taken to ensure no alcohol remains on the patient from the surgical prep and that there are no flammable products around (check for leaks from anaesthetic machines).

Cautery should be applied to small areas, preferably to individual small blood vessels: overuse of **cautery** causes necrosis of tissue and retards healing. Any excess blood or fluids should be removed with a gauze swab as this will decrease the effectiveness of **cautery**.

Having arrested any bleeding, consideration should be given to the total blood loss suffered by the patient. Should any appreciable blood loss have occurred (more than 10% of blood volume or approximately 100 ml for a 10-kg dog, 40–50 ml for a 4-kg cat), then the fluid administration rate should be increased and addition of colloid considered.

AVOIDING SKIN TENSION

Skin tension at the wound edge must be avoided as it reduces healing, makes accurate closure difficult and can cause problems of restriction of venous return (or even arterial supply) to distal areas if there is skin tension on a limb wound. Fortunately, the skin of dogs and cats is fairly elastic and so in most cases fairly large skin wounds can be closed by relatively basic techniques.

The most straightforward way of reducing skin tension during wound repair is to plan the repair properly. This means anticipating problems of wound closure before performing a **lumpectomy**, and making your incisions accordingly. Having a working knowledge of the direction of tension lines on the body or referring to a tension diagram before performing the surgery may all help. Figure 7.17 shows a simplified diagram of tension lines on a dog.

It is also a very good idea to have a back-up plan for wound repair as surgery doesn't always go as expected.

Prior to surgery, the skin around the intended wound should be picked up and stretched to find out how much spare tissue there is available for repair.

Various sophisticated techniques are available to reconstruct skin deficits, such as using flaps of skin together with their own blood supply (axial pedicle flaps), tubed pedicle flaps, tunnel grafts (pouch flaps) and inflatable tissue-expanders. However, these are not applicable to minor veterinary surgery and will not be covered in any detail here. The interested reader is directed to one of the more specialised reconstructive surgery texts.

For minor surgical intervention, there should be no reason to apply any technique more complex than undermining skin, suturing parallel to tension lines, using tension-relieving sutures and

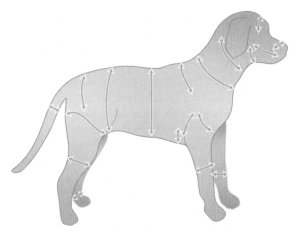

Figure 7.17 Approximate skin tension lines on a dog. To avoid tension on wounds, incisions should be made parallel to these lines.

stents, performing relaxing incisions or making use of nearby skin in the form of advancement flaps.

Undermining skin

This is the easiest way of reducing tension at the skin edge and should provide adequate skin for closure in most cases.

- The skin and panniculus muscle are bluntly dissected away from underlying tissue around the wound
- Occasional sharp dissection may be required to free tight bands of fascia
- Atraumatic thumb forceps (De Bakey) are used to attempt to **appose** the skin to see whether enough tissue has been undermined. Allis tissue forceps will damage the subdermal blood vessels and should not be used. Stay sutures are very useful for this purpose
- Enough undermining should be performed for the wound edges to **appose** without tension. This procedure may be combined with walking sutures (see later) to reduce the amount of skin undermining required
- The skin around a limb can be almost completely circumferentially undermined in order to free enough tissue to close a limb wound. The risk here is that closure of the wound may create a tourniquet around the limb and lead

to severe swelling of the distal limb or worse. Limb wounds are better closed by suturing in a plane perpendicular to the long axis of the limb

Tension-relieving sutures and stents

Placing sutures some way back from the wound edges will reduce tension at the edge itself. In this way, tension may be shared between various areas of a wound, rather than concentrated at one point, compromising blood supply.

- Walking sutures: sutures are placed in the sub-cuticular layer or deep dermis and in the fascia of the body wall so that the deeper sutures are closer to the wound edge (Figure 7.18). Tightening the suture draws or walks the skin forward, towards the wound edge, at the same time reducing tissue dead space. Simple horizontal mattress sutures of 3/0 absorbable synthetic suture material (e.g. polyglactin 910, polydioxanone, glycomer 631) are recommended. Walking sutures should be placed 3 cm apart within the wound to avoid leaving too much suture material behind. This should result in a wound which is easily **apposed** with little tension and which may now be routinely closed with subdermal and skin sutures. If correctly placed, little dimples may be seen on the skin surface: these usually disappear after 2–3 weeks
- Tension-relieving skin sutures: horizontal or vertical mattress sutures placed 1–2 cm back from the wound edges take tension away from the wound edge itself and are usually removed 3 days postsurgery. Vertical mattress sutures cause less compromise to skin blood supply and pressure from both sutures can be spread or reduced by the use of **stents** (rubber bands, buttons or **sterile** gauze swabs may all be used). Stents should be placed so as to max-imise the area over which pressure is applied; larger stents are preferred to small, hard ones (Figure 7.19). Specialised sutures (far-near-near-far and far-far-near-near) help reduce tension and improve apposition, but their use in minor surgery is limited

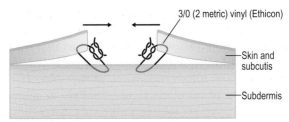

(a) Simple interrupted mattress sutures are placed near the middle of the wound into the subdermis/muscle/fascia layers and through the subcutis some distance away from the wound edge.

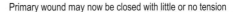

Primary wound may now be closed with little or no tension

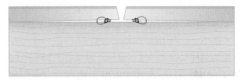

(b) As the sutures are tightened, dead space is reduced and the skin is drawn inwards to the centre of the wound.

Figure 7.18 Walking suture placement to reduce skin tension.

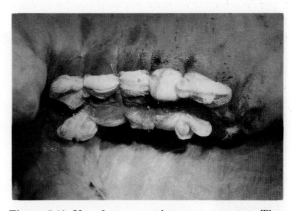

Figure 7.19 Use of stents to reduce suture pressure. The stent was placed following reconstruction of a large ventral skin deficit. It was removed 2 days following surgery.

Relaxing incisions

Although they are rather messy and should not be required for minor surgery provided adequate skin has been undermined, relaxing incisions are effective ways of reducing wound tension. Small

(1-cm) incisions are made in the skin approximately 1 cm away from the wound edge. The incisions should be placed 1–2 cm apart in a row. As the wound is closed, the relaxing incisions open up and allow expansion of the skin. If a single row of incisions is not enough to allow apposition, further incisions are made in a second row (staggering the incisions) or on the other side of the wound. Once sufficient incisions have been made, wound closure is performed. The smaller incisions are bandaged and allowed to heal by second-intention healing.

Advancement flaps

Flaps of skin may be raised and pulled forward to cover a deficit. This takes advantage of the frequent juxtaposition of loose elastic skin to areas of inelastic skin. A good example is on the head, where skin from the neck can be pulled forward to cover an area the size of the scalp without skin tension, or on the proximal limb, where skin from the torso can be moved to cover wounds (Figure 7.20).

The technique for making advancement flaps is outlined in Figure 7.21.

- The amount of skin needed to cover a deficit is measured and, preferably, a plan is drawn on the skin with a **sterile** skin-marking pen (Johnson & Johnson, or Aspen Surgical Products: they may be bought ready-sterilised). Triangular areas of skin (Bürow's triangles) are marked at the fixed end of the flap
- The skin is incised along the marked area and Bürow's triangles removed. Skin (and panniculus muscle) is undermined under the flap and beyond, to allow free movement of the flap to cover the deficit
- Walking sutures are placed to reduce dead space and allow advancement of the flap to the closure site. If the triangles have been estimated correctly, this should avoid the production of 'dog ears'
- Routine closure of subdermal tissue and skin is performed
- As a general guide, as long as the flap length is no greater than twice its width, there should be no problem with blood supply

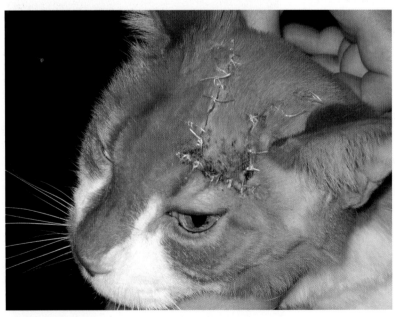

Figure 7.20 Following removal of a skin mass above the eye, the skin has been closed with an advancement flap to avoid deformation of the eyelid fissure.

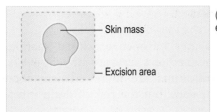

(a) Skin mass is excised.

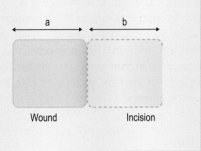

(b) Parallel incisions are made and subcutaneous tissue is dissected to make a flap.

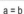

a = b

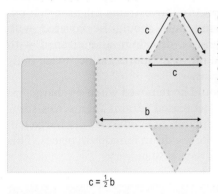

(c) Equilateral triangles of skin are removed from the fixed end of the flap to reduce 'dog ears'.

$c = \frac{1}{2}b$

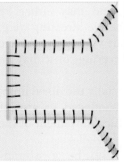

(d) The flap is advanced to cover the wound. Subcutaneous sutures are placed to reduce 'dead' space and skin is apposed with an interrupted or continuous suture pattern.

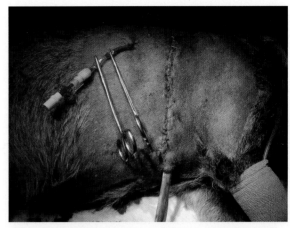

Figure 7.22 Drain placement. A Penrose drain has been placed below the ventral skin wound of this border terrier following thoracotomy. A chest drain has also been placed. The chest drain was removed after 8 h; the Penrose drain was removed 3 days after surgery.

SURGICAL DRAINS

Surgical drains are used to provide egress from a wound of fluids and air, thus reducing dead space in superficial wounds. They may be classified as passive or active, depending on whether they are allowed to drain in a dependent manner, or whether suction is applied to assist drainage (Figure 7.22).

The use of drains in minor surgery is limited. Drains are not a substitute for poor technique and should not be used as an alternative to proper surgical closure of dead space and adequate **lavage** and **debridement**. Infected wounds are treated more effectively by open wound management and delayed primary or secondary closure or second-intention healing. Drains themselves

Figure 7.21 Skin advancement flap technique. (a) The skin mass is excised, creating squared wound edges. (b) Parallel incisions are made from one end of the wound, extending to the same length as the wound. Skin is undermined to create a flap. (c) Equilateral triangles of skin are removed from the fixed end of the flap to remove potential 'dog ears'. (d) The flap is advanced to cover the wound. Subcutaneous sutures are placed to reduce dead space and skin is **apposed** using an interrupted or continuous suture pattern.

may create dead space by allowing air to be sucked into a wound. The presence of a drain in a wound predisposes to infection by allowing an entry hole for microorganisms and facilitates persistence of infection by the presence of a foreign body.

Passive drains

Penrose drains (soft latex tubes, e.g. Penrose tubing, Sherwood Medical) are most commonly used for drains in small-animal surgery. Although a small amount of fluid drains through the lumen of the tube, the outside provides the bulk of drainage. The capacity for drainage is therefore dependent on the surface area of the tube. Cutting fenestrations into Penrose tubing thus reduces the potency of this type of drain.

* Good-quality, radiopaque Penrose tubing should be used as it is less likely to leave remnants during removal and persistence of fragments may be detected by radiography
* Passive drains should be placed in a dependent area of the wound, so that gravity allows drainage. They should be placed through a separate drain hole and not exited through the surgical wound, as this is likely to cause wound **dehiscence** and may compromise the entire wound. The drain hole should be about 1.5 times the diameter of the tube (or about the width of the flattened tube)
* It is only necessary to have an exit hole for the drain: a second hole (usually placed near the top of the wound) does not increase wound drainage but does increase the risk of wound infection. The drain should be secured within the wound by a single suture (it is most convenient to tack the tubing on to deep fascia with a synthetic absorbable suture). The drain suture should only engage one wall and should be placed 4–5 mm from the edge
* Removal of the drain is accomplished by pulling sharply down on the Penrose tubing. The tacked edge should rip through cleanly. Alternatively, the drain may be sutured in place through the skin, and removed by removing the suture

Active drains

Active drains may be open or closed suction, depending on whether a separate air vent exists. Open suction drains are more efficient than closed suction ones, but the risk of drain infection is increased.

* As with passive drains, active drains are always exited through a separate drain hole and never through the surgical wound. Although it is not as important to place them in a dependent manner, doing so will decrease the risk of seroma formation once the drain is removed
* Active drainage is either provided intermittently by syringe or suction pump, or else by portable suction pumps

Care of drains

Drains should be checked twice daily for placement and to ensure active drains still have suction. The drain and hole should be covered with **sterile** absorptive dressings and cleaned with skin disinfectant (e.g. chlorhexidine) twice daily to reduce sepsis.

Drains should be removed when discharge has considerably decreased (drains themselves stimulate the production of exudate so discharge will never stop while the drain remains in place). This is usually 1–3 days postsurgery.

POSTOPERATIVE WOUND CARE

* If on the torso, the wound may either be covered with a self-adhesive dressing (e.g. Primapore, Smith & Nephew) or non-adhesive dressing with bandage covering, or it may be left uncovered
* Wounds to the limb, especially the distal limb, should be dressed and bandaged to protect against bumps and to reduce movement of the skin edges
* If the patient is known to be a wound-mutilator, it may be prudent to fit an Elizabethan collar (E-collar) or wound-protecting sock. Similarly, if the nature of the wound is such that any disruption would be disastrous (e.g.

the eyelids), the benefit of the doubt should not be given and an E-collar should be fitted

- The owners should be instructed on wound care (a fact sheet is useful) and what to do if the patient removes the dressing
- For clean surgical wounds, the dressings are removed after 24–48h and the wound examined for inflammation, discharge, loosening of sutures or signs of pain. It is worth reminding the owners that any swelling, redness or discharge should be reported
- Excess wetting will inhibit healing by interfering with formation of a fibrin plug. For this reason, the wound should be kept dry and any dried blood near the wound should be gently combed out or removed by dabbing with a moist swab or tissue
- The patient is most likely to interfere with a wound if it is painful or inflamed: this should be borne in mind and further analgesics or antibiotics considered if self-trauma to the wound occurs

SUTURE REMOVAL

Sutures are typically removed at 7–14 days postoperatively. At this stage, the wound has only approximately a quarter of the tensile strength of normal skin. However, this is usually sufficient strength to cope with most day-to-day abrasions and trauma and the underlying fascia takes much of the strain. If left in longer, suture reactions and infections are likely to occur, and scarring is increased. Occasionally, staged suture removal is recommended; for example, a long axilla injury. The skin here is subject to much movement and removing every other suture at 10 days postoperatively and the rest at 14 or 18 days may reduce scarring significantly but provide further support for the wound.

Sutures on the pinna as a treatment for aural haematomata are traditionally left in place for 14–21 days: the additional time probably increases the degree of scarring within the ear and reduces the likelihood of recurrence.

It is good practice to wear disposable gloves when removing sutures, and to wash your hands before and after.

Sutures should be removed with suture scissors or suture blades (although, if suture blades are used, care should be taken not to injure the patient, client or yourself!). Simple interrupted or cruciate sutures may be grasped at a free end with a pair of dressing forceps or fingers and traction applied to lift them away from the skin. The suture is best cut at the junction of the skin, to reduce the risk of debris being dragged along the suture tract by the material. Ford interlocking sutures are easily removed in sections by cutting at every second or third pass.

Surgical staples should be removed using the dedicated staple-removing tool (Royal skin staple remover, Vetoquinol).

The wound should be carefully examined to ensure that no sutures are missed, or that no fragments of sutures remain in the wound. It is not uncommon to see a little swelling or discharge around the sutures themselves: provided the swellings are only 1–2mm and there is no pyrexia, the skin should return to normal within 2–3 days.

Sutures that have been placed too tightly or are covered in wound exudate may present a problem in removal: these can sometimes be deeply embedded in tissue and it may be frustrating to procure a free end, especially if the patient finds it painful and is difficult to keep still! The application of a little local anaesthetic cream will usually numb the site enough for a little probing.

8 Common surgical procedures

SKIN WOUND CLOSURE

The preparation of skin wounds to facilitate primary (or delayed primary) closure has been discussed previously (Chapter 6). Bacterial swabs should be taken for culture and sensitivity. The patient should be anaesthetised and the wound prepared for aseptic surgery. Full **sterile** theatre apparel should be worn (hats, masks, gown, gloves) and **sterile** drapes should be placed.

The surgical kit should include a minimum of equipment:
- Scalpel holder
- Scissors (Mayo, Metzenbaum)
- Thumb forceps (dressing and tissue, e.g. De Bakey)
- Needle holders (Olsen-Hegar or Mayo-Hegar: if Mayo-Hegar holders are used then a separate pair of suture scissors should be included, to save wear on the dissecting scissors)
- Needles (curved or half-curved reverse-cutting, selection of sizes)
- Two pairs of haemostatic forceps (Halstead Mosquito, Kelly or Crile)
- **Sterile** gauze swabs (count!)

And consumables should include:
- Scalpel blade: no. 10 or 15 is suitable for most procedures
- Synthetic absorbable suture material for sub-cutaneous tissues (e.g. 3/0 (2 metric) or 4/0 (1.5 metric) glycomer 631 (Biosyn, Veto-quinol), polyglactin 910 (Vicryl, Ethicon), lactomer 9-1 (Polysorb, Vetoquinol) or poly-dioxanone (PDS II, Ethicon))
- Synthetic non-absorbable suture material for skin sutures (e.g. 3/0 (2 metric) or 4/0 (1.5 metric) polypropylene (Prolene, Ethicon),

nylon (Monosof, Vetoquinol) or polyamide (Surgilon, Davis & Geck))

Holding skin with atraumatic forceps, the edges should be brought into apposition, following skin tension lines (see Figure 7.17). Any necessary skin undermining should be performed by gentle blunt dissection using a pair of Metzenbaum scissors. The wound is then closed as follows (Figure 8.1):

- Any dead space is closed with synthetic absorbable suture with simple interrupted sutures
- If the wound is deep, subcutaneous tissues are closed using a simple continuous suture pattern. A left-handed surgeon will find it easier to suture from left to right, a right-handed surgeon from right to left. If preferred, simple interrupted sutures may be used to close the subcutaneous layers
- A simple laceration that does not gape may be repaired by a single continuous suture through the subdermal layer or an appropriate skin suture pattern (simple interrupted, cruciate or Ford interlocking may all be used)
- A gaping wound, or a circular wound, is best apposed initially with widely spaced interrupted sutures (simple or mattress) through the subcuticular (subdermal) layer. This helps spread the tension around the wound edges and reduces the formation of 'dog ears'. A larger circular wound may be closed completely at the centre and converted to a cross-shaped wound (Figure 8.2). Alternatively, it may be converted to an oval wound that closes with the formation of untidy triangles of spare tissue. Any 'dog ears' remaining after subdermal closure should be cut off with a scalpel prior to skin suture placement

Postoperative care should include antibiotics for wounds treated after the 'golden period' (6 h following injury) and **sterile** dressings and pressure bandages as necessary. Small wounds to the torso and proximal limb (less than 10 cm) do not tend to require dressings, whereas wounds to the distal limb and large or infected wounds elsewhere do require dressings.

For uncomplicated wounds, postoperative checks should be arranged for 48–72 h postoperatively and sutures are generally removed at 10–14 days. Owners should be instructed not to allow the wound to get wet until sutures are removed, and to restrict exercise or movement as necessary, depending on the nature and position of the wound.

For complicated wounds or wounds with dressings requiring regular changes, consideration should be given to hospitalising the patient. Dressing changes must be carried out under aseptic conditions and it is unlikely that many owners have the necessary equipment at home. If the patient is to be sent home, the owners should be given clear instructions on care of bandages and, ideally, a fact sheet should be prepared (see Figure 5.10).

SKIN AND PERCUTANEOUS BIOPSY TECHNIQUES

Skin biopsy is indicated to investigate any focal or generalised skin change, such as masses, inflammatory lesions, hair loss or discoloration. Biopsy technique will depend on:
- Preference of surgeon
- Nature of skin change
- Reason for biopsy
- Temperament of patient
- Likelihood of obtaining a definitive result
- Laboratory/pathologist's recommendation

Biopsy techniques will either yield a grossly visible sample, which should be investigated by a histopathologist (surgical biopsy/tissue-core biopsy), or else only microscopic samples may be collected on a slide and investigated by cytological methods (fine-needle aspiration biopsy or FNAB).

Surgical skin biopsy

Almost without exception, this should be performed on anaesthetised patients, observing strict aseptic technique throughout.
- For investigation of surface skin changes, or changes affecting all skin layers including superficial layers, full skin preparation is not carried out, as shaving and application of skin

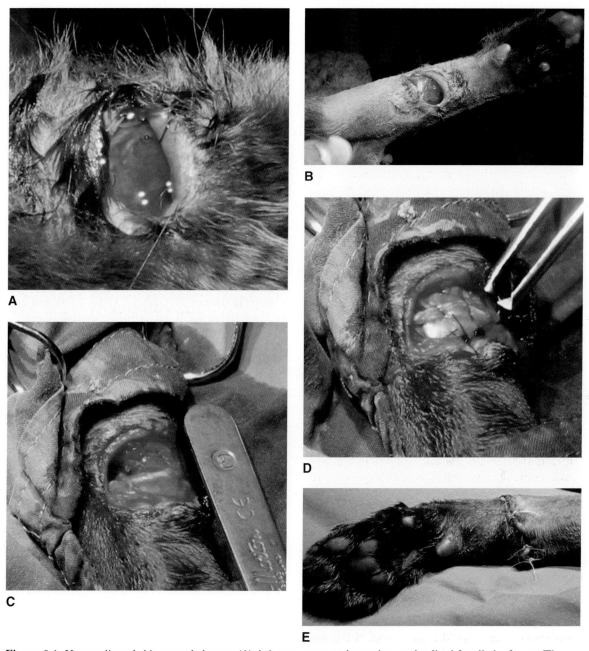

Figure 8.1 Uncomplicated skin wound closure. (A) A 2-cm transverse laceration on the distal fore limb of a cat. The wound is less than 2 h old and thus well within the 'golden period'. The wound has been filled with KY gel to reduce contamination with hair during the surgical clip. (B) The limb has been clipped for surgery and the wound can now be better assessed. The whole limb is examined for further wounds. The limb can now be prepared for aseptic surgery and flushed with copious amounts of **sterile** saline. (C) The limb is draped and the wound edges are debrided. Any visible debris is removed using forceps and **sterile** gauze swabs. The wound is flushed again with **sterile** saline. Haemorrhage is slight, but fresh blood can be seen issuing from the wound edges. (D) Subcutaneous tissue is closed to reduce dead space. The suture material used here is 4/0 (1.5 metric) PDS II (Ethicon). (E) Finally, the skin edges are apposed with 3/0 (2 metric) nylon (Ethilon, Ethicon) in a cruciate pattern. The wound is closed perpendicular to the long axis of the limb to reduce skin tension. A light dressing (non-adherent dressing, padding, conforming and cohesive layer) is then applied.

(a) Skin undermined and brought together from four 'corners'. N.B. Dead space must be reduced by suturing subcutis to subdermal layers.

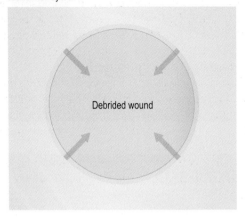

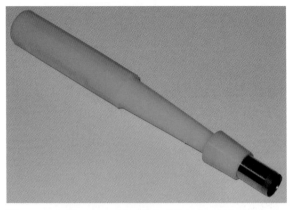

Figure 8.3 Biopsy punch (Global Veterinary Products).

- For all other skin biopsies, routine preparation of the surgical site is carried out (clipping, skin prep with antimicrobial soaps, covering with **sterile** drapes)
- A small surgical kit (similar to that used in wound suturing, see above) is appropriate
- A single-use, disposable biopsy punch (Global Veterinary Products, Figure 8.3) may be used to remove round skin biopsies. The punch should be placed perpendicular to the skin and, applying gentle pressure, rotated forwards and backwards to cut into the skin. Care must be taken to avoid the punch going too deep and damaging deeper tissues. Applying pressure with a **sterile** gauze swab for 5 min usually controls any bleeding. Any larger vessels may be caught with a pair of haemostatic forceps and ligated or clamped for 5–10 min. The skin biopsy may come away with the punch, in which case a pair of thumb forceps may be used to grasp the subcutaneous tissue and remove it. Otherwise, a fine pair of atraumatic thumb forceps should be used to lift the biopsy from the wound and the fascial connections snipped
- Alternatively, the biopsies may be performed using a scalpel. A fine blade is preferred for this: either a no. 11 or no. 15. An elliptical or oval incision is made, being careful to enter the skin at a perpendicular angle. The skin is separated from the subcutaneous tissue as above
- If a skin mass is biopsied, one sample is usually enough, provided it is a large enough sample.

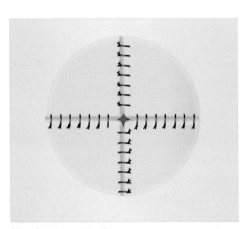

(b) Skin edges sutured together.

Figure 8.2 Closure of a circular wound by conversion to a cross-shaped wound.

disinfectants may disrupt pathological changes and reduce the investigative yield. In these cases, hair may be cut shorter using scissors and gentle vacuuming used to remove loose debris. However, this should not be taken as an excuse to neglect aseptic precautions: **sterile** gown and gloves, mask and hat should be worn to reduce **nosocomial** infection. **Sterile** drapes should also be used to reduce the risk of infection by microorganisms present on other areas of the patient

Punches yield fairly small sections and it may be wise to include several samples. Biopsies for generalised skin conditions should include normal-appearing skin, skin from the centre of a lesion and skin spanning the junction between normal and abnormal tissue. Samples should be placed into formalin with saline (formal-saline) and water added to bring the final concentration of formal-saline to 10%. N.B.: for some special histological stains, different methods of fixing are required; this should be confirmed with the laboratory prior to biopsy

- The skin incisions should then be closed. With small biopsies (less than 1–2 cm) a simple interrupted skin suture should suffice. With larger biopsies, subcutaneous or subcuticular sutures may be placed
- Provided the surgery was carried out under strict aseptic conditions, no antibiotics are necessary
- A disadvantage of skin biopsy to investigate skin **neoplasia** is that, if a malignancy is discovered that requires removal with a large free margin, the margin must now be measured from the limit of the biopsy incision, thus requiring a larger area of excision. There is also a risk that the biopsy procedure may cause spread or seeding of the **neoplasia**

Fine-needle aspiration biopsy

FNAB is a very quick, reliable and underused method for obtaining a biopsy of a skin or subcutaneous mass. Although only a small number of cells may be obtained, it is usually sufficient to distinguish between inflammation and **neoplasia** and may give a definitive diagnosis in most cases.

Information from FNAB may be used to decide whether removal of a mass is necessary, or whether another modality of treatment may be more appropriate. A cytological diagnosis of a particular type of **neoplasia** will direct the surgeon to include an appropriate surgical margin around the mass.

- Since no anaesthesia or sedation is required (exceptions being intractable or vicious patients or masses near the eye), FNAB may be safely performed on geriatric or ill patients
- Any masses discovered during a consultation period may be readily aspirated in the consultation room, or the patient may be removed to a treatment room for the procedure to be carried out, if more convenient
- Multiple masses on a patient are far more readily assessed by FNAB than by surgical biopsy
- The technique requires very little equipment and is inexpensive to perform
- FNAB should always precede excision of a skin **tumour** as it may help decide size of margin
- In a hospital or practice where laboratory staff are competent at examining cytological samples, FNAB may be used intraoperatively to reassess margins

Equipment required:
- 5-ml **sterile** syringes
- 23 G ¾-inch **sterile** hypodermic needles
- Cleaned and polished microscope slides
- Slide/glass marking pen
- Slide container

Technique (Figure 8.4)
- No skin preparation is required
- A 23 G hypodermic needle is attached to a 5-ml syringe and held (preferably in the **dominant hand**)
- The skin or subcutaneous mass is held in the other hand to keep it steady
- The needle is inserted into the mass and the syringe plunger pulled back (to about 4 ml). The syringe and needle should be redirected within the mass to sample several areas of the mass, while retaining the vacuum
- Blood appearing in the hub usually indicates penetration of a blood vessel. The sample is unlikely to be useful and the FNA should be repeated in another area. If blood is consistently sampled, it may be that the mass truly is blood-filled, or else that there is sampling error; it is worth sending the sample off for examination in any case

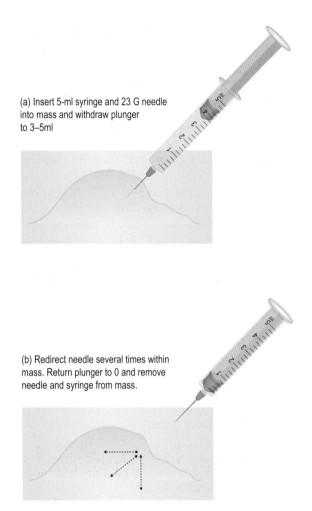

(a) Insert 5-ml syringe and 23 G needle into mass and withdraw plunger to 3–5ml

(b) Redirect needle several times within mass. Return plunger to 0 and remove needle and syringe from mass.

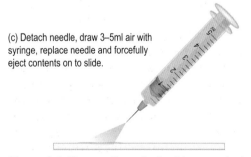

(c) Detach needle, draw 3–5ml air with syringe, replace needle and forcefully eject contents on to slide.

Figure 8.4 Fine-needle aspiration biopsy method.

- Having redirected the needle within the mass, the plunger should be slowly released and the syringe and needle withdrawn from the mass. The needle is removed and held while 3–4 ml of air is drawn into the syringe. The needle is then replaced and the air is forcefully ejected from the syringe, aiming over a clean glass slide. A few droplets may be seen on the slide, or else a large amount of material may be ejected. A second glass slide should be used to smear the sample and the slides should be waved about to air-dry them
- The process is repeated to get three to four samples. Any bleeding from this method is usually minimal and may be blotted away with clean cotton wool or a gauze swab
- An alternative method is to use the needle without a syringe attached: this method is easier for small masses, when it may be difficult to sample accurately with a bulky syringe on the end of the needle. The needle is used to stab the mass gently several times. Having sampled the area, a 5-ml syringe (already charged with 4 ml air) is added to the needle and the sample ejected on to the slides as above
- The slides are labelled and sent to a laboratory specialising in veterinary cytological examination

Tissue-core biopsy

This combines the convenience of FNAB with the larger sample size of surgical biopsy. Specially designed instruments are used, which have a sharp central needle with variable-sized trough or sample collection site and a sleeve with a sharpened end (Figure 8.5). The whole ensemble is used to penetrate the area of interest and the inner needle is advanced to the centre of the mass. The outer sleeve is then advanced, cutting the slice of tissue that has fallen into the sample collection trough as it does so. The biopsy device is then removed, with the sleeve preventing the sample from falling off.

- Very small biopsies are obtained by this method, size depending on needle gauge and trough length. However, the architecture of

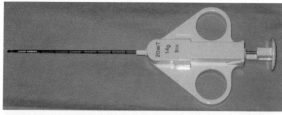

A

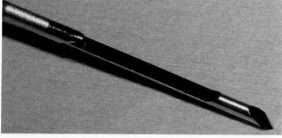

B

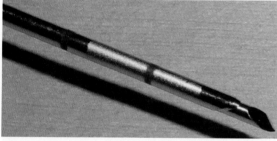

C

Figure 8.5 Tru-cut biopsy needle. (A) Tru-cut biopsy needle, 14 G (Global Veterinary Products). (B) Close-up to show biopsy recess (sheath withdrawn). (C) When fired, the sheath shoots forward to cut tissue and trap it in the biopsy recess.

the sample is usually preserved, allowing for a histological rather than cytological biopsy
- There is reportedly an increased risk of seeding **tumour** cells along the biopsy tract when compared with FNAB. If the subcutaneous mass is manipulated as close to the skin as possible, so that interceding tissues are pushed out of the way, this is less likely to be a problem. It is also good practice to make the biopsy approach perpendicular to the skin directly above the mass. In this way, the biopsy tract will be removed during excision of the mass

- Rotating the device slightly once the central needle is extended helps to cut fascial connections from the sample
- Spring-loaded biopsy devices (e.g. Tru-cut biopsy needle, Global Veterinary Products) are easier to use one-handed than manual devices. They often provide better biopsies as a result
- Removal of the tissue core from the biopsy instrument can be simply accomplished by rinsing with **sterile** saline from a 5-ml syringe. The use of hypodermic needles or scalpel blades to remove the sample should be discouraged as this can cause damage to the delicate biopsy
- The sample should be placed into 10% formal-saline and sent to a laboratory used to dealing with tissue-core samples
- Most tissue-core biopsy devices are only designed for single use and should be discarded. Sterilisation by autoclave tends to melt the plastic and blunt the needles. *They should never be used to biopsy more than one mass on a patient:* this may well result in spreading of **tumour** cells

SKIN-SURFACE TUMOURS AND SUBCUTANEOUS GROWTHS

In terms of minor veterinary surgery, removal of these masses with a minimum of clear margin (1 cm) is termed **lumpectomy**. This is a fairly misleading term and is open to a lot of interpretations. A 5-mm benign skin mass is clearly removable by **lumpectomy**, but a football-sized mass of the same histological type of **tumour** is obviously not as straightforward to remove.

Strictly, a **lumpectomy**:
- Should be restricted to masses that have been identified as benign, thus requiring minimal clear margins, or else palliative removal of malignant masses, where complete excision is not possible or spread has occurred, and removal of the mass by **lumpectomy** will increase the patient's comfort
- Should require a small enough incision to be amenable to closure by routine means, not requiring flaps, or other reconstructive techniques

Table 8.1 Common skin and subcutaneous tumours of the dog and cat

Skin tumours	Subcutaneous tumours
Mast-cell tumour (M)	Lipoma (B, M rarely (liposarcoma), but may be infiltrative)
Squamous cell carcinoma (M)	Haemangioma (B)
Histiocytoma (B)	Haemangiosarcoma (M)
Lymphoma (M)	Haemangiopericytoma (B, but recurrence likely)
Melanoma (B, M)	Lymphoma (M)
Basal cell tumour (B)	Mast-cell tumour (M)
Sebaceous adenoma (B)	Sarcoma (M)
Sebaceous adenocarcinoma (M)	
Trichoepithelioma (B)	
Papilloma (B)	
M, malignant; B, benign.	

- Should involve masses within the skin or immediate subcutaneous tissue
- Should not involve masses on or near delicate structures, as the removal of such lumps may cause damage or distortion to those structures (for example, eyelid, nasal planum, penis or anal masses). Even with a small benign mass in these areas, surgery is complicated by requiring delicate, precise reconstruction of the wound

Chapter 1 discusses the scope of the schedule 3 Amendment to the Veterinary Surgeons' Act 1966 in more detail, with regard to performance of minor surgery by qualified and listed veterinary nurses.

Skin and subcutaneous tumours can be of a variety of tissue types and degrees of malignancy. Table 8.1 lists some common skin and subcutaneous tumours. N.B.: the list is not exhaustive, but is merely presented to indicate the variety of **tumour** types present.

Many skin masses may have a characteristic shape, size or colour, or they may be found more commonly in certain breeds and ages. However, this cannot be relied upon to suppose a certain **tumour** type is present. Mast-cell tumours (MCT) have often been described rather whimsically as 'the great pretender', and may resemble many types of **tumour**, often presenting as the most benign-looking mass.

The author has twice removed 'fatty lumps' that appeared to be benign lipomata (plural of lipoma), to discover on **histopathology** that the masses were anything but benign: one was found to be a highly malignant haemangiosarcoma, the other an MCT.

MARGIN OF EXCISION

Without knowing whether a skin or subcutaneous mass is benign or malignant, the clear margin or margin of excision cannot be decided upon. This is the area of tissue surrounding a mass that must be removed to make sure that all **tumour** cells that may have migrated from the mass have also been removed (Figure 8.6).

With removal of malignant masses, the best chance of removing all **tumour** cells is with the first surgery. The reason for this is that if the **histopathology** demonstrates cells extending to the margin of the excision, surgery should be repeated to take a bigger margin. The problem is that the new margin must be measured from the wound site, not the original mass, and must include margins from all sides (including deep to the mass). If a long, deep wound was made in the initial surgery, a longer, deeper wound must be made for the second attempt, and so on, until margins are clear (Figure 8.7). In fact, a much

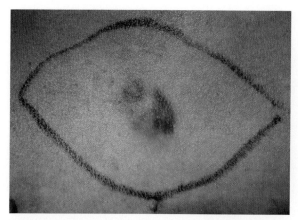

Figure 8.6 Use of skin-marking pen to plan margin of excision – in this case, a cutaneous haemangioma on the ventral abdomen of a dog.

wider and deeper margin must be made, because the excision must take into account fascial planes that were divided and disrupted during the first surgery.

To reduce the chance of this happening, and to give the best care to your patient:

- All skin or subcutaneous masses should be biopsied (preferably by FNAB) prior to removal
- Regardless of the results, *all* masses should be sent for definitive histopathological examination, including skin margins

In order to help locate the mass at surgery, several steps may be taken:

- The location and a brief description of the mass(es) should be entered in the clinical notes at the time of initial consultation. This not only provides a good memory aid for finding the mass again, but also enables some appreciation of change in size or shape of the mass, which may give a further indication as to its nature. It also avoids disputes with the owner regarding the mass
- If surgery is to be performed very soon, the hair overlying the mass may be shaved or cut short. This may also make FNAB easier to perform
- On admission, the owner should be asked to point out the location of the mass or masses.

If these are easily found, a brief note of their size and location may be made on the consent form. If the lumps are small and difficult to find, the application of a little correction fluid to the overlying hair may help. The client should always be asked to confirm the location in case an additional lump has been found. In this case, it is best to delay surgery until FNAB has been performed on the new lump

Prior to surgery, the mass should be methodically examined and palpated with regard to the full extent, depth and likely subcutaneous attachments.

Removal of skin-surface tumours

Assuming FNAB has suggested a benign mass, amenable to **lumpectomy,** and the patient is otherwise fit for surgery:

- The patient is anaesthetised and the surgical site is prepared for aseptic surgery
- The surgical personnel are prepared for **sterile** surgery and full aseptic procedure is followed (hats, masks, gowns, gloves and full **sterile** draping of patient)
- For most **lumpectomies,** a simple operating kit will suffice (see above)
- An oval skin incision is made around the mass, allowing at least a 0.5-cm margin (1 cm is preferred). Incision is made easier if the finger and thumb of the opposite hand are used to apply a little tension to the skin and hold the mass in place. Care should be taken that the scalpel is held perpendicular to the skin. This ensures that the margin is accurately maintained. Wherever possible, the incision should follow the line of skin tension in that area (Figure 8.8)
- The incision should be extended to the subdermis. At this level, the skin suddenly springs apart, improving visualisation of subcutaneous tissues. Any blood vessels should be avoided or clamped if transection is necessary to extend the incision. The incision should be continued in this way all around the mass
- If the mass is superficial on the skin, the subcutaneous tissue may be dissected free from

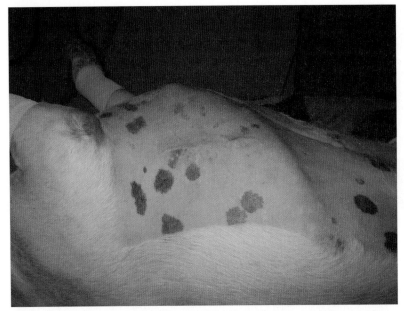

A

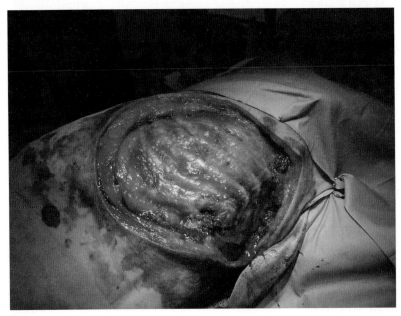

B

Figure 8.7 Consequences of inadequate margins of surgical excision. (A) A malignant skin **tumour** was removed from this English bull terrier 2 months previously. Inadequate margins of excision were taken and the **tumour** has recurred along the surgical incision site. A reddened, raised mass on the sternum was aspirated and malignant cells were seen. (B) Surgical excision included skin, subcutis and muscle layers. Closure required extensive skin undermining and reconstruction.

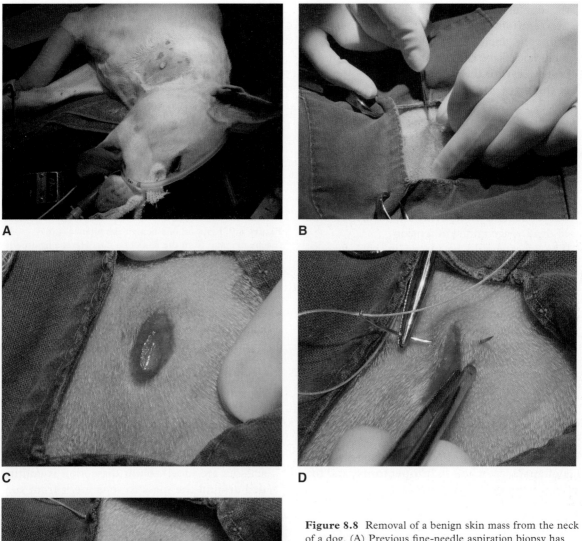

Figure 8.8 Removal of a benign skin mass from the neck of a dog. (A) Previous fine-needle aspiration biopsy has identified this skin mass as benign. Hair is clipped from the area and the site is prepared for aseptic surgery, in this case with povidone-iodine. (B) An elliptical skin incision is made around the mass. The incision is extended to the subcutis. The margin of excision is approximately 0.5–1 cm. A no. 15 scalpel blade has been used in this case. (C) The mass has been removed and sent for confirmatory **histopathology**. The wound is small in this case and there is little dead space. (D) A curved cutting needle is used to **appose** the skin edges with 3/0 (2 metric) nylon (Ethilon, Ethicon). (E) The first suture has been placed. In this case, a simple interrupted suture pattern has been chosen. Two to three more sutures will be sufficient to close this wound. There is no need for a dressing.

the skin at this stage using scissors (Mayo or Metzenbaum). If the mass is deeper within the skin, the incision should be deepened to include excision of the subcutaneous tissue. It is very easy for the incision to reduce in width at this stage and some care should be given to avoid this. The excised tissue should be snipped free from its fascial connections and removed

- Any bleeding should be controlled by application of **sterile** swabs or haemostats (see Chapter 7) and the wound should be closed in a routine manner by closure of the subcutaneous tissues and skin, paying attention to closure of dead space and skin tension
- The mass should be placed in 10% formalsaline and sent for **histopathology**
- If multiple masses are to be removed from a patient, it is recommended that a separate kit and fresh **sterile** gloves be used for each one to avoid the risk of spreading a **tumour**
- Provided surgery time is short and strict aseptic technique has been observed throughout, there is no need for antibiotics

Removal of subcutaneous masses

As above, assuming FNAB has suggested a benign mass, amenable to **lumpectomy,** and the patient is otherwise fit for surgery:
- The patient is anaesthetised and the surgical site is prepared for aseptic surgery
- The surgical personnel are prepared for **sterile** surgery and full aseptic procedure is followed (hats, masks, gowns, gloves and full **sterile** draping of patient)
- A simple operating kit will suffice (see above) for most subcutaneous **lumpectomies**. However, a pair of small Gelpi self-retaining retractors can improve visualisation within the wound
- A straight skin incision is made over the mass, parallel to skin tension lines. Applying a little tension to the skin with the thumb and forefinger of the opposite hand will make the incision easier to make and more accurate
- The incision should be allowed to extend just beyond the margins of the mass

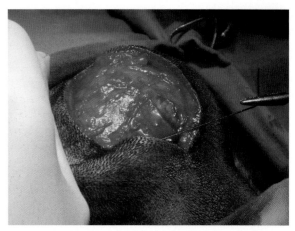

Figure 8.9 Removal of a benign subcutaneous mass (haemangioma) from the flank of a dog. Here, a ligature is placed on one of the disconcertingly large blood vessels.

- Any subcutaneous blood vessels should be clamped with fine haemostatic forceps and transacted (Figure 8.9), or carefully dissected around and pushed to one side
- Some subcutaneous masses have a fine capsule surrounding them. Where possible, this should be left intact to provide a layer of protection reducing likelihood of recurrence of the mass
- Using fine dissecting scissors (Metzenbaum scissors are ideal), blunt dissection is continued around the mass to separate it from surrounding connective tissue and fascia. Any connecting blood vessels are clamped and ligated. It is preferable to use instruments (toothed thumb forceps) rather than hands to manipulate tissue. Allis tissue forceps are rarely helpful in holding **tumour** tissue, tending to cause tearing of the **tumour** capsule, and should never be used to hold skin. For small, well-circumscribed masses (i.e. those with a clearly defined capsule), application of a little pressure on either side of the skin wound can often aid exteriorisation (they may pop out of the wound), but excessive force should not be used as this may lead to crushing of the mass and dispersal of **tumour** tissue
- Certain tumours, which feel well-circumscribed prior to surgery, may turn out to have

indistinct borders. The classic example of this is the infiltrative lipoma. Although not malignant, these tumours tend to grow and extend along fascial planes between muscle bodies and are often impossible to excise completely. They are not possible to distinguish from well-encapsulated lipomata on the basis of FNAB and even careful palpation of all surfaces of the mass through the skin may not reveal the infiltrative nature of these masses. Large-scale, complex dissection through several muscle layers does not fall into the remit of minor surgery or of **lumpectomy** and nurses performing these removals should request veterinary assistance

- Having removed the mass, subcutaneous tissues should be closed, being particularly careful to reduce dead space, and skin sutures should be placed
- Provided surgery time has been short (less than 1 h) and provided strict attention has been paid to aseptic technique throughout, no antibiotics are necessary
- The mass should be placed into 10% formal-saline and sent for **histopathology**

Mammary lumpectomy

In human surgery, the term **lumpectomy** is reserved for the removal of small mammary lumps with a minimal margin. Many veterinary surgeons use the same definition of **lumpectomy**.

Mammary tumours are the most common **tumour** type in female dogs (accounting for approximately one-third of all tumours in dogs). Almost 50% are malignant in dogs and almost all are malignant in cats. Early neutering of bitches and queens dramatically reduces the risk of mammary **neoplasia**, with an almost 100% reduction in incidence for bitches spayed before their first season. Subsequent oestrus cycles increase the risk of **neoplasia**, with little or no reduction if the bitch is spayed after her third season.

There are many different types of mammary masses, ranging from benign mammary **hyper-**

plasia to the highly malignant inflammatory carcinomas. They may present as tiny (1-mm) nodules or massive pedunculated or dangling growths. They may have little or no skin change or be ulcerated and secondarily infected. The latter group usually carries a poorer prognosis (Figure 8.10).

Initial work-up should include FNAB. Routine bloods and biochemistry should be included (to

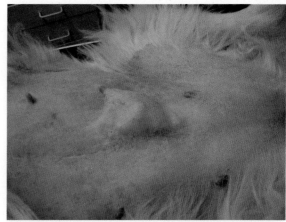

A

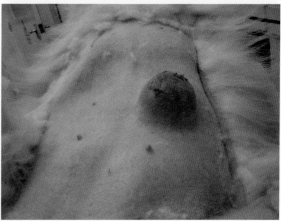

B

Figure 8.10 Examples of mammary masses. (A) A benign mammary adenoma on a 12-year-old Shetland sheepdog. Removal of this mass provided a cure. (B) Mixed mammary adenocarcinoma on a 7-year-old Samoyed. Metastasis had already occurred at the time of excision. The bitch survived for another 4 months, prior to euthanasia.

rule out concomitant age-related disease). Radiography of the chest (together with radiography and ultrasonic examination of the abdomen) should be carried out to investigate **metastatic** disease, although this can be carried out on the day of surgery if required. Inguinal and axillary lymph nodes should be examined for any sign of involvement (increase in size).

If the cytology results are suggestive of benign growth, and the mass is reasonably small (less than 0.5 cm), it may be removed by **lumpectomy**.

- A margin of excision of 1 cm or more is taken
- The surgery is performed in the same way as excision of a skin mass, making an elliptical or oval incision and deepening this by a mixture of blunt and sharp dissection, keeping the wound edges parallel to ensure that the margin of excision is maintained
- Special attention should be given to identifying and ligating the cranial or **caudal** superficial epigastric vessels that supply the mammary glands
- It is often easier to remove an entire mammary gland (including nipple), as this avoids the risk of secretions such as milk and lymph causing wound irritation
- **Lavage** of the wound may be necessary if there has been much bleeding or if there is a lot of fat or tissue debris in the wound
- The subcutaneous tissues and skin should be closed as above, being careful to reduce dead space, and the mass is sent for **histopathology**
- Any larger mammary mass or any mass diagnosed as malignant by aspiration cytology should not be classed as minor surgery and should be performed by a veterinary surgeon

SURGICAL MANAGEMENT OF ABSCESSES

Abscesses are accumulations of purulent exudate within an organ or tissue, usually associated with direct trauma or puncture, but can also occur secondary to **haematogenous** spread of bacteria. With minor surgery we are most concerned with subcutaneous abscesses or oral abscesses (see Chapter 9 for treatment of oral abscesses).

Abscesses (cat-bite abscesses, CBA) are one of the most common reasons for cats presenting at veterinary clinics and almost always result from fights with other cats, although foxes, squirrels and rats are often unfairly blamed!

Cats usually present pyrexic (temperature often in excess of 40°C) and may be inappetant or anorectic. There is often a history of known cat fights one or several days earlier. In general, abscesses are not hard to find: if on the face they may result in facial asymmetry or a very noticeable lump. If on a limb, they are usually associated with lameness. The tail or perineum is another common site for a CBA.

The treatment for abscesses is to lance, flush and drain, as well as providing antibiotic treatment and **analgesia**. There are important considerations in the treatment of abscesses, however, and treatment will depend to a large extent on:

- The previous and present health status of the animal: elderly patients or ones with pre-existing illness may be nutritionally embarrassed or dehydrated. Anaesthetising (or sedating) these patients, or using certain drugs (e.g. non-steroidal anti-inflammatory drugs or NSAIDs) may exacerbate renal insufficiency or other disease. Consideration should be given to hospitalisation and intravenous (IV) fluid therapy for these patients for 24 h prior to anaesthesia for surgical management of the CBA
- The position and condition of the **abscess**: abscesses in a dependent position are more likely to continue draining after lancing than non-dependent CBA. For example, an **abscess** above the zygomatic arch may not drain as well as an **abscess** near the ramus of the mandible. Repeated flushes or a more intense surgical curettage of the **abscess** may be required in the former case. Similarly, abscesses which are pointing (i.e. which have an area of obviously very thin, soft skin signifying the **abscess** is about to burst) may be amenable to lancing immediately, whereas abscesses deep within the subcutaneous tissue may need to be left overnight, with or without hot pads being applied to draw the infection
- The temperament of the patient: some cats are very placid and may allow a CBA to be shaved,

lanced and flushed under only very mild sedation or local anaesthetic. Others may be vicious, frightened and in pain and require sedation within a crush cage even to examine the **abscess**

- Client factors and considerations: often clients will have dealt with cat abscesses before, and will have seen them treated in a certain way. Some owners have cats that present monthly with **abscesses** from new fights! It is difficult in these cases to promote a different form of treatment (which may be more expensive) when, in their experience, a course of antibiotic tablets has sufficed. Good communication is required. Remember, it is up to us to advise on the best form of treatment; it is then up to the client to decide whether or not to accept that advice

Analgesia

Abscesses are painful and it is a combination of pain and bacterial toxaemia that causes the morbidity associated with abscesses. NSAIDs are extremely effective analgesics for CBA, but should not be used in dehydrated patients due to increased renal toxicity. Young cats that are moderately pyrexic but are eating and drinking should not be at any increased risk and will benefit from NSAID use, but older cats, or cats that have not eaten or drunk for 24–48 h, may be moderately dehydrated and may be at risk of kidney damage from NSAID use. Other analgesics (e.g. buprenorphine) should be considered until drinking resumes, or IV fluid therapy should be instigated. Local anaesthesia (e.g. Emla cream) is unlikely to provide appreciable **analgesia**, but may be useful as adjunct pain relief for surgical management of CBA.

Antibiotics

Bacteria commonly associated with CBA include: *Staphylococcus* spp., *Pasteurella multocida*, *Streptococcus* spp., *Escherichia coli* and various anaerobes, although rarely other bacteria and fungi may be involved.

Broad-spectrum antibiotics, active against many Gram-positive and Gram-negative bacteria, should be selected. A good initial choice for most cases is a clavulanate-potentiated amoxicillin (e.g. Synulox, Pfizer) 12.5–25 mg/kg BID.

Sedation/general anaesthesia

Lancing and flushing abscesses is a painful procedure and should be performed with appropriate **analgesia**. In addition, the patient may be difficult to handle or aggressive. In most cases, therefore, some degree of sedation or general anaesthesia is warranted. This not only provides a greater degree of control over **analgesia**, but also allows time for a more rigorous flushing and curettage of the **abscess**.

It may be argued that a routine antibiotic injection, followed by 6 days of oral antibiotics, will resolve most abscesses, whether or not they are lanced. This may well be appropriate for small **abscesses**: however, any **abscess** with an attendant toxaemia and appreciable amount of pus should really be flushed to reduce the bacterial load as quickly as possible, thus reducing the toxaemic effect on the organs.

Medetomidine–butorphanol sedative combinations are safe to use and provide good levels of **analgesia** (see Chapter 3), but it is important to remember that reversal of the sedative using atipamazole also removes the analgesic activity of the α_2-agonist.

Surgical treatment of abscesses

The patient is sedated or anaesthetised according to preference, having ensured that fluid balance is reasonable. IV fluid therapy should be considered in all cases and should be used routinely for general anaesthesia (see Chapter 4).

- The skin surrounding the **abscess** is clipped and prepared for aseptic surgery (why risk introducing new bacteria to the **abscess**?). **Sterile** drapes should be placed over the patient. Water-repellent drapes are useful as they prevent the patient becoming soaking wet during the flushing procedure

- Full aseptic technique should be observed (masks, gloves, hats) for several reasons:
  - To reduce the risk of introducing additional infectious agents into the **abscess**. As methicillin-resistant *Staphylococcus aureus* (MRSA) becomes more prevalent in the veterinary world, this becomes more important
  - To reduce the risk of acquiring infection from the patient. Most bacteria in abscesses are widespread commensals. However, occasionally unusual bacterial or fungi are isolated and these may have zoonotic potential
  - Wearing full aseptic regalia helps to focus the mind to perform the procedure, following good surgical practice
- It is a good idea also to wear goggles or safety spectacles to reduce the risk of spattering bacteria into the eyes
- Using a no. 11 scalpel blade, a stab incision is made in the skin overlying a dependent area of the **abscess**. This should result in release of purulent exudate. The incision should be extended to allow free drainage of purulent material. A useful technique is to remove a triangle of skin approximately 0.7–1 cm wide. The incision may be extended to improve drainage if necessary
- Purulent exudate is squeezed out of the **abscess**, using firm but gentle pressure on the skin surrounding the **abscess**
- Using a 20-ml syringe and 19 G needle, the **abscess** is flushed with warmed **sterile** saline or Hartmann's solution. At least 500 ml should be used. Dilute chlorhexidine (0.05%) may be added if desired (a 1-in-40 dilution of stock solution)
- For chronic abscesses with a thick fibrous capsule, a surgical curette (e.g. Volkmann curette, or a Spratt bone curette) may be used to scrape the fibrous lining and so debride the **abscess**. Flushing should be repeated following curettage
- The wound is usually left open to drain, although large wounds with much dead space may be partially closed and a Penrose drain placed. If partial closure is to be performed, an absorbable monofilament suture material

should be placed. The knot should have the minimum number of throws placed to reduce bacterial persistence
- The wound may be left open to drain, or a dressing placed. A suitable dressing would be Intrasite gel (Smith & Nephew) or Allevyn (Smith & Nephew). If a dressing is placed, it should be changed regularly (at least daily, occasionally twice daily) until no further exudate is seen. The wound should be flushed daily, using sedation or general anaesthesia as required, until granulation tissue is seen, indicating resolution of infection
- Antibiotics and analgesics (e.g. NSAIDs) should be continued for at least 1 week, or until healing is complete

For smaller abscesses, instructing the client to perform saline bathing of the wound at home may be sufficient aftercare following **debridement** and flushing. The **abscess** wound should go on to heal uneventfully.

Treatment of complicated abscesses

If an **abscess** fails to heal following the procedure outlined above (i.e. if resolution is not seen within a week or two) or if there is recurrence, then an underlying cause should be suspected.
- Bloods should be taken for haematology and biochemistry to investigate the presence of metabolic disease such as renal or hepatic disease or endocrinopathy (e.g. diabetes mellitus). Feline leukaemia virus (FeLV)/feline immunodeficiency virus (FIV) status should be investigated
- A bacterial swab should be collected from deep within the **abscess** for culture and sensitivity
- Radiography should be considered to look for evidence of foreign material within the wound
- If no obvious cause is forthcoming, a full surgical exploration of the **abscess** should be made, extending to the underlying body cavity if necessary. Wound closure, using omentum as a natural drain, can be considered

Feline leukaemia virus/feline immunodeficiency virus

FeLV and FIV are chronic immunosuppressive retroviruses that may be transmitted by bites and scratches. Cats with CBA are therefore at risk of contracting infection or passing these viruses on. Several effective vaccines exist for FeLV and it is hoped that this will be the case for FIV (at the time of writing, there is no vaccine available in the UK against FIV). Cat owners should be informed of the risks of infection through fighting and vaccination protocols followed appropriately.

FIV or FeLV infection is widespread and should be suspected in any ill cat, especially where there is a history of fighting; serological testing should be carried out on these animals.

Following a cat bite from a cat infected with either of these viruses, a transient viraemia may result, with clinical signs, which may be indiscernible from routine CBA (pyrexia, inappetance). Seroconversion (time taken for the virus to be detectable by serological means) may take 60 days or so. It is important, therefore, that any cats testing negative for FIV/FeLV following CBA are retested 2–3 months later.

Surgical management of abscesses in rabbits

Rabbits present a particular challenge in terms of treatment of **abscess**. Abscesses in this species are especially difficult to treat because:

- The exudate (pus) is very thick and sticky. It therefore doesn't drain very well and persists in infected wounds
- The most common **abscess** in rabbits occurs on the face, secondary to dental disease. It is very difficult to resolve the dental disease completely, thus the abscesses are also difficult to resolve
- The bacteria involved have a great tendency to invade bone and cause inflammation and bone abscessation. Penetration of antibiotics into these areas is frequently poor, leading to bacterial persistence

- The bacteria may be present in several pockets of tissue, making it difficult to flush all parts of an **abscess**. In addition to this, bacteria may seed abscesses in other parts of the body
- Our choice of antibiotics is limited in this species due to susceptibility to fatal enteric microbial derangement

For these reasons, rabbit abscesses often carry a poor prognosis and more often than not result in euthanasia.

The bacteria most commonly isolated from rabbit abscesses are *P. multocida* and *S. aureus* and it is not unusual to find pure growths of these organisms in the **abscess**. Even so, culture and sensitivity should be routinely performed to facilitate correct choice of antibiotic.

Every rabbit presenting with an **abscess** should be given a full clinical examination, including, most importantly, oral examination to document dental disease. Bloods should be taken for routine haematology and biochemistry and X-rays should be considered to check for lung abscessation.

The rabbit should be anaesthetised (paying particular attention to **analgesia**) and the **abscess** treated as above.

- Several packing agents have been proposed to increase the chance of resolution of infection (calcium hydroxide dental paste, Intrasite gel with or without combined antibiotic, honey, antibiotic-impregnated polymethylmethacrylate (AIPMMA) beads)
- The use of wound irrigation through a drain may also increase the chances of curing rabbit abscesses. Recently, addition of proteolytic enzymes (e.g. trypsin) to liquefy the pus and aid in **debridement** has been suggested
- Provided a clear margin can be obtained, treating the **abscess** as a **tumour** and removing it by en bloc excision may provide the best means of treatment. This is unlikely to be successful for dental abscesses as it is difficult to remove all infected tissue
- In any case, antibiotics (e.g. enrofloxacin 5–10 mg/kg orally BID) should be used for extended periods of time, usually 2–3 months

NASOLACRIMAL DUCT FLUSHING

The nasolacrimal duct runs from the lacrimal puncta on the upper and lower palpebrae to the ventral surface of the nasal cavity in dogs and cats (Figure 8.11). The puncta or duct openings are between 0.5 and 1 mm in diameter. They are thus just visible to the naked eye, although magnification is recommended when examining these structures.

Flushing of nasolacrimal ducts is indicated to resolve blockage of the ducts and to treat infection of the nasolacrimal sac (dacryocystitis). Such conditions tend to be characterised by chronic epiphora (tear staining) and recurrent conjunctivitis. Another indication for nasolacrimal catheterisation is in maintaining patency of puncta after surgical treatment of stenotic puncta.

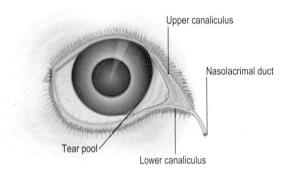

Upper canaliculus

Nasolacrimal duct

Tear pool

Lower canaliculus

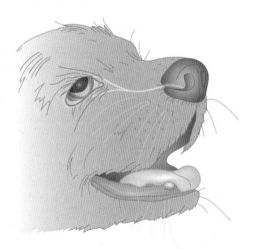

Figure 8.11 Nasolacrimal duct in the dog/cat.

Although well-behaved and calm patients may be flushed conscious, it is often necessary to utilise some sedation. A premedication dose of acepromazine and buprenorphine is usually sufficient for dogs: cats may require deeper sedation (see Chapter 3). It can be very frustrating to have the patient shake its head just after the cannula has been inserted; there is also the concern about **iatrogenic** damage to the cornea with an improperly restrained animal.

- A few drops of topical (local) anaesthetic should be applied to the eye (e.g. amethocaine 0.5% drops (Minims, Chauvin Pharmaceuticals)) and 1–2 min allowed for it to take effect. An injection of NSAID may also help reduce postoperative discomfort in the case of dacryocystitis
- A brief surgical hand-wash should be performed and **sterile** gloves worn. It is impossible to perform the procedure in a **sterile** manner, but it is good practice to avoid risk of **nosocomial** infection wherever possible
- It helps to prepare an instrument trolley with the necessary equipment: **sterile** trolley drape, **sterile** irrigating cannula or nasolacrimal cannula (irrigating cannula, Portex, medium (pink, 0.91 mm outside diameter (OD)) and small (blue, 0.76 mm OD)), warmed **sterile** saline or Hartmann's solution, 5-ml syringes
- Stretching the eyelids between thumb and forefinger, the dorsal and ventral lacrimal puncta are identified. It may be helpful to evert the eyelid slightly using atraumatic thumb forceps (e.g. De Bakey)
- The irrigating cannula is inserted into the punctum. This can be difficult to do, the commonest difficulty being that the cannula slides over the opening. This can be made easier by cutting the cannula a little shorter and bevelling the end somewhat (i.e. cutting the cannula at an angle). This should be done with fine scissors and the resulting point smoothed off or rounded by careful cutting to avoid production of sharp edges
- If one punctum proves difficult to catheterise, then the other punctum should be tried. If that proves difficult, due to scar tissue or inflammation reducing the punctum diameter,

then a 2–3-cm length of stiff, fine monofilament suture material (2/0 (3 metric) PDS II is ideal) may be used to gain access to the duct. The irrigating cannula may then be slid over the suture material. Due to the risk of damage to the punctum, the use of a hypodermic needle is not recommended

- Having catheterised the duct, a 5-ml syringe, preloaded with **sterile** saline, is attached to the luer-end and gentle pressure exerted on the plunger. A drop of dye (e.g. fluorescein dye 1%, Minims, Chauvin Pharmaceuticals) may be added to the saline: this helps visualisation of the flush solution as it exits the nose. It may be necessary to use a reasonable amount of force to unblock the lacrimal sac: a 5-ml syringe is unlikely to produce sufficient pressure to cause damage to the duct itself
- 20–30 ml of saline is used to flush the duct: some workers recommend flushing a little ophthalmic antibiotic prior to removal of the cannula (e.g. gentamicin eye drops, Tiacil, Virbac Laboratories)

Care should be taken that no damage occurs to the eye after flushing: the local anaesthetic remains active for some while and may diminish the blink reflex, leaving the eye susceptible to trauma.

Nasolacrimal duct flushing in rabbits

Rabbits are prone to dacryocystitis. It usually occurs in this species as a result of impaction of molar teeth causing inflammation and direct pressure on the duct as it passes through the maxillary bone and nasal chambers overlying the cheek teeth.

As with the cat and dog, epiphora is the main presenting sign. Pressure on the lacrimal sac at the medial canthus of the eye frequently results in the expression of whitish purulent exudate. Examination of the cheek teeth may demonstrate abnormal wear and spur production; radiographs may be necessary to demonstrate root impaction. A combination of nasolacrimal duct flushing, topical and systemic antibiosis and molar rasping/extraction is required to treat this condition, but recurrence is likely.

Nasolacrimal flushing is carried out in much the same way as it is for dogs and cats, except that rabbits only have a single nasolacrimal punctum, on the medial aspect of the lower eyelid.

EAR SURGERY AND AURAL HAEMATOMA

Wounds to the ear should be treated like any other wound, by prompt surgical attention (remember the 'golden period') and **debridement** as necessary. Having an appreciation of the direction of blood supply to the ear helps to make decisions regarding repair of wounds: wounds running perpendicular to blood flow are more liable to wound **dehiscence**. It is always a good idea to warn owners of any cosmetic consequences of ear surgery: this should not affect the surgical decision, but can avoid any misunderstanding or upset!

Suturing wounds to the ear

- Preanaesthetic clinical examination of the patient should be performed and any necessary blood tests run. **Analgesia** should be administered. Due to the relatively lower blood flow to the ears, antibiotics should be administered (at the time of surgery and for 3–5 days thereafter). General anaesthesia is necessary for ear surgery
- The pinna is clipped and prepared for **sterile** surgery. It can be difficult to prepare the pinna aseptically: one good way is to hold the base of the pinna to prepare the tip, then to have a scrubbed assistant wearing **sterile** gloves hold the tip of the pinna while the base is prepped. Alternatively, having scrubbed the tip of the ear it can be held with **sterile** atraumatic tissue forceps, such as Babcock forceps (do not use Allis tissue forceps!). The pinna is then laid on to a **sterile** drape and other **sterile** drapes are used to cover the base of the ear and the rest of the patient. Feline ears are rather easier to prep, as they are not pendulous: once prepared, they can be covered by a fenestrated drape

- Any loose flap of skin should be tacked back on to the ear using a full-thickness suture in a vertical mattress formation (i.e. in line with the ear)
- Lacerations only involving the skin may be repaired with simple interrupted sutures of 3/0 (2 metric) or 4/0 (1.5 metric) synthetic non-absorbable material. Monofilament suture material is preferred (e.g. Monosof, Vetoquinol). Wounds that involve the skin and cartilage can usually be sutured in the same way (i.e. simple interrupted through the skin only), but long incisions involving the cartilage may lead to a loss of support from the cartilage and bending of the pinna. Vertical mattress sutures engaging the skin and cartilage are best used in these cases. Full-thickness wounds to the ear should be sutured by a line of vertical mattress sutures engaging skin and cartilage on one side and a line of simple interrupted sutures through the skin on the other side

Small wounds may be left uncovered, but wounds larger than 2 cm should be dressed with a non-adhesive dressing and an ear bandage (see Chapter 5) to prevent the wounds opening or leaking if the patient shakes its head. An Elizabethan collar may be used to prevent self-trauma if needed.

Removal of ear tumours/pinnectomy

Any skin **tumour** can occur on the skin of the pinna (Table 8.1); in addition, ceruminous gland adenoma/adenocarcinoma is exclusive to the pinna. Auricular masses are usually initially seen as small raised nodules. These masses should be treated as any other skin mass (investigated by FNAB and removed with a margin of excision as directed – the cartilage may be taken as an effective margin since it is unusual for **neoplasia** to cross a cartilage border).

Squamous cell carcinoma, preceded by actinic keratosis, is the most common pinna neoplasm of cats, occurring most often on the ears of white cats. Resulting from ultraviolet damage from exposure to sunlight, the early lesions may appear as alopecia of the ear tips, accompanied by a

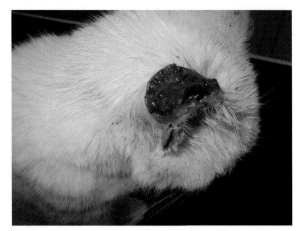

Figure 8.12 Squamous cell carcinoma on pinna of cat: this **tumour** had been present for at least 2 years prior to surgery. Fortunately, pinnectomy proved curative and no recurrence was seen 5 years after surgery.

slightly flaky appearance to the skin. In time, the ear tip deforms and ulcerates, developing ultimately into destructive erosive lesions on the ears (Figure 8.12).

- White cats (or cats with white ears) should have restricted access to direct sunlight, or else the pinna should be covered with total-block suncream (a human paediatric form is best as these tend to be of low toxicity)
- Any progressive change to the tip of the ear should be dealt with by early amputation of the pinna tip
- Pinnectomy is carried out using Mayo dissecting scissors and dealing with any blood vessels by electrocoagulation or crushing with fine haemostats. Ligatures should be kept to a minimum as they often result in local wound breakdown
- The skin edges are apposed and sutured by a line of horizontal mattress or simple continuous sutures (4/0 (1.5 metric) synthetic non-absorbable suture material should be used – Monosof (Vetoquinol) is appropriate). The skin on the dorsal (or convex) aspect of the ear is less closely attached to the auricular cartilage than that of the ventral (concave) aspect at the base of the ear. This makes it easier to move the convex pinna skin over the wound to **appose** skin

- A non-adhesive dressing and ear/head bandage should be placed for 48–72 h following surgery and sutures removed after 7–10 days
- Resected tissue should be sent for **histopathology**. The level of amputation depends on the staging of the **neoplasia**/preneoplastic change. For solar dermatitis (actinic keratosis), a 0.5–1-cm margin should be sufficient. For any ulcerative lesions suggesting a progression to **neoplasia**, the whole pinna should be removed

Aural haematoma

Although most commonly seen in dogs, aural haematoma also occurs in cats. It is usually caused by self-trauma (scratching the ear and head-shaking). This is usually secondary to infection or inflammation of the ear canals, so any animal presenting with aural haematoma should have a meticulous otoscopic examination.

Bleeding from the branches of the great auricular artery that supply the cartilage of the pinna causes the haematoma. The cartilage splits in two like a beer mat and a seroma forms. If left, fibrosis and wound contracture will occur and the seroma will resolve. Unfortunately, this usually results in a misshapen ('cauliflower') ear. Other than looking cosmetically unappealing, this can also lead to an increased incidence of **otitis externa**, due to the altered microclimate of the vertical ear canal.

Treatment is thus warranted to drain the seroma and allow repair of the cartilage in its normal anatomical arrangement.

Several methods are regularly used:

- Conservative: the seroma is drained by (aseptic) needle aspiration and a pressure bandage placed. This is rarely successful and most cases recur. The placement of a small teat cannula into the haematoma, and maintenance of drainage for 2–3 weeks, can be effective in treating this, but it is difficult to keep the cannula in place for so long
- Conservative/medical: various techniques have been described for draining the haematoma and injecting corticosteroids to reduce

recurrence of the seroma. The most successful method in the author's hands involves injecting 0.04 mg/kg betamethasone (Betsolan, Schering-Plough Animal Health) intramuscularly (IM) 72 h prior to (aseptically) aspirating the haematoma. At the time of aspiration 0.2 ml (8 mg) of a depot-acting methylprednisolone (Depo-Medrone, Pharmacia Animal Health) may be injected directly into the seroma cavity. The seroma generally recurs 3–5 days after aspiration and then resolves after 2–3 weeks with a minimum of disfigurement of the pinna. Although reasonable results may be obtained with this and other 'medical' treatments for aural haematoma, the risks of **iatrogenic** hyperadrenocorticism and inducement of hypoadrenocorticism by suppressing the pituitary–adrenal axis are very high. This method should therefore be used with caution, and the owner made aware of possible complications (the steroid usage is 'off-label')
- Surgical: a variety of surgical methods have been suggested to deal with aural haematoma. A simple method is described below

Surgical treatment of aural haematoma

- The patient is anaesthetised and the ear prepared for aseptic surgery, with the patient in lateral recumbency. Ear surgery is very painful, so consideration should be given to the best forms of **analgesia** (check whether corticosteroids have been administered prior to administering NSAIDs)
- The concave (inner) surface of the pinna is incised over the length of the haematoma. An S-shaped incision is less likely to result in twisting of the ear during healing (Figure 8.13)
- The haematoma is drained and a sharp-edged curette (e.g. a Spratt bone curette) is used to remove all fibrin from the haematoma cavity and the cavity is flushed with **sterile** saline
- Leaving the wound gaping slightly (2 mm) to provide drainage, the ear is sutured. This is the most crucial step in the surgery. Two staggered lines of mattress sutures are placed on

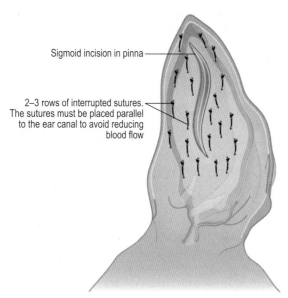

Sigmoid incision in pinna

2–3 rows of interrupted sutures. The sutures must be placed parallel to the ear canal to avoid reducing blood flow

Figure 8.13 Surgical treatment of aural haematoma.

either side of the incision, so that the sutures run parallel to the line of incision (synthetic non-absorbable suture material, e.g. Prolene, Ethicon, may be used). The suture material does not need to be thick: 4/0 (1.5 metric) is suitable, as long as the sutures are not placed too tightly. The tips of the needle holders should be able to be inserted under the suture when correctly placed, to allow for postoperative swelling. Orientation of the sutures perpendicular to the plane of incision results in interruption of blood supply to the wound and delays healing. Excessively tight sutures cause a lot of postoperative pain and may lead to wound breakdown
- Stents may be placed under the sutures to distribute pressure more evenly and prevent cutting through of the sutures. Historically, buttons were used, or else pieces of X-ray film. Stents may be difficult to sterilise and often increase postoperative discomfort by providing niches for bacterial growth. Provided the sutures are not placed too tightly, there should be no need for stents
- A non-adherent dressing and ear/head bandage is placed and the patient is fitted with an Elizabethan collar

Box 8.1

Any treatment of aural haematoma must take into account the resolution of underlying otitis externa.

Box 8.2

Regular check-ups and early detection of otitis externa are key to successful management.

- Provided strict aseptic technique has been observed, there is no need for antibiotics, but **analgesia** should be continued for at least 5 days
- The bandage is changed after 2–3 days and the sutures are removed between 7 and 10 days postsurgery (Box 8.1)

Otitis externa

Otitis externa in dogs and cats is a complex disease, resulting from the interaction of microorganisms and the inflammatory status and microclimate of the external auditory canal (Box 8.2). Table 8.2 lists the most common factors associated with canine and feline **otitis externa**.

Bacterial and fungal involvement in otitis is usually secondary, the microbes colonising an already damaged and inflamed ear canal. Clinical signs associated with **otitis externa** are head-shaking, head tilt, malodour and pain on ear examination.

Diagnosis of **otitis externa** involves:
- Otoscopic examination of the canals to look for ulcers, foreign bodies, growths, stenosis and damage to the tympanum
- Isolation of primary infectious agents, e.g. parasites. Usually otoscopic examination is sufficient to demonstrate the presence of these organisms
- Microscopy of swabs/smears of ear canals to identify the presence of pathogens and to

Table 8.2 Factors associated with otitis externa cases in dogs and cats

Factor	Species affected
Hypersensitivity	
Atopy	Dog
Food hypersensitivity	Dog
Contact allergy (to ear preparations)	Dog
Foreign bodies	Dog
Anatomical factors	
(stenotic canals, pendulous ears)	Dog
Immune-mediated disorders (e.g. pemphigus)	Dog, cat
Neoplasia	Dog, cat
Bacteria	
Pseudomonas aeruginosa	Dog, cat
Staphylococcus spp.	Dog
Streptococcus spp.	Dog
Pasteurella multocida	Cat
Proteus spp.	Dog, cat
Escherichia coli	Dog, cat
Fungi	
Malassezia pachydermatis	Dog, cat
Parasites	
Otodectes cyanotis	Cat, dog
Demodex canis	Dog
Neotrombicula autumnalis (harvest mite)	Cat, dog

quantify them (in order to stage the infection and follow progression)
- Culture and sensitivity of bacterial swabs
- Radiography (or computed tomography) of the head to evaluate the external and internal auditory canals and investigate the presence of **otitis media**
- Investigation of underlying factors (**neoplasia**, hypersensitivity). This is the crux of management of **otitis externa** and may involve routine blood tests, serology (e.g. for panels of immunoglobulin E) to demonstrate hypersensitivities, intradermal skin testing, food trials and biopsies

The treatment of **otitis externa** involves:
- Flushing the ear canals to remove debris which will otherwise interfere with penetration of topical medication to the canal

- Appropriate antimicrobial (antifungal, antibiotic, antiparasitic) medication. Numerous combination products exist, which vary in their active ingredients, ceruminolytic properties and frequency and duration of application
- Regular use of ear-cleaning agents to reduce the build-up of wax and debris and to reduce the likelihood of microbial build-up
- Identification of primary cause and management. It is rarely possible to cure the primary factor, and so most treatments are aimed at reducing the impact these have on the microclimate of the ear. Management may involve food trials for hypersensitivity, judicious use of corticosteroids, surgical correction of anatomical anomalies (e.g. stenotic canals)
- Regular appraisals of response to treatment. This is most important and is the primary reason for the perpetuation of **otitis externa**. Excellent client communication is crucial for the management and treatment of **otitis externa**. Owners must be made aware of the likely requirements for long-term treatment of their pet and the need for regular consultations and ear examinations

Ear-flushing as a treatment for otitis externa

As mentioned, one of the most important initial stages in the treatment of ear infections is the removal of debris (purulent exudate, wax, necrotic tissue) from the external ear canal. This facilitates proper examination of the canal and tympanum and makes the application of topical medication far more effective.

Several machines are available for flushing ears and these are very effective when used correctly. However, manual flushing remains the most common way of cleaning the ears. Dogs usually suffer no ill effects of ear flushing. Cats, however, have a high incidence of (usually) reversible complications. Most common is Horner's syndrome, damage to the sympathetic nerves passing the inner ear, resulting in drooping eyelid, widening of pupil and protrusion of the third eyelid (secondary to sinking in of the eye). Another common temporary effect of ear flushing in cats is a head tilt. These complications generally resolve in a few days, although they can sometimes persist for several weeks. Damage to the tympanum may occur during the procedure, or the tympanum may need to be purposefully ruptured (myringotomy). Having controlled infection, the eardrum usually heals uneventfully. Owners must be made aware of the potential for complications and the necessity for treatment.

- Equipment needed: otoscope and earpiece, 10-ml syringe, catheter (4 F gauge tom-cat catheter is suitable), a mild ceruminolytic ear cleaner (e.g. Leo Ear cleaner, VetXX (previously Leo Laboratories), Epi-Otic Ear Cleaner, Allerderm/Virbac), warm **sterile** saline or Hartmann's solution. Ear loops and alligator forceps may also help in the removal of large pieces of debris
- The patient should be anaesthetised and the endotracheal tube inserted with the cuff inflated (in case of reflux of infected debris along the eustachian tube). Sedation is rarely sufficient for ear flushing and is likely to result in paroxysmal head-shaking whilst performing the procedure
- The key to successful ear flushing is to be patient and gentle. Ideally, the procedure should be performed under direct visualisation of the ear canal at all times; however, this is rarely possible due to the narrow field of vision and the difficulty of balancing many instruments in the ear. Far better to concentrate on gentle flushing and make frequent checks
- The ear canal is examined carefully and any large pieces of debris are carefully removed with ear loops or alligator forceps. Cotton-tipped sticks (cotton buds or Q-tips, Johnson & Johnson) should not be used as they tend to compact wax and debris and can cause tympanic rupture
- The catheter is inserted as far down the ear canal as can be visualised and gentle pressure on a 10-ml syringe is used to flush the canal. Warmed saline should be used until the integrity of the tympanic membrane can be confirmed. Having done this, a weak ceruminolytic solution can be used (not recommended in

cats – saline only in this species) to loosen debris and soften waxy deposits. There are various ways of flushing: back-and-forth flushing, using the syringe to suck up the flush solution and debris, is the most effective method, but care must be taken not to allow the end of the catheter to contact the wall of the ear canal during suction as this can cause a lot of inflammation. The author prefers simply to flush via the catheter and remove dirty flush solution at the entrance of the ear canal with another syringe or cotton-wool pads
- The flush is continued until the canal is visibly clean. This can take quite a long time (45 min or so) and unless the saline is warmed it can result in appreciable cooling of the patient
- Provided the tympanum is intact, a topical medication may be instilled into the ear and the patient woken up

The owners should be given clear instructions as to the frequency of application of topical medications and the patient should be re-examined 24–48 h later. An ear-cleaning solution should be used daily or every other day as required until the debris remains cleared.

Removal of foreign bodies (grass awns) from ears

Springer and cocker spaniels, with their pendulous, hairy ears are the breeds most commonly troubled by grass awns and other foreign bodies in the ear canals, though the problem can occur in any breed, and should be suspected in any animal presenting with head tilt or head-shaking in the late summer months.

Any foreign body in the ear is intensely painful due to direct trauma to the canal and inflammation elicited by the presence of foreign material. If the foreign body remains there for any longer than 24–48 h, secondary infection occurs and the chronic **otitis externa** may result. The pain caused by grass awns makes it difficult and often impossible to examine the ear canal adequately in a conscious patient. Sedation or even general anaesthesia is required. NSAIDs should be

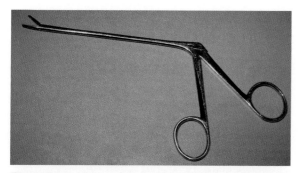

Figure 8.14 Alligator forceps are useful for removing awns and other foreign bodies from ears.

Box 8.3

Having discovered a grass awn in the ear, always check the paws and elsewhere on the body for more awns.

used prior to anaesthesia to reduce postoperative pain.

Grass awns are generally removed fairly easily with alligator forceps (Figure 8.14); in larger dogs these may be passed down the otoscope earpiece and directly visualised. In smaller dogs and cats, it is not possible to fit the alligator forceps into the lumen of the earpiece. In these cases, the alligators are passed alongside the otoscope. It is helpful to have an assistant provide traction on the pinna to open up the ear canal and increase visibility.

Once the grass awn has been extracted, the tympanum should be carefully examined for damage and the ear gently flushed with warmed **sterile** saline to remove any remaining debris (Box 8.3).

TAIL AMPUTATION FOR TRAUMA OR DISEASE

There is considerable controversy regarding tail amputation and tail docking in all countries. A popular misconception is that tail docking is distinct from amputation as it is carried out at an early age. The terms 'docking' and 'amputation' are synonymous in this situation and there is considerable evidence to show that removal of a tail at any age results in a great deal of pain and can have an effect on the subsequent growth rate of the puppy. The argument that tail docking is done for prophylactic reasons is a fatuous one: the vast majority of docked dogs are not working animals and the majority of working dogs that do not have amputated tails do not suffer as a result.

The Royal College of Veterinary Surgeons has made the situation clear by stating that the amputation of a dog's tail for any reason other than *truly* therapeutic or prophylactic is capable of amounting to disgraceful professional conduct.

The docking of tails by a layperson has been illegal in the UK since July 1993. Similar bans exist in many other countries in Europe.

Tail amputation for trauma or disease is occasionally required, and is indicated in situations including chronic osteomyelitis (or other infection that is non-responsive to medical treatment) of the tail, neurological damage (i.e. following a road traffic accident or tail-trapping), degloving injuries and **neoplasia**.

Generally, as little of the tail should be removed as is necessary to treat the condition (partial caudectomy). Removal of the entire tail (total caudectomy) is subject to potential complications and does not fall within the remit of this book.

Partial caudectomy (Figure 8.15)

- The patient should be anaesthetised and placed into lateral or sternal recumbency (Box 8.4). The tail should be clipped and prepared for aseptic surgery. The tail tip may be covered with cohesive bandage and suspended from a drip stand to facilitate surgical preparation. Good attention to **analgesia** is very important and may prevent self-trauma following surgery. NSAIDs should be administered, and it may be worth considering the use of local anaesthetics
- **Sterile** drapes are used to provide a **sterile** surgical field and strict aseptic technique is adhered to throughout. The tail tip should be covered with a **sterile** bandage or drape
- If desired, a tourniquet of Penrose tubing or **sterile** bandage material may be placed one to

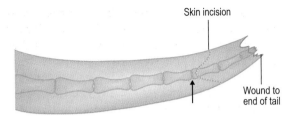

Skin incision

Wound to
end of tail

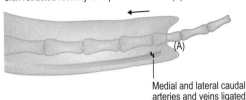

Skin retracted rostrally to expose articulation (A)

(A)

Medial and lateral caudal
arteries and veins ligated

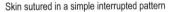

Skin sutured in a simple interrupted pattern

Figure 8.15 Partial caudectomy.

Box 8.4 Use of local analgesia during partial tail amputation

- The tail should be examined and the amputation site decided
- 1–3 ml mepivacaine (Intra-epicaine, Arnolds) should be injected (via a 25 G needle) subcutaneously around the circumference of the tail, at the level of the intervertebral space immediately proximal to the site of amputation. The syringe should be aspirated first to avoid accidental intravascular injection. Injection should be performed aseptically and it may be wise to wait until the surgical prep has been carried out
- The needle is then directed into the intervertebral space and a further 0.5–1 ml local anaesthetic is injected, aspirating first to avoid intravascular injection
- The main innervation of the tail is the cauda equina. However, branches of the coccygeal nerve may supply the base of the tail

from the vertebral body. The tail may then be removed by transection through the intervertebral joint with a scalpel blade

- The tourniquet should be loosened slightly to test the effectiveness of the ligatures. If bleeding is still seen, then a ligature may be placed around the entire vertebral body
- The subcutaneous tissue and muscle should be apposed with simple interrupted or mattress sutures of synthetic absorbable material (3/0 (2 metric) or 4/0 (1.5 metric) PDS II, Ethicon, is recommended)
- The skin should be apposed and may be trimmed as necessary to avoid excessive flaps. Simple interrupted sutures of synthetic non-absorbable (4/0 (1.5 metric) Ethilon, Ethicon; Monosof, Vetoquinol) or subcuticular sutures of synthetic absorbable (4/0 (1.5 metric) PDS II, Ethicon; Biosyn, Vetoquinol) may be used. Skin sutures are preferred to subcuticular sutures as the latter may act as a nidus for bacterial growth and increase the incidence of self-trauma

two vertebrae proximal to the amputation site
- A V-shaped incision is made through the skin on each side of the tail, starting laterally just proximal to the intervertebral space at the level of amputation and extending to the mid vertebral body on the dorsal and ventral tail surfaces
- Blood vessels run ventrally and laterally to the tail vertebrae. These should be identified and ligated immediately proximal to the transection site (the intervertebral space)
- The soft tissues just distal to the intervertebral space should be incised and dissected away

- A non-adherent wound dressing (e.g. Melolin, Johnson & Johnson) and tail bandage (see Chapter 5) should be placed and an Elizabethan collar may be used to prevent self-trauma
- Provided strict aseptic technique has been followed there should be no need for antibiotics (except in cases of tail amputation due to chronic infection). NSAIDs should be continued for 3–5 days postsurgery
- The dressing should be changed or removed 3 days after surgery, but the Elizabethan collar should be kept in place until sutures are removed 7–10 days postsurgery

Complications from partial caudectomy include wound **dehiscence** and infection, which should be dealt with according to the principles of wound management discussed in Chapter 6. Occasionally, chronic irritation and self-trauma may be seen following amputation. Repeating amputation slightly more proximally usually resolves this.

DEWCLAW AND NAIL REMOVAL

At the time of writing, dewclaw removal is not covered by the same regulations that prohibit tail docking and consequently dewclaws may be removed by a layperson without any anaesthetic provided the dog is less than 1 week old.

A veterinary surgeon may only remove dewclaws where, in the opinion of the veterinary surgeon, injury to the animal is likely to occur during normal activity. The removal of dewclaws for cosmetic purposes, or if the client requests it for any reason other than treatment or true prophylaxis, may constitute unethical behaviour.

Certain breeds of dog have rather vestigial dewclaws that are liable to become torn and caught. Oddly enough, one such breed is the Bernese mountain dog, which has double dewclaws in the hind limb. This is a breed standard and offering to remove one or both dewclaws is likely to be met with some degree of hostility from the breeder! The author has yet to see a torn dewclaw on a Bernese mountain dog and so the importance of dewclaw removal in general is questionable.

However, it is the responsibility of the veterinary profession to ensure that this procedure is carried out as humanely as possible. Dewclaw removal may be divided into removal in puppies less than 1 week of age and those older than 1 week of age. Details of both procedures are included, although the author would like to state that he does not carry out the procedure in puppies less than 1 week of age, preferring to wait until the animal is older and potential problems with the dewclaw can be assessed more accurately.

The procedures below describe removal of the dewclaw from the hind limb, as the fore-limb dewclaw is less commonly removed. For the fore limb, the technique is exactly the same, but for metatarsophalangeal joint read metacarpophalangeal joint.

Dewclaw removal in puppies less than 1 week of age
(Figure 8.16A)

- Although the procedure may be performed without anaesthesia, this should not preclude the use of analgesics. NSAIDs should be used at the low end of the dose range (e.g. meloxicam (Metacam, Boehringer Ingelheim) 0.1 mg/kg; carprofen (Rimadyl, Pfizer) 2 mg/kg). Local analgesics (mepivacaine (Intraepicaine, Arnolds) may be injected directly into the skin around the dewclaw (0.2–0.8 ml is usually sufficient). A sedative (acepromazine–buprenorphine at the lowest doses) may increase **analgesia** and aid in restraint
- The medial hind paw should be prepared for aseptic surgery. It is usually quite difficult to clip hair at this age, and this should not prove a problem provided aseptic technique is otherwise adhered to
- An assistant should restrain the patient and extend the paw. Using **sterile** Mayo scissors, the dewclaw should be amputated through the metatarsal bone or at the metatarsophalangeal joint
- Haemorrhage is usually minimal and should be controlled with pressure. Skin may be apposed using a single suture of synthetic

(a) Puppies less than 1 week old

(b) Puppies over 1 week old

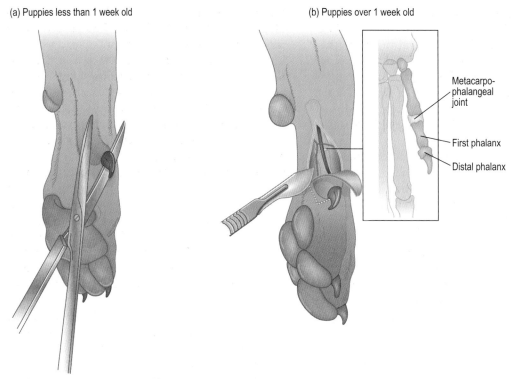

Metacarpo-
phalangeal
joint

First phalanx

Distal phalanx

Figure 8.16 Removal of dewclaws.

non-absorbable material or tissue adhesive (e.g. Vetbond, 3M)

Dewclaw removal in puppies older than 1 week of age (Figure 8.16B)

- It is recommended that puppies be left until at least 3 months of age. A general anaesthetic is required, which should include NSAID premedication. The patient is placed in lateral recumbency and the paws are clipped for aseptic surgery (the hanging-limb technique may be used to prep the paws, or they may be raised by placing a sandbag at the elbow). One limb is prepared first; when the dewclaw has been removed, the dog is rotated and the other side is prepared
- Local anaesthetic (e.g. 0.5% mepivacaine) may be used to provide additional **analgesia** and 1–2 ml may be infiltrated around the

dewclaw and into the metatarsophalangeal joint
- The metatarsophalangeal joint of the dewclaw is palpated and an elliptical incision made to encompass this and the dewclaw itself. A mixture of sharp and blunt dissection is used to separate the dewclaw from the underlying connective tissue
- Any blood vessels (dorsal and ventral) should be located, clamped with fine Halstead mosquito forceps and ligated proximal to the metatarsophalangeal joint
- The muscle and tissues around the proximal phalanx should be dissected free to expose the joint and this should be transected with a scalpel blade. If preferred, bone cutters may be used to cut the proximal phalanx at about one-third of its length
- 4/0 (1.5 metric) synthetic absorbable suture material (e.g. Vicryl, Ethicon; Biosyn, Vetoquinol) should be used to close subcutaneous tissues around the stump and to close

the dead space. The skin should be apposed with 4/0 (1.5 metric) synthetic non-absorbable suture material (e.g. Prolene, Ethicon) in a simple interrupted or cruciate pattern. If desired, tissue adhesive may be used

- Non-adherent dressing (e.g. Melolin, Johnson & Johnson) is applied to the wound and held in place by a foot bandage (with plenty of padding)
- Provided strict aseptic technique has been adhered to, antibiotics are not necessary. However, **analgesia** in the form of NSAIDs should be administered for 3–5 days following surgery
- The bandage is removed 3 days following surgery and another dressing placed if necessary (e.g. if the dog is very bouncy). Sutures are removed 7–10 days following surgery
- It is unusual for complications to occur following this surgery. The usual risks of wound **dehiscence** or infection are possible if asepsis is not maintained or if Halstead's principles are not followed. Cutting the phalanx, rather than disarticulation, tends to produce a less favourable cosmetic result and can cause splitting of the bone, leading to postoperative pain

Nail removal (onychectomy)

Nail removal may only be performed for therapeutic purposes in the UK. Elective onychectomy to prevent damage to furniture is considered unnecessary mutilation and unethical. Indications for therapeutic onychectomy include chronic nail bed infections (e.g. **onychomycosis**, caused by *Trichophyton mentagrophytes*) or **neoplasia** (e.g. squamous cell carcinoma, soft-tissue sarcomas and osteosarcomas), although it is more usual to perform digit amputation in the latter cases. Due to the small margins obtained by this amputation, it may be best reserved as a biopsy technique, with a view to extending the excision to a digital amputation on the basis of **histopathology**.

The claw or nail is produced from the germinal cells in the distal portion of the third phalanx

and so the whole (or most) of this bone is removed along with the nail. If several nails are to be removed, it is recommended that a regional nerve block be performed, details of which may be found in a more detailed surgery tome. For single onychectomy, infiltration of local **analgesia** (0.5–1 ml 0.5% mepivacaine) into the digit and distal phalangeal joint is possible using a 25 G needle and should be sufficient, provided opioid **analgesia** and NSAIDs are also used.

- The patient is anaesthetised and placed in lateral recumbency. The paw is clipped and prepared for aseptic surgery. It may be difficult to scrub the underside of the claws adequately – a nailbrush helps the cleaning process. **Sterile** drapes are placed (the paw may be inserted through a fenestrated drape)
- Local anaesthetic is injected into the digit (see above)
- A tourniquet or tightly wound bandage placed below the elbow helps reduce blood loss. Alternatively, a blood-pressure cuff may be used to occlude arterial flow (see Chapter 7)
- The claw is extended by pressing the base of the digital pad or by grasping the nail with a pair of Allis tissue forceps. The claw is removed by cutting around the thin skin at the base of the claw and transecting the deep digital flexor tendon, the common digital extensor tendon, the dorsal elastic ligament (cats), the lateral and medial collateral ligaments and the joint capsule. Alternatively, for cats, a guillotine-type nail clipper (metal ones may be sterilised by autoclave) is placed at the level of the distal phalangeal joint and used to amputate the claw (Figure 8.17). Using the latter method, it is not possible to remove the distal phalanx completely: a small ventral portion remains. However, this is usually sufficient to remove diseased tissue. Since the deep digital flexor tendon inserts at this point, it may help maintain support for this digit. The nail is sent for fungal culture or **histopathology**, as required
- The skin is apposed with 4/0 (1.5 metric) synthetic non-absorbable suture material (e.g. Monosof, Vetoquinol) or tissue adhesive (e.g. Vetbond, 3M) and a non-adherent dressing (e.g. Melolin, Johnson & Johnson) is

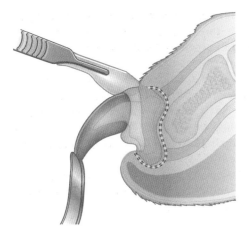

(a) Onychectomy using scalpel

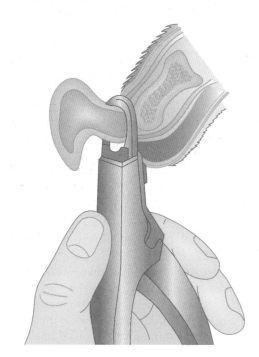

(b) Onychectomy using guillotine nail clippers

Figure 8.17 Onychectomy.

placed and covered with a soft, padded foot bandage
- Antibiotics are not necessary unless the claw is removed for reasons of bacterial infection. NAIDs are administered for 3–5 days following surgery and the dressing is removed at 3 days following surgery

- A small amount of wound breakdown is not uncommon after this procedure and this is best treated by open wound management and application of clean dressings. Complications such as **plantigrade** stance and lameness are more likely to occur if several nails are removed. The author reiterates that this procedure should only be used therapeutically or for biopsy purposes

DIGIT AMPUTATION

Amputation of the digit is the natural progression from onychectomy and is performed in cases of severe degloving or fracture injury, **neoplasia** (osteosarcoma or soft-tissue sarcoma, squamous cell carcinoma, malignant melanoma and MCTs are the most common) or chronic infection (bacterial or fungal onychitis, osteomyelitis). The technique is relatively straightforward, prime difficulties being positioning the patient to allow the easiest approach to the digit and ensuring asepsis in the preparation phase (the nail beds and interdigital webbing being difficult to scrub). The outermost digits (3 and 4) should only be removed if there really is no alternative, as loss of one or both of these digits causes persistent lameness. Due to the practical difficulties of the dissection and the potential for causing persistent lameness, this procedure should not be considered suitable for minor surgery. It is included in this book for completeness.
- The patient is anaesthetised, placed in lateral recumbency and the foot is clipped and prepared for aseptic surgery (the hanging-limb technique may be used, or else the foot may be suspended over the edge of the operating table). A tourniquet (or inflated blood-pressure cuff) is placed below the elbow. The paw is draped
- In addition to opioids and NSAIDs, local anaesthetic (0.5% mepivacaine) may be used to provide further **analgesia**. Infiltration anaesthesia is usually insufficient for this procedure and a suitable nerve block for the sensory innervation of the paws is required. This is beyond the scope of this book and the interested reader is directed to a specialised volume. IV antibiotics (e.g. cefuroxime

(Zinacef, Glaxo) 20–50 mg/kg IV) may be administered

- A circumferential incision is made around the digit, angling proximally on the dorsal aspect to form an ellipse and extending this with a single dorsal incision to form an inverted Y (Figure 8.18). The circumferential incision is centred about level with the middle of the first phalanx (depending on the level of amputation) and the dorsal incision should extend to the distal metatarsus (metacarpus)
- The digital blood vessels are located, grasped with haemostatic forceps and ligated (4/0 (1.5 metric) Biosyn, Vetoquinol, or Vicryl, Ethicon are both suitable)
- The subcutaneous tissues, ligaments and tendons (deep digital flexor and common digital extensor tendons) are transected just distal to the metacarpo(metatarso)phalangeal joint. The joint capsule is cut, disarticulating the digit. Alternatively, bone cutters may be used to cut through the proximal phalanx, although this can cause bone splintering
- Subcutaneous tissues are apposed to cover the stump and dead space is closed. 3/0 (2 metric) or 4/0 (1.5 metric) synthetic absorbable suture material (e.g. PDS II or Vicryl, both Ethicon) may be used for this. The tourniquet is removed and any bleeding dealt with
- Skin edges are apposed with 3/0 (2 metric) or 4/0 (1.5 metric) synthetic non-absorbable

suture material (e.g. Monosof, Vetoquinol) in a simple interrupted or cruciate pattern

- A non-adherent **sterile** dressing (e.g. Melolin, Johnson & Johnson) is applied to the wound and covered with a soft padded bandage
- NSAIDs are continued for at least 5 days postoperatively. Further antibiotics are usually not required, provided the surgical time has been short and asepsis has been maintained throughout
- The dressing is changed 3 days postoperatively and dressings and sutures are removed at 10 days after surgery

JUGULAR AND INTRAOSSEOUS CATHETER PLACEMENT

The placement of catheters into peripheral veins is described in Chapter 3. Patients with reduced cardiac output or low peripheral venous pressure (e.g. due to dehydration or shock) may have collapsed peripheral veins that are difficult to catheterise. In these situations, the jugular vein may be chosen as a more central IV access, or else an intraosseous catheter may be placed. Although a regular 22 G over-the-needle IV catheter (e.g. Angiocath, BD Medical) may be used for short-term jugular vein placement and a spinal needle (e.g. 22 G spinal needle, Terumo) may be used for intraosseous placement in small or young animals, the techniques are best performed with specialised and dedicated equipment (Box 8.5).

Jugular vein placement

- Sedation is usually not required and may be contraindicated if the patient is dehydrated or otherwise unstable. The animal is placed in lateral recumbency and gently restrained
- The jugular vein is palpated and a reasonable area of skin overlying it is clipped and aseptically prepared (a 10-cm square is sufficient in most cases). A **sterile** fenestrated drape is placed over the vein. A bleb (0.2–0.4 ml) of 0.5% mepivacaine or lidocaine is injected subcutaneously over the proposed site of

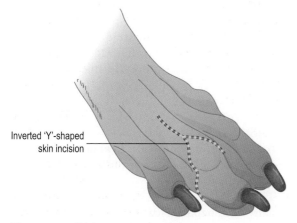

Inverted 'Y'-shaped skin incision

Figure 8.18 Digit amputation.

Box 8.5 Recommended needles for jugular and intraosseous placement

Jugular

Peel-Away Jugular catheterisation system: Global Veterinary Products (formerly Cook Veterinary Products). Sizes available: 15 G, 17 G (dogs), 19 G (cats, young animals).

Sledinger catheterisation system: sizes as above.

Intraosseus

Disposable intraosseous needle, Global Veterinary Products (formerly Cook Veterinary Products). Sizes: 14 G, 16 G, 18 G (dogs), 20 G (cats, young animals).

catheterisation and 2–3 min are allowed for the local analgesic to take effect. Hand-scrubbing should be performed and **sterile** gloves worn

- Using a no. 15 scalpel blade, a cut down on to the jugular vein is performed. The skin is held taut by one hand while the other uses the scalpel blade to make an incision approximately 0.3–0.7 cm long directly over the jugular vein. The incision is deepened by gently brushing the scalpel against the underlying tissues until the vein is visualised
- In thin animals, the jugular vein may be easily visualised through the skin and a cutdown may not be necessary. However, it may still be helpful to make a small incision through the skin with a scalpel blade or the bevelled edge of a 22 G hypodermic needle to reduce drag on the cannula sheath
- The technique for placement will now depend on the choice of jugular catheter. The two methods described below are for the peel-away catheter and the J-wired catheters (the Sledinger technique)
- Placing a peel-away catheter (e.g. Global Peel-Away jugular catheter): the sheath needle is introduced into the vein (usually away from the head). Correct placement is confirmed by occluding the jugular vein as though one were collecting a jugular blood sample. Blood should appear in the needle hub. The sheath

is slid into the lumen and the needle removed. This is a potentially risky time as air embolism can occur. Pinching the end of the sheath between thumb and forefinger as the needle is removed reduces the risk. The catheter is introduced into the lumen of the vein by passing it down the sheath. The sheath is then peeled away by grasping the two toggles and gently pulling. This part of the procedure is much aided by a gloved assistant holding the catheter in place to prevent it being pulled out as the sheath is torn away

- Placing a jugular catheter by the Sledinger technique: these are technically very easy to place, despite the bewildering array of components to the **sterile** pack! The contents of the packs are as follows: one metal, thin-walled IV cannula (introducer needle), one J-wire with plastic wire guide, one short plastic dilator, one latex or silicon jugular catheter with suture holes. The thin-walled cannula is introduced into the jugular vein; placement is confirmed by the presence of blood in the hub as above. The J-wire is passed down the cannula (using the wire guide) for at least the length of the jugular catheter. The IV cannula is removed from the vein by sliding it off the wire. The J-bend holds the wire in place in the jugular vein and prevents it from slipping out easily. Next, the widener is threaded on to the wire and passed along it into the jugular vein, turned slowly and then removed. This step is optional, but makes passage of the IV catheter easier. Finally, the soft, flexible catheter is threaded down the wire, sutured in place and the wire is gently pulled out (Figure 8.19)
- The catheter is then flushed with 2–5 ml heparinised saline, a **sterile** injection cap is placed (or else a giving set is linked to the catheter) and the catheter is sutured to the skin with 4/0 (1.5 metric) synthetic non-absorbable suture material
- An adherent dressing (e.g. Primapore, Johnson & Johnson) is placed over the catheter and the neck is bandaged
- The catheter should be flushed four times daily with heparinised saline and the dressing changed daily to allow inspection of the catheter placement

Rates of fluid administration are similar to those used for peripheral IV placement (see Chapter 3).

Intraosseous catheter placement

This procedure is associated with a reasonable amount of pain, so care should be taken to provide adequate **analgesia**. Local anaesthetics are suf-ficient if administered appropriately, or else sedation may be considered.

Intraosseous needles are available in a variety of sizes and may be placed at various sites (medial aspect of proximal tibia, greater tubercle of the humerus, dorsal iliac wing), although the most common placement is in the trochanteric fossa of the proximal femur.

- The patient is placed into lateral recumbency and the site of intraosseous needle placement

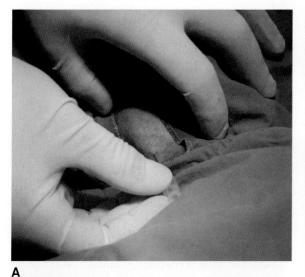

A

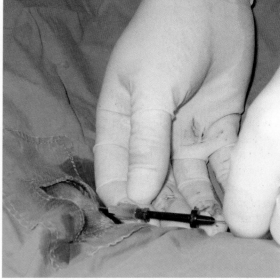

B

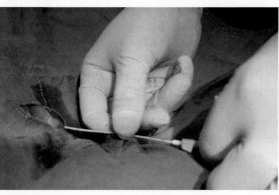

C

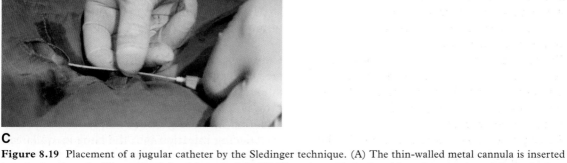

Figure 8.19 Placement of a jugular catheter by the Sledinger technique. (A) The thin-walled metal cannula is inserted into the jugular vein. The patient's head is to the left. (B) The wire guide is placed into the cannula and the J-wire is passed through the cannula into the vein. (C) The cannula is removed and the jugular catheter is threaded over the wire and into the jugular vein. Once passed, it is sutured in place. (D) Placement of intravenous cannula into the marginal vein of a rabbit. Blood can be seen in the hub of the needle, confirming accurate placement. (cont'd)

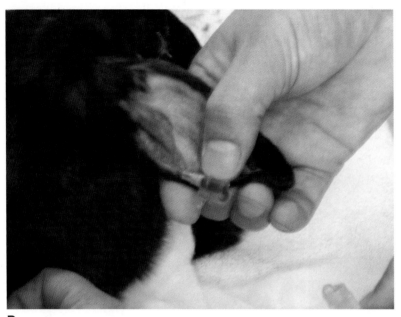

D

Figure 8.19 (Continued).

is palpated (immediately dorsal and medial to the greater trochanter of the femur). The site is clipped and aseptically prepared and a **sterile** drape is placed. Hand-scrubbing should be performed and sterile gloves worn

- 0.5 ml of 0.5% mepivacaine or lidocaine is injected subcutaneously at the site of catheterisation. The needle is advanced until bone is reached and a further 0.5 ml local anaesthetic is injected into the **periosteum**. Allow 3–5 min for the local **analgesia** to take effect
- A small stab incision is made in the skin overlying the site and an intraosseous needle and stylet is introduced. The needle should enter parallel to the axis of the femur. A gentle twisting motion, coupled with firm downward pressure, should allow the needle to penetrate the bone cortex. When placed properly, there should be little swaying motion of the needle
- The stylet is then removed and the needle should be flushed with 1–2 ml heparinised saline. An injection cap or giving set should then be connected and the catheter sutured in

place with 4/0 (1.5 metric) synthetic non-absorbable suture material
- An adherent dressing is placed over the catheter and a padded bandage should be placed to prevent pain or dislodgement of the catheter with the patient's movement. The catheter should be flushed four times daily with heparinised saline
- The needle should only remain in place for 3 days, after which another site for placement must be found

Care must be exercised if intraosseous catheters are used in neonates or skeletally immature animals, as it is relatively easy to damage the growth plates by incorrect placement. Strict attention must be given to aseptic technique, as introducing infection into the bone medulla can be disastrous.

Rates of fluid administration are similar to those for IV placement (see Chapter 3), but it is recommended that the rate should not exceed 11 ml/min for gravity flow systems.

Catheterisation of the ear vein(s) in rabbits

IV catheterisation can be achieved in rabbits using the cephalic or median saphenous veins, in the same way as in dogs and cats. The marginal ear vein can be used, but due to the risk of ear tip necrosis as a result of thromboembolism of the vein or overzealous bandaging of the catheterised ear, this placement should be reserved for cases that are difficult to catheterise using the limbs.

Good restraint is a must as, apart from being frustrating, the ear vein can be ruined by ill-timed movement of the patient. Sedation is optional and may be recommended for excitable bunnies (ketamine (35–40 mg/kg) and medetomidine (0.25–0.5 mg/kg) IM or subcutaneously). A handy tip is to apply a little topical local anaesthetic to the ear (Emla cream, AstraZeneca). This numbs the ear slightly and improves visualisation of the vein. Shining a low-wattage bulb through the ear (e.g. hand-held ophthalmoscope on low setting) also helps visualisation.

- The rabbit is restrained in sternal recumbency (or sedated)
- Emla cream is applied to the **caudal** ear margin. Having allowed 3–5 min for the local anaesthetic to take effect, the ear is clipped and surgically prepped. **Sterile** gloves should be worn
- A 25 G **sterile** over-the-needle IV catheter (e.g. Angiocath, BD Medical) is selected. With an assistant applying a little pressure to the base of the ear to raise the vein, the catheter is introduced into the marginal ear vein approximately halfway along the ear. As soon as blood is seen in the hub of the needle, the catheter is advanced over the stylet and allowed to enter the vein completely (Figure 8.19D). Some texts advise pre-flushing the catheter with a little heparinised saline. In the author's experience this makes it slightly difficult to observe backflow of blood, and should not be necessary provided placement is fairly swift
- Once the catheter is placed, a little sticky tape (e.g. Durapore tape, 3M) is wrapped loosely around the ear to prevent the catheter becoming dislodged. A 1-ml syringe is used to flush the catheter with 0.2–0.5 ml heparinised saline (a larger syringe may 'blow' the vein with undue pressure)
- A **sterile** injection bung or IV giving set is attached to the catheter and a padded bandage is used to support the ear against the body. Care must be taken when bandaging rabbits: it is easy to apply too much tension in the cohesive bandage layer, restricting the rabbit's breathing

The cannula should be flushed four times daily with heparinised saline and the bandage checked for placement regularly. The catheter should not be left in for any longer than 72 h, as this will increase the risk of ear tip necrosis. The catheter should be removed immediately if any inflammation or skin discoloration is seen around the placement site.

ACTING AS THE SCRUBBED ASSISTANT IN MAJOR SURGERY

The benefits of having a scrubbed assistant for major surgery cannot be overstated. We have already discussed how a spare pair of **sterile** hands can be useful in holding limbs, tails and ears during the aseptic scrub procedure in order to provide a means of keeping sterility until draping is complete. Other useful functions of a scrubbed assistant include:

- Providing retraction of tissues or organs. This is especially useful when performing surgery in body cavities. Omentum has a knack of encroaching on to a ligature placement and an assistant keeping the way clear not only speeds up the surgery, but also improves the security of ligature placement. Orthopaedic surgery is greatly facilitated by a second 'surgeon' presenting a limb at the correct angle for a procedure, or providing retraction of muscles, nerves or other soft tissues out of the way of orthopaedic power tools (Figure 8.20). Hand-held retractors such as Army-Navy or Hohmann retractors are usually placed by the surgeon and then held in place by an assistant. Alternatively, the gloved hands may be used to

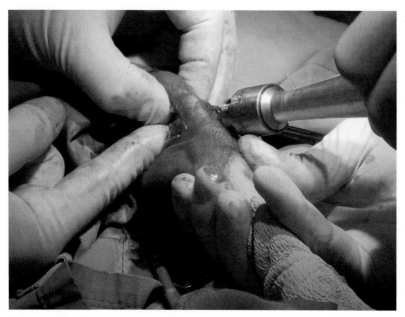

Figure 8.20 Tibial crest transposition made much easier with a scrubbed assistant.

push or hold organs or tissues out of the way. Gelpi retractors are exceptionally useful for holding skin and muscle edges apart, but they can only do this in one plane. A gloved assistant can retract in three planes. When performing nephrectomy, approach to the kidney is made much easier by having an assistant hold the abdominal wall muscles apart and pushed down slightly, to reduce the depth of the surgical field

- Temporarily occluding blood flow. Certain surgical procedures (e.g. nephrotomy) are aided by short-term cessation or reduction of blood flow through vessels. Although specialised clamps (e.g. Johns Hopkins or De Bakey bulldog clamps) are more correctly used for this, a well-placed thumb and forefinger clamp may well suffice for very short-term occlusion. Should inadvertent cutting or tearing of a blood vessel occur during surgery, having a gloved assistant on hand to apply pressure (either directly on the vessel, or else proximally to the site of bleeding) gives the surgeon more time to clamp and ligate the vessel
- Acting as bowel clamps for intestinal surgery. Doyen tissue forceps are commonly used to occlude the lumen of small and large bowels

for enterotomy or enterectomy. They may be used with or without rubber tubing covers (these are used to increase clamping action of the forceps, whilst spreading the contact area of the clamps to reduce trauma. However, pressure on tissues is often much higher with the rubber tubing in place and tissue trauma is more likely to occur: the jaws are designed to be relatively atraumatic in any case). Holding the intestines between the first and second finger is an extremely atraumatic method of occluding the lumen, and has the advantage that the assistant can lift and turn the gut to facilitate suture placement for the surgeon. Occluding the intestine between thumb and first finger, however, is more tiring for the assistant and is more likely to result in leakage of gut contents and pressure damage

- Passing instruments. This is probably the main role for a scrub nurse or other aseptically prepared assistant. Passing instruments in a **sterile** manner when requested means that the surgeon does not have to release his or her hold on tissue and is less likely to lose sight of a bleeding vessel. A good assistant will anticipate the surgeon's needs and be ready with the correct instrument, returning used

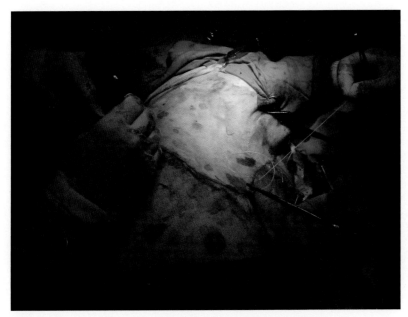

Figure 8.21 Reduction of operative time by use of suture assistant.

instruments to the trolley in a tidy manner so that they may be found again more readily. It is the responsibility of the scrub assistant to keep a swab count and account for all instruments at the end of surgery

- Using suction or irrigating devices. Surgical suction is underused in general practice. It is an extremely useful tool for improving visibility in the surgical field or removing flush solution or waste liquids (urine, bile). The units are usually foot-operated and fitted with **sterile** hoses to which are fitted suction tips (e.g. Yankauer or Poole suction tips). A scrubbed assistant can direct the suction to where it is needed, leaving the surgeon free to operate. Similarly, some surgery requires irrigation or flushing of the surgical site; either to provide cooling (in certain orthopaedic or spinal procedures) or to remove debris from the surgical site. Whilst a non-scrubbed assistant can perform this by leaning over the operating area, it is far better to carry out this technique in an aseptic manner, to avoid any breaches in sterility

- Suturing the skin. Asking a scrubbed assistant to suture the skin wound following invasive

surgery allows the veterinary surgeon to perform other tasks, thus allowing more efficient use of time. It may alternatively be useful to have a second person suturing a large wound to reduce operative time (Figure 8.21)

The main quality expected of a scrubbed assistant is patience. Although there will be times of activity (but hopefully not frenzy!), much of the surgical time involves waiting until needed. It is important to remain aware at all times so that the surgeon's requests can be granted immediately and accurately. This requires a high degree of knowledge of the surgical procedure and, of course, instrumentation. Gloved hands should be held together at chest height, whilst waiting, to minimise the risk of breaches in sterility.

Prior to surgery, the entire surgical team should be briefed about the intended surgery, special equipment needed (and how to operate it) and any likely complications. Although this may be fairly time-consuming at first, once experience is gained it becomes a matter of routine and improves morale and teamwork, as well as improving surgical outcome.

9 Dental and oral surgery

NORMAL DENTITION OF THE DOG AND THE CAT

Dogs and cats have teeth of similar structure and development to human teeth, being brachydont, or short crowned teeth (in distinction to rabbits and ruminants, which have teeth with high crowns and are termed hypsodont). Puppies and kittens are born toothless (edentulous) and develop a set of temporary (primary or deciduous teeth) between the first and second months of life. These primary teeth are replaced (in the order: incisors, premolars, canines and molars) by permanent teeth between 2 and 7 months of age in most animals.

A dental formula may be used to describe the anatomic location of each type of tooth:

Dog:
Deciduous teeth

$$\frac{3i\ 1c\ 3p}{3i\ 1c\ 3p} = 28\ \text{Teeth}$$

Dog:
Permanent teeth

$$\frac{3I\ 1C\ 4P\ 2M}{3I\ 1C\ 4P\ 3M} = 42\ \text{Teeth}$$

Cat:
Deciduous teeth

$$\frac{3i\ 1c\ 3p}{3i\ 1c\ 2p} = 26\ \text{Teeth}$$

Cat:
Permanent teeth

$$\frac{3I\ 1C\ 3P\ 1M}{3I\ 1C\ 2P\ 1M} = 30\ \text{Teeth}$$

i, I = Incisors; c, C = Canines, p, P = Premolars, m, M = molars

By convention, lower-case letters are used to represent primary teeth whereas upper-case letters represent permanent teeth. Teeth numbers above the line relate to maxillary teeth, and mandibular teeth are below the line. Only one side of the dental arcade is included.

Individual teeth may be identified using the anatomic formula system, using a series of superscripts and subscripts:

^1I = upper left first permanent incisor
p_3 = lower right third deciduous premolar
M^2 = upper right second permanent molar
^1C = upper left permanent canine

Alternatively the teeth may be identified using a shorthand method:

URI1 = upper right (permanent) incisor 1
LLp2 = lower left (deciduous) premolar 2

and so on.

A further way of identifying individual teeth for dental records is to use the modified Triadan system. In this system, each tooth is given a unique number. The teeth are numbered from the middle incisor caudally (towards the back of the mouth) from 01 to 11.

The numbers are prefixed:

1. Right maxilla
2. Left maxilla
3. Left mandible
4. Right mandible

In the modified Triadan system, the upper right second premolar in a dog would thus be 106, the lower left third incisor would be 303, and so on. This system has the advantage of brevity, but the disadvantage that cats have 'missing' numbers due to the fact that certain teeth are not present. The system is thus not intuitive and must be remembered or copied into a chart.

Figure 9.1 shows the permanent dentition of the dog and cat, together with the various dental numbering systems.

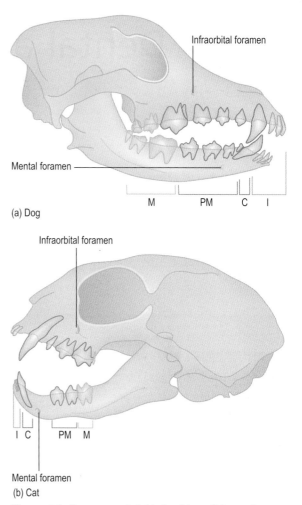

(a) Dog

(b) Cat

Figure 9.1 Permanent (adult) dentition of dog and cat.

Tooth structure

The structure of a permanent tooth is shown in Figure 9.2. For simple dental purposes, teeth may be divided into crown and root. The junction between crown and root is the neck.

The crown is defined by the covering of **enamel**, which imparts the tremendous tensile strength of the tooth. The rest of the tooth comprises dentine (similar to bone in structure) with a central core (the pulp cavity).

The tooth root is attached to the underlying **alveolar bone** by the **periodontal** ligaments, which affix to the dentine of the root via cementum (a bony substance produced by the **periodontal** ligaments). There may be one, two or three roots depending on the tooth type (Table 9.1). It is important to know the number of roots each tooth has in order to extract teeth. The junction between two roots is called the furcation.

The oral mucosa immediately surrounding the tooth is known as the **gingiva**, which forms a seal over the **periodontal** space and protects the **periodontal** ligament and **alveolar bone**.

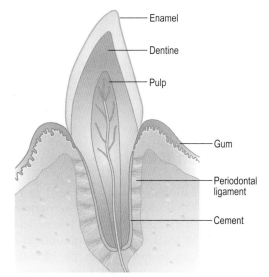

Figure 9.2 Structure of a permanent tooth.

(Labels from top to bottom: Enamel, Dentine, Pulp, Gum, Periodontal ligament, Cement)

Table 9.1 Root structure of canine and feline teeth

Tooth	Number of roots	
	Dog	**Cat**
Upper teeth		
Incisor	1	1
Canine	1	1
Premolar 1	1	1
Premolar 2	2	2
Premolar 3	2	3
Premolar 4	3	–
Molar 1	3	1
Molar 2	2	–
Lower teeth		
Incisor	1	1
Canine	1	1
Premolar 1	1	2
Premolar 2	2	2
Premolar 3	2	–
Premolar 4	2	–
Molar 1	2	2
Molar 2	2	–
Molar 3	1	–

Carnassial teeth

The temporomandibular joint of dogs and cats allows very little side-to-side movement, acting almost solely as a hinge joint. The premolars and molars therefore do no chewing, but rather have a scissor action. This is most notable in the upper fourth premolar and the lower first molar of dogs (108/P^4/URP4; 208/^{4}P/ULP4; 309/$_1$M/LLM1 and 409/M_1/LRM1). These are the largest cheek teeth of dogs and are called carnassial teeth. When the jaws are closed together, the carnassials exhibit a very strong shearing action that effectively cuts meat (in cats the carnassial teeth are the upper third premolars and the lower first molars (108/P^3/URP3; 208/^{3}P/ULP3; 309/$_1$M/LLM1 and 409/M_1/LRM1)).

Nerve supply to the teeth

The trigeminal nerve (cranial nerve V) is responsible for sensory innervation of the teeth.
- The trigeminal nerve is divided into the ophthalmic, maxillary and mandibular nerves
- The maxillary nerve provides sensation to the upper teeth via two branches: the pterygopalatine and the infraorbital branches
- The inferior alveolar branch of the mandibular nerve provides sensation to the **caudal** mandibular teeth. A branch of the inferior alveolar nerve, the mental nerve, supplies the lower canines and incisors

DENTAL AND PERIODONTAL DISEASE

Dental disease in dogs and cats can be divided into:
- Congenital/developmental
- Metabolic/nutritional
- Traumatic
- Neoplastic
- Infectious/inflammatory

Congenital/developmental

The mandibular teeth of dogs and cats usually lie just medial to the maxillary teeth when the jaws are closed ('scissor bite'). Protrusion of the mandibular incisors so that they lie in front of the maxillary incisors is known as undershot jaw and is common (and the breed standard) in many **brachycephalic** breeds of dog and cat (Figure 9.3). The converse condition, known as overshot

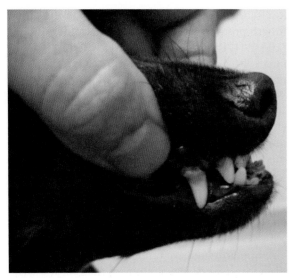

Figure 9.3 Undershot jaw in a cross-breed terrier.

jaw, occurs when the maxillary teeth protrude excessively in front of the mandibular teeth (excessively is usually taken to be more than 2–3 mm). This tends to occur more frequently in **dolicocephalic** breeds. It is rare for undershot or overshot jaws to cause much of a problem, but severe malformations can result in poor growth if suckling or eating is compromised. Any deformations of tooth arcade anatomy tend to result in abnormal wear on teeth and abrasional injuries to crown **enamel**. Additionally, food and debris can build up in gaps and crevices between uneven teeth and contribute greatly to inflammatory gum disease.

Retained primary teeth tend to occur more often in toy breeds of dog (e.g. cavalier King Charles spaniels) and can also occur in the cat, with the canine teeth being particularly predisposed. Food debris and **plaque** tends to accumulate between the retained primary and the permanent tooth, leading to gingivitis and more serious **periodontal** disease.

Other developmental dental problems include impaction of teeth, oligodontia (absence of one or more teeth) and **enamel hypoplasia** (usually caused by distemper virus infection in young puppies). In addition, various drugs (e.g. tetracycline) cause permanent staining of teeth if administered to young animals or pregnant bitches and queens.

Treatment of the above is by removal of primary or impacted teeth and good ongoing prophylactic dental care. Tetracycline staining is permanent, but not associated with any problems of mastication.

Metabolic/nutritional

Advanced renal disease in cats can lead to the syndrome of renal secondary hyperparathyroidism. This is a disease of calcium homeostasis and may result in leaching of calcium and phosphorus from bones. In severe cases, the **alveolar bone** is affected to such an extent that the normal rigid support is lost and the teeth become loosened ('rubber jaw'). This is quite uncommon, especially given the wide range of renal support diets available, but it should be borne in mind when extracting teeth from elderly cats. The main oral/dental problem seen in cats with renal disease is uraemic **ulcer** formation on the **gingiva** and tongue. This can mimic (or worsen) primary **periodontal** disease and must be considered a differential in any aged cat with sore gums.

Complete lack of certain vitamins or severe malnutrition may cause dental and oral disease: hypovitaminosis A results in bleeding gums, hypovitaminosis D causes nutritional secondary hyperparathyroidism (see above) and any chronic anorexic state is likely to result in inflammation and worsening of any gingivitis.

Traumatic

Abrasion (wearing away) of teeth is commonly seen in dogs, especially dogs that like to carry stones and sticks, or those that chew on cages. The damage to teeth can be quite dramatic, with some dogs having completely flattened occlusal surfaces by 2–3 years of age. Usually, as the tooth is worn the pulp recedes and is replaced by tertiary dentine. However, if wearing occurs quickly then the pulp may become exposed, leading to painful teeth and the possibility of pulpitis (infection and inflammation of the pulp cavity).

In contrast, attrition is the normal age-associated wearing of teeth. It is hastened by a poor diet and by malocclusion.

Fractures of the teeth are very often seen in dogs and cats. They may be caused by chewing or biting, fighting, malicious blows and kicks, falls or road traffic accidents. The seriousness depends on the extent and position of the fracture. Small fractures involving the crown **enamel** only are often inconsequential. Although initially the exposed dentine may be sore, this sensitivity decreases over a few weeks. The patient may be given non-steroidal anti-inflammatory drugs (NSAIDs) to decrease pain in the sensitive period. Occasionally it is necessary to file or rasp sharp edges to reduce tongue or cheek trauma. Larger fractures may expose the pulp cavity or produce cracks that extend to the roots. These may remain painful for considerably longer periods of time and may allow infection to track down the tooth to the root and **alveolar bone**. These fractures are best treated by dental extraction.

Neoplastic

Many tumours affect the oral cavity, with some deriving from **alveolar bone** and tooth directly. Oral **neoplasia** is discussed later on in the chapter.

Infectious/inflammatory

Periodontal disease, resulting from infection and inflammation of the oral cavity, is one of the most common clinical diseases of companion dogs and cats and probably accounts for almost half of the anaesthetic caseload of a practice.

The normal dog and cat mouth is home to many bacteria, notably *Pasteurella multocida* in the cat and dog, *Staphylococcus* spp., *Streptococcus* spp. and Enterobacteriaciae and various anaerobic bacteria (e.g. *Bacteroides* spp.). All of these have the potential to cause infection, but do not tend to cross an intact epithelium. The production and advancement of **plaque** subgingivally cause damage to the **gingiva** and allow infection

to occur. At first, mild gingivitis results, which is noted by a reddening of the gum margins. As the disease worsens, the gums recede (draw back from the teeth) and **alveolar bone** is resorbed. Ultimately, if not treated, pus is produced and the tooth becomes loosened.

Periodontal disease (gingivitis, **periodontitis**) is usually divided into four stages:

- Stage 1: early or mild gingivitis. There is a small build-up of **plaque** and **calculus** and reddening of the gum margins. This stage is completely reversible, and prompt dental treatment will return the periodontium to a healthy state
- Stage 2: chronic gingivitis. There is moderate to heavy build-up of **calculus** and **plaque** on the teeth and subgingivally. The gums are reddened and visibly swollen. At this stage, there are no radiographic changes and this stage is also reversible
- Stage 3: mild or early **periodontitis**. The normal smooth contour of the gum margins is lost at this stage due to gum recession and oedema. The gums bleed easily and pockets may be present between the gum and the tooth, exposing the roots slightly. Radiographs demonstrate loss of **alveolar bone**. This stage is not reversible, but may be stabilised by treatment to delay progression to stage 4
- Stage 4: established **periodontitis**. This is the end-stage of **periodontitis** and is characterised by loosening of the teeth, well-established **periodontal** pockets with pus oozing, much bone loss and severe inflammation. Radiography will show loss of bone, cavitation or alveolar pockets and irregularity of the surfaces of the roots. This stage is irreversible and extraction is required (Figure 9.4)

In addition to gingivitis and **periodontitis**, other inflammatory dental diseases include:

- Tooth-root abscesses (periapical **abscess**): these usually occur as complications of established **periodontitis**, although they can occasionally follow traumatic insertion of a foreign body (e.g. stick) into the **periodontal** space. In mild to moderate cases swelling and redness are seen at the base of the tooth; in more severe cases the swelling may be substantial

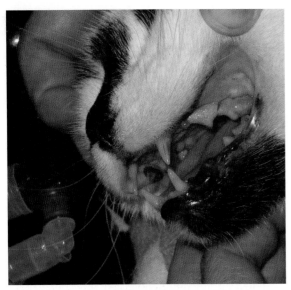

Figure 9.4 Stage 4 **periodontitis** in a cat. There is severe **calculus** visible and the first upper premolar has been severely eroded by an odontoclastic resorptive lesion.

Box 9.1 Oral antibiotics for dental disease

Amoxicillin–clavulanate (Synulox, Pfizer)
Dogs, cats: 20 mg/kg (combined) BID
or
Clindamycin (Antirobe, Pharmacia)
Dogs, cats: 11 mg/kg BID

---

and cause a noticeable lump on the side of the face or the mandible, or even protrusion of the eye if the maxillary molars are involved. If not treated, the **abscess** can burst through the **gingiva** or side of the face and form a fistula. Treatment involves a combination of antibiotics (Box 9.1) and tooth extraction
- Odontoclastic resorptive lesions (OCRL, or odontoclastic lesions, OCL): although primarily seen in cats, dogs may occasionally present with these destructive tooth lesions. OCRLs typically appear as moth-eaten tooth, usually at the crown–root junction and subgingivally. There is often gingivitis at the affected tooth, and, of course, the rest of the mouth may have

concurrent **periodontal** disease. The cause is uncertain, and various factors (diet, breed, etc.) have been postulated. Treatment involves extraction of affected teeth and dental prophylaxis
- Chronic **stomatitis** (also called ulcerative **stomatitis** or faucitis): this is mainly seen in cats, but can also occur in immunocompromised dogs. There are two forms. The first is associated with feline leukaemia virus (FeLV)/ feline immunodeficiency virus (FIV) infection or other immunocompromising disease. The cause for the second form has yet to be determined, but it is sometimes called lymphocytic plasmocytic **stomatitis**. In either case, the clinical signs are similar. There is an intense gingivitis with proliferation and inflammation of the gums. The fauces (the gums at the back of the mouth beyond the last molars) are often most severely affected. The condition is extremely painful, so cats tend to present as anorexic and may even claw at their mouths. Diagnosis is made by culture and sensitivity of biopsy samples, **histopathology** and serology to rule out FIV/FeLV. Treatment can be unrewarding, although in some cases edentation (extraction of all teeth) may help; other cases may respond to a combination of antibiotics and long-term corticosteroids

DENTAL INSTRUMENTATION

In addition to good technique and a methodical approach, the success of dental treatment is greatly influenced by choice of instrumentation. Dental equipment may be divided into power tools and hand tools (Box 9.2).

Power tools (Figure 9.5A–C)

- Dental scalers: these may be sonic or ultrasonic: the ultrasonic type are used more frequently. They rely on high-frequency vibration dislodging gross **calculus** from the teeth. There are various types available, which differ in their design and in the means of ultrasound production (magnetostrictive (cavitron-like) or piezoelectric). The water jet transmits the

Box 9.2 Dental instruments

Power tools
- Dental scalers
- Drills/burrs
- Suction
- Three-way syringes (water/air-blowers)
- Polishers

Hand tools
- Calculus removal forceps
- Dental gags
- Dental chisels/hand scalers/curettes
- Periodontal probes/explorers
- Gingival retractors/periosteal elevators
- Dental elevators
- Extraction forceps

Box 9.3

Hand dental tools can be cold-sterilised by immersion in a chlorocresol–triethanolamine solution (e.g. Novasapa, Fort Dodge) for 1 min at room temperature.

ultrasound wave and flushes the debris away effectively. Most machines have a choice of tip and newer machines have very small tips which allow subgingival descaling
- Drills/burrs: dental drills may be electrically driven or air-driven. Electric drills tend to overheat very easily. They also have a lower maximum speed than air-driven drills. Air-driven drills are preferred, as the higher speed and air-cooling both tend to produce less thermal injury to tissues. In addition, most air-driven handpieces also have water-coolant jets integrated, which further decrease thermal injury and help clear debris. The disadvantage is that they require a separate compressor unit, which is often bulky and requires more maintenance. Air-driven handpieces require regular maintenance (cleaning and lubrication) to maintain performance and prevent wear and tear
- Suction: dental suction units help reduce the risk of aspiration of dental debris and improve visualisation of the oral cavity. Suction tips may be reusable or disposable
- Three-way syringes (water/air-blowers): these are available on most compressor dental machines and provide a jet of water or air. They are extremely useful for flushing the oral cavity during dental procedures to remove debris; they are also useful for drying teeth

prior to application of medications and to improve visualisation of **calculus** deposits
- Polishers: these are usually available as separate polisher handpieces for the drill units. They should be used at a lower speed than drills and do not have water jets. A new disposable rubber or latex cup (prophylactic or polishing cups) should be used for each patient as they may be a considerable source of infection

All power-tool handpieces should be sterilised after each patient. Some handpieces may be autoclaved; most need to be cold-sterilised using the manufacturer's recommended sterilising agent (Box 9.3). Drill bits should be examined for wear and sterilised after each use. Worn or blunt drill bits may cause stalling of the drill and increase the risk of thermal injury to the tooth. Water bottles should be topped up before each procedure to ensure that the coolant water does not run out during drill use. Seals on bottles should be checked and replaced at regular intervals to make sure there is no loss in water delivery pressure.

Before use, handpieces should be lubricated and any joints tightened: loose joints may result in the handpiece not working or the handpiece cogs wearing out or breaking. Compressors should be serviced regularly and the leads checked for water or air leaks.

Hand tools (Figure 9.6)

- **Calculus** removal forceps: these are designed specifically for the rapid removal of gross **calculus** prior to ultrasonic scaling. They have sharp ends and can damage gums and crown

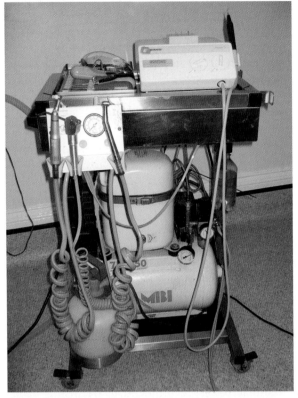

A

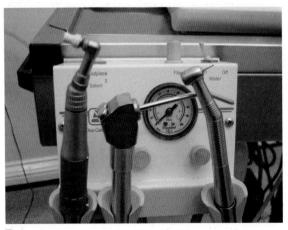

B

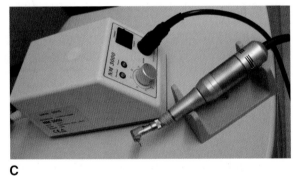

C

Figure 9.5 (A) A typical dental station, comprising air compressor for dental dril! and polisher. An ultrasonic scaler fits nicely on to the top of the station. (B) Detail of the dental station handpieces: left to right: polisher, three-way syringe and drill. (C) Electric dental drill: it is very easy to cause overheating of teeth using this machine, due to the lower speed and lack of water coolant.

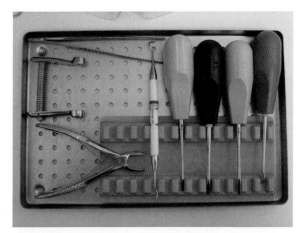

Figure 9.6 A selection of hand dental tools. Left column, top to bottom: thumb forceps, small dental gag, extraction forceps. Right row, left to right: subgingival curette, selection of **periodontal** elevators/luxators.

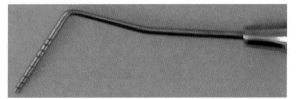

Figure 9.7 Dental probe.

enamel unless used very carefully. They are seldom used, as extraction forceps provide a reasonable alternative for cracking **calculus** from teeth

- Dental gags: these are spring-loaded devices and come in two or three sizes. The smaller ones are suitable for cats and toy dogs, while the larger ones are designed for dogs of varying sizes. Depending on the type, they are placed unilaterally on the canines or behind both upper and lower canines. The unilaterally placed gags can be infuriating to place when wearing disposable gloves, as the gloves have a habit of becoming caught in the spring. It is important not to apply too much retraction: the jaws should be opened wide enough to permit adequate visualisation. Over-retraction of the jaws can lead to masseter muscle pain postoperatively

- Dental chisels/hand scalers/curettes: these are used in combination with or instead of ultrasonic scalers to remove **calculus** from teeth. The dental chisels (or hoes) should only be used above the gum line (supragingivally), whereas the smaller curettes may be used both supra- and subgingivally. They are especially useful for removing small deposits of **calculus** from grooves on crowns. They must be regularly sharpened and should be stored on instrument trays to avoid damaging the tips

- **Periodontal** probes/explorers: dental probes have blunt ends and are often notched at 1–3-mm intervals (Figure 9.7). They are used to assess the degree of gum recession and **periodontal** pocket formation. They are prone to breaking (especially notched ones) and should be stored carefully. **Periodontal** explorers are often called 'shepherd's hook' explorers due to their shape. They are used to search for any irregularities in the supra- or subgingival tooth surface. They should not be used to remove **calculus** as this can damage the tips and the **enamel**

- Gingival retractors/periosteal elevators: these are used for the production of mucoperiosteal and gingival flaps for surgical closure of extraction sockets. They may also be used for shaving off small sections of **alveolar bone** to reshape the gum surface prior to closure of sockets. They have a sharp, concave side and a smoother convex side: the convex side should face the soft tissues to reduce tissue trauma. They must be sharpened regularly and should not be used as dental elevators as this can bend and blunt them

- Dental elevators: also called luxators (although technically, luxators are a different type of tool, being somewhat narrower), these are used to break down the **periodontal** ligament attaching the tooth to the **alveolar bone**. There are many different types and they differ in size, angle of blade, tip shape, whether they are serrated or not and whether the edges flare out (winged) or not. Elevators are used in a rotating, twisting and levering way. In order to be as effective as possible and to reduce tissue trauma, the sides and the end must be kept honed (sharpened in such a way as to maintain the correct blade angle). Considerable torque and leverage can be produced using these instruments and it is possible to cause substantial damage to teeth and to surrounding bone with improper use

- Extraction forceps: designed primarily to grasp teeth for extraction, they are also commonly used to remove gross **calculus** from teeth before ultrasonic scaling. There are several types, differing in size and conformation of the head (straight or angled). The jaws are tube-shaped, facilitating a better grasp on the teeth, and many extraction forceps have ribbing or serrations on the jaws to reduce slipping. Very fine, triangular-ended extraction forceps are available to remove fragments from deep within the alveolus. As with other hinged instruments, the hinge loosens with time and the jaws (or beaks) should be checked periodically for alignment
- Dental mirrors: these can help visualise the backs (or **lingual** surfaces) of teeth and are also handy lip retractors. They can be used to reflect light to the far side of a tooth to improve visualisation

All hand tools should be cleaned and sterilised between patients. Although all (except mirrors) are suitable for autoclave sterilisation, this can take a long time and cause delays to the surgery list. Cold sterilising agents (Box 9.3) act rapidly to disinfect and may be used to reduce turnaround time for dental procedures in busy practices. Otherwise, it is necessary to purchase several sets of dental instruments. All instruments should be regularly sharpened, using a sharpening stone (e.g. Arkansas stone). Most of these require a lubricating oil to sharpen effectively, and some practice is required to produce a perfect finish.

PREPARATION OF DENTAL PATIENT

Dental treatment always requires a general anaesthetic, for several reasons:

- The procedure is painful: even subgingival probing in a reasonably healthy mouth can be very painful
- There is a great risk of getting bitten!
- It is impossible to perform an adequate dental on a conscious patient. It is of very little benefit

to the patient to have a small amount of **calculus** picked off in the consulting room: without polishing, this is likely to build up again very quickly. It is not possible to clean subgingivally on a conscious animal, or to probe for dental disease (such as OCRL)

- It is not possible to examine **caudal** molars adequately in a conscious patient
- Movement of the improperly restrained patient may result in trauma to the oral cavity (e.g. fracturing teeth, tearing the gums)
- In short, although it may seem as though performing a limited dental on a conscious patient will save the owner money and reduce anaesthetic risk, the patient is likely to suffer and there will be little or no improvement in the short-term management of the teeth and absolutely no improvement in the long-term state of the teeth

A full clinical examination should be carried out several days before admission for dental surgery. As patients presenting for dental treatment are often elderly, there may well be concurrent disease. Common concurrent illnesses seen in animals presenting for dental treatment include:

- Renal failure: the animal may or may not have increased thirst and/or urine production (polyuria or polydipsia), may have lost weight or in severe cases may have uraemic breath and mouth ulcers
- Cardiac disease: there may be a murmur present, cough, weight loss or dyspnoea. History may reveal reduced exercise tolerance or episodic collapse
- Hyperthyroidism in cats: cats are likely to have lost weight, have poor coat condition and intermittent diarrhoea and often show altered behaviour (usually becoming 'stressy' or hyperactive). Heart rate is usually elevated (220 beats/min or faster). A thyroid nodule may be palpable in the ventral neck
- Other age-related illnesses include arthritis, bronchitis (or other lung changes) and **neoplasia**

Preoperative blood *and* urine tests should be performed in all elderly animals before dental surgery. Any abnormal results should be investigated as directed. Any medical problem (e.g. hyperthyroidism) should take precedence over routine dental surgery, but the opportunity to provide some form of ameliorative care in the form of antibiotics and home dental care should not be passed up. Dental surgery results in aerosolisation of huge numbers of oral bacteria, and the release of large numbers of bacteria into the blood stream (bacteraemia). These bacteria are unlikely to cause a problem in otherwise healthy animals, although valvular endocarditis (infection of the heart valves) is occasionally seen. However, it is not appropriate to consider **sterile** surgery at the same time as dental treatment. Removal of skin tumours or other minor surgical procedures should therefore be scheduled separately (Box 9.4: although fine-needle aspiration biopsy (FNAB) may be carried out at the time of dental surgery, it may be more sensible to investigate any masses prior to anaesthesia as malignant tumours will of necessity take precedence over dentistry).

Intravenous fluid therapy (IVFT) should be performed as routine for dental surgery in an elderly patient (see Chapter 4) due to the risks of renal insufficiency, poor perfusion and possibly poor food and water intake. Anaesthetic times are often fairly long for dental procedures and IVFT will help maintain fluid and electrolyte balance. For details of anaesthetic drug combinations, see Chapter 4.

Provided there is no renal or hepatic disease, NSAIDs should be administered prior to anaesthesia. The use of antibiotics is discussed elsewhere.

The anaesthetised patient should have a cuffed endotracheal tube placed and the cuff inflated (cats should have a non-cuffed endotracheal tube fitted: see Chapter 4). The patient should be placed in sternal recumbency (Box 9.5) with the neck and anterior chest raised so that the pharynx drains towards the front of the mouth. This is usually achieved by placing a sandbag under the neck. A plastic or metal tray (with a metal grill tray) should be placed under the patient's head, unless a specialised 'tub table' or dental table is used. A sponge (or several swabs) soaked in water is used to pack the pharynx to reduce the risk of blood, debris and fluids entering the trachea during the procedure. The gag should be placed gently to avoid damaging the larynx or forcing the cuffed tube down the trachea. It is a good idea to place a tie of some sort around the packing material, to facilitate removal. Wrapping the end of the tie around the endotracheal tube not only keeps it out of the way, but also helps ensure the packing is not left in by mistake once the endotracheal tube has been removed!

Any monitoring devices (pulse oximeter, capnograph, electrocardiograph) should be placed and tested. A warming device, such as a covered electric blanket or warm-flow water bed, is recommended, the patient should be covered with a fleece or blanket and it may be worth considering wrapping the paws in foil or using some other heat-saving technique to prevent hypothermia.

Box 9.4

Dental surgery should not be performed at the same time as sterile surgery: there is an increased risk of wound breakdown and potentially life-threatening infections.

Box 9.5

An anaesthetised dental patient should always be turned dorsally over ventrally (i.e. with the nose pointing down) to avoid fluid running into the pharynx.

Operator safety

Scalers, drills and polishers propel **contaminated** debris for considerable distances. This, coupled with the aerosolised bacteria, poses a risk for the vet or nurse performing the dental. For this reason, and to comply with health and safety directives, when performing (or assisting with) a dental procedure, safety glasses and masks *must* be worn. Disposable gloves should also be worn.

CLEANING AND POLISHING TEETH

There are various stages in dental treatment:

- Gross scaling
- Ultrasonic and hand scaling
- Probing
- Subgingival curettage/root planing
- **Gingivectomy**
- Extracting
- Polishing
- Oral irrigation

Gross scaling

This involves removing the larger deposits of **calculus** from the teeth, to improve visualisation of the **periodontal** structures.

- If **calculus**-removing forceps are used, the longer jaw is placed on the tip of the crown and the shorter, sharp jaw is positioned near the gum margin. Dental extractor forceps may be used in a similar way. The jaws are closed, cracking off the **calculus**
- Care should be taken not to twist the tools while squeezing the handles together, as this can

fracture the tooth. Care should also be taken not to scratch the **enamel** or tear the gums

- It is not necessary to remove all **calculus** completely in this way, but if most is removed that will reduce the time spent on ultrasonic scaling
- Any teeth with odontoclastic lesions below the neck should be left as there is a great risk of fracturing these teeth and complicating extraction

Ultrasonic and hand scaling

Having removed the gross **calculus**, the ultrasonic scaler and hand scalers or curettes may be used to remove remaining **plaque** and debris.

- There is potential for causing a tremendous amount of thermal and mechanical damage to teeth using an ultrasonic scaler. They must always be used delicately
- The side of the ultrasonic scaler tip should be applied to the tooth. There should be only the smallest amount of pressure applied (as though one were pushing a marble along a flat surface) (Figure 9.8)

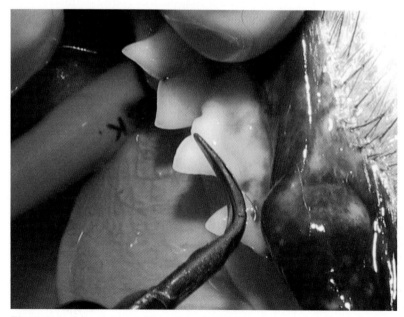

Figure 9.8 Correct use of ultrasonic scaling tool.

- The scaler tip should be moved continuously to avoid thermal damage and not more than 20 s at a time spent on a tooth (if any deposits are missed, the tooth can be returned to later)
- The power setting should be set according to the manufacturer's recommendations. If these are not known, then the power should be adjusted and reduced to the lowest possible setting that knocks **plaque** off. The water jet should be high enough to flush away debris and cool the tip
- The scaler should not be used subgingivally, unless a special subgingival tip is fitted. Routine tips do not have adequate water cooling at the tip to prevent thermal injury occurring
- All surfaces of every tooth should be scaled. This seems obvious, but it is easy to miss teeth unless one is regimented about the process. The most commonly missed teeth include the **lingual** face of the premolars and the **caudal** molars. A dental gag should be used to improve visualisation, but the tooth on which the gag is placed should not be forgotten
- If the patient is in right lateral recumbency, it is best to clean the **buccal** side (closest to the cheek) of the left arcades and the **lingual** side (closest to the tongue) of the right arcades. The patient may then be turned into left recumbency and the process repeated. Alternatively, a dental mirror may be used
- A hand scaler should be used to remove sub-gingival **plaque** and any **calculus** that remains on the crowns. As with ultrasonic scalers, the side of the tip should be used and the instrument should be placed parallel to the tooth
- To remove subgingival **plaque**, the curette should be introduced into the **periodontal** space and the sharp edge held lightly against the tooth whilst slowly and steadily scraping the curette up towards the neck of the tooth. Scratching noises and a rough feel during movement will demonstrate any remaining **calculus**. Meticulous attention to detail is required: unless all subgingival **plaque** is removed, the treatment is a waste of time (Box 9.6)

Box 9.6

Good lighting (spot lights, dental lights) is essential for dentistry. It is worth investing in a ceiling-mounted high-intensity lamp to improve visualisation.

- Typically, this stage of a dental takes anywhere between 20 min and an hour to perform properly
- Air-drying the teeth often helps to make any remaining **calculus** more visible. An alternative is to use a disclosing solution (e.g. First Sight, CET). This is applied to the teeth with a cotton bud or swab, and the oral cavity is rinsed to remove excess stain. Any missed **plaque** or **calculus** stains pink and can be easily visualised. These stains are a very useful training tool to help improve scaling technique
- The level of **plaque** build-up on each tooth should be recorded on the dental chart

Probing

A combination of sharp and blunt probing is used to identify problem teeth.
- The notched or graded end of a blunt probe is used to explore the **periodontal** space of each tooth, walking the probe around the tooth and being careful to test all around the tooth
- There is usually between 1 and 3 mm depth between each tooth and gum margin. Any depth greater than 5 mm constitutes a **periodontal** pocket and must be treated by curettage, **gingivectomy** or extraction, depending on the state of the tooth
- Next, a sharp probe (or explorer) is used to examine the neck of each tooth. Due to the springy nature of the steel, any irregularities or cavities will be easily felt and with practice this procedure becomes much quicker to perform. By tapping the neck of the tooth with the point of the explorer it is possible to feel for softening of the dentine and any OCRL lesions

175

- All multi-root teeth should be carefully examined at the furcation and the probe used to ascertain the degree of gum and bone recession. A healthy tooth should have no exposure of the furcation: if it is possible to insert the probe between two roots, then there is moderate gum and **alveolar bone** resorption. The tooth may still be salvageable with good curettage and **gingivectomy**. If the probe passes easily from one side of the tooth to the other, this is bad news for the tooth and it should be extracted
- All findings (normal and abnormal) should be recorded on the dental chart

Subgingival curettage/root planing

Where there is thick **calculus** on the surface of the root, or gingival recession to 5 mm or less, then subgingival scaling will not be sufficient to retard or reverse **periodontal** disease. In this case, the surface of the exposed root can be planed back using a dental curette to remove all pitting and **calculus** deposits. The gingival tissue is also scraped to debride diseased tissue and allow for second-intention healing to improve gingival attachment to teeth. Any pockets deeper than 5 mm are unlikely to benefit from this technique and it may be more appropriate to extract these teeth.

Gingivectomy

This is indicated when there is **hyperplasia** of the gums. The most overtly representative breed for this condition is the boxer dog, where the teeth have virtually disappeared under a mound of hyperplastic gum by the age of 5–6 years.
- It should not be used to treat deep **periodontal** pockets, since there is unlikely to be sufficient healthy gum remaining to provide good healing
- The **periodontal** space should be carefully probed and the depth noted
- The probe can be used to mark the line of **gingivectomy** (by creating a series of perforations along the gum). There should be at least 2 mm of healthy gum remaining after excision
- Using a scalpel (or electrocoagulation unit) the excess gum should be excised. The cutting angle should be such that the gum slopes down from the tooth, rather than cutting at right angles to the tooth
- If an electrocoagulation unit is used, care should be taken not to set the power too high or to touch the tooth root. Both of these will result in thermal injury and may cause gum or tooth necrosis
- If using a scalpel blade, haemorrhage, though appearing dramatic, is usually brief and may be controlled by pressure via a moistened swab. Haemostatic dressings may be applied, though these are difficult to retain in position

Extracting

This is a complicated procedure and is covered later in this chapter. Having extracted a diseased tooth, the neighbouring teeth should be carefully re-examined by sharp and blunt probing to ensure no aspect was missed previously and that the tooth has not been injured by the extraction procedure.

Polishing

Polishing the teeth not only provides an acceptable cosmetic finish to the dental procedure, but also reduces rough surfaces on the teeth, which may otherwise act as foci for **plaque** build-up. It is therefore an important part of the procedure and care must be taken that each and every tooth is attended to, on all sides.
- Thermal injury can easily occur during polishing, so various steps should be taken to avoid this:
  - The polisher should be set to a low speed
  - Plenty of prophylactic polisher paste (prophy paste) should be used to act as lubricant
  - The lightest of touches should be applied: a soft rubber polishing tip or cup should be used as this flares with minimal pressure

- The polisher should be kept moving at all times and no more than 2–3 s spent on a tooth at any one time (the tooth can always be returned to later)
- All surfaces of the tooth should be polished, being careful to include the subgingival area

Oral irrigation

Flushing the oral cavity following dental treatment serves several purposes:

- It removes debris and blood from the oral cavity which may serve as potential sources of infection or aspiration hazard to the patient, as well as being unpleasant and unprofessional
- It improves visualisation of the oral cavity and facilitates examination to ensure no teeth have been neglected and no oral trauma has occurred. It also allows assessment of **haemostasis**
- The removal of debris decreases postoperative inflammation and increases patient comfort
- The addition of 0.1% chlorhexidine to the water (or use of a ready-made oral irrigation solution) reduces bacterial load and may help decrease postoperative inflammation, although it is unlikely to be of any long-term benefit

Most compressor-style dental machines have a water syringe (usually combined with an air jet). Each tooth should be sprayed, until all traces of blood, debris and prophy paste are removed.

Finally, the oral cavity is dried to reduce risk of aspiration of fluid and the pharyngeal packing swabs are removed. If the procedure has been lengthy, requiring several extractions, **opioid** analgesic injection may be repeated and the patient is woken up. The neck support should be kept in place until the patient is able to raise its head, so that any fluid in the pharynx will drain forwards out of the mouth.

DENTAL RADIOGRAPHY

Radiography of teeth and **alveolar bone** is woefully underused in practice. This is undoubtedly due to reluctance to increase the cost of an already costly dental procedure. However, radiography should always be offered and is very important for several reasons:

- The extent of dental lesions may not be apparent by examination of the erupted portion of the tooth. Radiography will highlight **alveolar bone** resorption, root decay and even abscesses that may not be otherwise visible (Figure 9.9)
- Spaces between teeth may represent absent teeth, impacted teeth or remnants of fractured or resorbing teeth. Again, it is not possible to discern this without radiography
- Occasionally, radiography may pick up signs of other disease; for example, **neoplasia** (e.g. osteosarcoma) or metabolic disease (nutritional or renal secondary hyperparathyroidism leading to thinning of the bone)

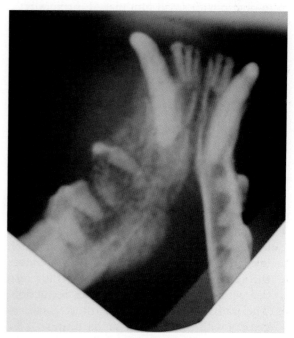

Figure 9.9 Intraoral radiograph of the mandible of a cat, using screened film within a flexible light-proof case (often mistakenly called 'non-screen film'). The cat presented with severe **periodontal** disease and gingivitis. The destructive nature of the radiographic lesion is suggestive of **neoplasia**. However, biopsy demonstrated an inflammatory process and 6 weeks of antibiotics led to a resolution of clinical signs.

- Radiographs taken before and after dental extraction will confirm complete extraction of the correct tooth, provide a permanent record of the procedure and may be useful evidence in the case of litigation
- A crown fracture may also have fractures extending farther down the tooth: this will be missed without radiography

Dental radiography requires the use of fast/slow/ contrast films and, although it can be performed adequately using a regular-sized cassette and normal practice X-ray machine, there is no doubt that the use of a dedicated dental X-ray unit and dental film confers several advantages:

- Positioning and collimating are much easier with a dedicated dental radiography unit and dental film than trying to manipulate the patient's skull to obtain a view on a regular cassette. Indeed, some views are only possible to obtain with small film placed intraorally
- There is a huge amount of waste using a normal X-ray machine, as only a small percentage of the film contains the desired view. Dental film is much smaller and most of the film is usable. This also has a bearing on storing the films, as dental film takes up less space
- It is possible to approximate dental film with the teeth much more so than with a larger cassette. This not only reduces scattering, increasing resolution and operator safety, but also means that post object magnification is decreased
- A dental X-ray unit may be placed much closer to the patient (the film focal distance is much lower than a standard X-ray unit). This reduces the required amount of radiation, thus also decreasing scatter and improving resolution. The radiation controls are thus easier to comply with than with a standard unit
- The increased costs associated with buying a separate unit, films and a dedicated developer are usually offset by improved image quality and lower chemical (and film) costs

Using dental film, between six and 10 views are required to obtain survey radiographs of the whole mouth. Any lesions may then be investi-gated more thoroughly by centring and collimat-ing over the region of interest. Using a regular, extraoral cassette, fewer views are required to radiograph the entire mouth, but the radiographs are much more difficult to interpret and less informative due to angular distortion of the radio-graphic anatomy and superimposition of other structures.

EXTRACTIONS

At the time of writing, veterinary nurses are per-mitted to remove very loose teeth requiring no cutting of the **periodontal** ligament. This is a straightforward task and involves relatively gentle pulling of the tooth, having grasped it with a pair of extraction forceps. The tooth can be rotated about its long axis carefully, but care must be taken not to apply too much torque as this can break the root. Occasionally it is necessary to use a sharp dental elevator or scalpel blade to sever attachments between the tooth and the gum, usually on the **lingual** aspect of the tooth. There may be considerable bleeding, even from extremely loose teeth, and this is best managed by applying pressure with a saline- or water-soaked gauze swab. If haemorrhage does not stop within a couple of minutes, an alginate haemo-static product (e.g. Kaltostat, ConvaTec) or bone wax (Ethicon) may be applied.

Teeth that are not loose need to be surgically extracted, and this may be done in a number of ways:

- By patient and methodical breaking down and tearing of the **periodontal** ligament using a dental elevator. This technique works best for single-root teeth
- By sectioning the tooth with a drill or burr to isolate each root and then removing the tooth by the above method
- By creating a **buccal** gingival flap and remov-ing **alveolar bone** with a drill or burr to remove the tooth through the side of the gum. This technique is the method of choice for removal of large, well-attached canine and multi-root teeth

Dental extractions are associated with a fair degree of postoperative pain and so careful attention should be paid to **analgesia**. Local anaesthesia is a very useful adjunct to **opioid** and NSAID use and should be considered.

Lidocaine has only a short duration of action and is unlikely to provide **analgesia** for the duration of the procedure. Bupivacaine is longer-lasting and can be injected around the gingival margin and into the **periodontal** space to provide a degree of pain relief. Much more effective are nerve blocks: the mental and infraorbital nerves may be blocked by the injection of 2 ml/kg bupivacaine around the nerves as they exit the mental and infraorbital foramina. The procedure is technically demanding to perform and great care must be taken to avoid intravascular injection, but the increase in **analgesia** is tremendous.

Removal using a dental elevator

The dental elevator should be sharp and free from rough or bent edges. It is difficult to overstate the joy of using a really well-crafted high-quality luxator and it is well worth investing in several sets of different sizes (Figure 9.10).

- The elevator should be used primarily to cut the **periodontal** ligament and to act as a lever to loosen teeth. The initial entry to the **periodontal** space should be made by cutting the attachment between tooth and gum with a no. 11 scalpel blade

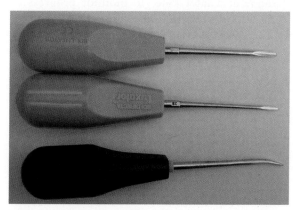

Figure 9.10 Selection of dental elevators. The upper and lower elevators are suitable for dog extractions, whereas the middle one is ideal for cats.

- The elevator is introduced into the **periodontal** space and some pressure is used to force the instrument towards the root (apex). The elevator should then be tilted slightly away from the tooth and held for 10–20 s. This stretches and tears the **periodontal** ligament. Alternatively, the end of the luxator may be rotated slightly side to side, allowing the sides of the tool to sever the ligamentous attachment
- Leverage may be applied by twisting or rotating the elevator, but in either case, it is better to apply a small amount of leverage for a few seconds than to apply a lot of leverage and risk breaking the tooth or the **alveolar bone**
- Some teeth will loosen after only a few minutes of repeated leverage and repositioning of the elevator; other teeth may take a longer time (Box 9.7). However, perseverance will eventually ensure that most of the alveolar ligament is broken down. The tooth may then be grasped by the dental extraction forceps and a moderate degree of force, coupled, if necessary, by a slight twisting motion, will break the remaining fibres and allow the tooth to be removed
- If the tooth will not pull out, do not use excessive force: continue elevation to break down the **periodontal** ligament
- The alveolar socket (alveolus) is curetted to remove any fragments of bone or tooth and to debride any infected tissue
- The alveolar socket is flushed with **sterile** saline or 0.05% chlorhexidine solution
- The **gingiva** may then either be sutured or left open to organise and repair by second intention. Both options have merits and potential complications. Unless all infected tissue is removed, wound breakdown is a potential complication of suturing. However, sutured gums will heal more quickly and there is a risk

Box 9.7 Golden rule
The golden rule of tooth extraction is slowly, slowly! Patience will be rewarded; impatience is likely to result in a fractured tooth or worse.

of food impaction into the socket of non-sutured gums. If suturing is performed, a 4/0 (1.5 metric) synthetic absorbable suture such as polyglytone 6211 (Caprosyn, Vetoquinol) is ideal

Removal by sectioning the tooth

Teeth with divergent, multiple roots are more easily removed in this way:
- A scalpel blade is used to cut the attachment between tooth and gum and a dental elevator (or periosteal elevator) is used to retract the gum from the tooth to enable visualisation of the furcation
- A side-cutting burr is used to section the tooth. The next stage is made easier by using the burr to widen the gap between both sections enough to permit entry of a dental elevator
- A dental elevator is used as above to break down the alveolar ligament. The elevator can be slipped between the tooth fragments and used to apply leverage to help loosen the teeth further. Again, it is worth applying a small amount of leverage for 10–20s to allow time for the ligaments to break down, rather than applying more leverage for a shorter time and risking tooth fracture
- Having loosened the tooth sufficiently, extraction forceps are used to remove each section of tooth
- The alveolus is curetted and flushed and then either sutured or left to heal by second-intention healing, as above

Removal by creation of a buccal flap

This is the most technically demanding technique for tooth extraction and can result in large gingival deficits if not performed properly. It is not regarded as minor surgery and is included here for completeness only:
- A no. 11 scalpel blade is used to cut the attachment between tooth and gum and a dental (or periosteal) elevator is used to reflect the gum margin from the tooth

- An incision is made in the **buccal** aspect of the gum **rostral** and **caudal** to the tooth. The incision should be down to the **periosteum** of the underlying **alveolar bone**. The incision should extend to the depth of the apex of the roots (as determined by radiography)
- A periosteal elevator is used to reflect the **buccal** mucosa away from the **alveolar bone**, thus creating a flap of mucosa. Care must be taken not to damage the mucosa, as this will affect the viability of the flap
- A cutting burr or drill is used to remove the **alveolar bone** surrounding the tooth. The tooth is removed by a combination of **alveolar bone** removal and disruption of **periodontal** ligament using a dental elevator
- Having removed the tooth, the alveolar socket is curetted to remove any debris and a dental burr is used to remove any protruding edges of **alveolar bone**
- The alveolus is flushed with **sterile** saline or 0.05% chlorhexidine solution and the **buccal** mucosal flap is used to close the **gingiva**: 4/0 (1.5 metric) synthetic absorbable suture material (Caprosyn, Vetoquinol) is ideal for this

DENTAL CHARTS AND RECORDS

For every dental procedure, a dental chart should be completed, for several reasons:
- They provide a record of the state of the teeth and oral cavity and enable comparisons to be made at a later date (to monitor progress of disease, success of home care, etc.)
- They provide a legal record of procedures performed and reduce any chance of misunderstanding and disagreements (e.g. over bills)
- They provide a focal point to discuss ongoing dental care with the owner
- They improve dental care by promoting methodical technique and reminding one to perform certain procedures
- They make it easier to remember what work has been done when working out the dental bill

There are various commercial dental record forms available, and they differ in the amount of information needed to complete the form and in the layout. Some forms are designed for use on the same patient on subsequent dentals, while others are for single use only. Figures 9.11 and 9.12 show examples of dental charts for dogs and cats, respectively.

In the examples, each tooth is represented both by Triadan position and by a picture of the tooth to make it easier to orient oneself. The form may be filled in using whatever shorthand the practice prefers, but it is a good idea wherever possible to use recognised dental shorthand to eliminate ambiguity. The picture of the tooth may be drawn over to illustrate treatment, or else a comment made in the relevant box. Important notes to make are:

- Presence and degree of gingivitis (and any gum **hyperplasia**)
- Amount of **calculus** and **plaque**
- Presence and degree of OCRLs
- Absent teeth or retained primaries
- Extractions
- Presence, position and degree of fractures
- Presence and degree of gum recession, **periodontal** pockets and furcation exposure

At first, dental charts are time-consuming and bothersome to complete, but with practice they can be filled in very quickly. If an assistant is available, it becomes a very easy matter to call out each tooth and any problems noted.

COMPLICATIONS OF DENTISTRY

Unfortunately, many complications of dentistry result from rushed or sloppy technique and lack of client communication. Owners should be made aware of the risks of dentistry, such as anaesthetic risks, and given a comprehensive estimate, including likely numbers of extractions if possible. Many clients find it difficult to accept that veterinary dentistry is important for the general health of their pet rather than just as a treatment for halitosis, and so it is worth spending time explaining the medical problems associated with chronic **periodontitis**.

Dental complications involve:
- Anaesthetic problems
- Iatrogenic damage

- Recurrence of dental disease
- Other problems

Anaesthetic problems

Provided a thorough clinical examination has been performed and IVFT is instigated, the dental patient should not be more at risk from the anaesthetic procedure than other minor-surgery patients. However, there are several important considerations with perioperative care:

- Most dental patients are elderly. They may thus be less able to regulate body temperature and fluid balance and may suffer from concurrent diseases. Anaesthetic problems are more likely in this group of patients
- Dental procedures take a long time (usually more than 1 h, often much longer). Body temperature will decrease during anaesthesia. Additionally, the frequent use of flushing solutions in the mouth will effectively decrease body temperature. Hypothermia is therefore likely to be a problem unless stringent methods are adopted to counter this
- Unless the cranial thorax is raised on sandbags and the pharynx is packed, aspiration of flush fluid, blood and debris into the trachea may be a problem during anaesthesia. The oral cavity and pharynx must be emptied of all fluid before the endotracheal tube is removed. Ongoing haemorrhage and salivation can cause aspiration problems or even laryngeal blockage, so patients must be monitored post-anaesthesia until they are able to support themselves in sternal recumbency with their heads raised
- Inadequate attention to **analgesia** can cause patients to become only lightly anaesthetised during dental anaesthesia. The usual response to this is to increase the concentration of volatile anaesthetic. This can lead to severe respiratory and cardiac depression and is responsible for increased anaesthetic deaths and postanaesthetic morbidity in dental patients. Proper use of balanced **analgesia** (especially local **analgesia**) should reduce this complication

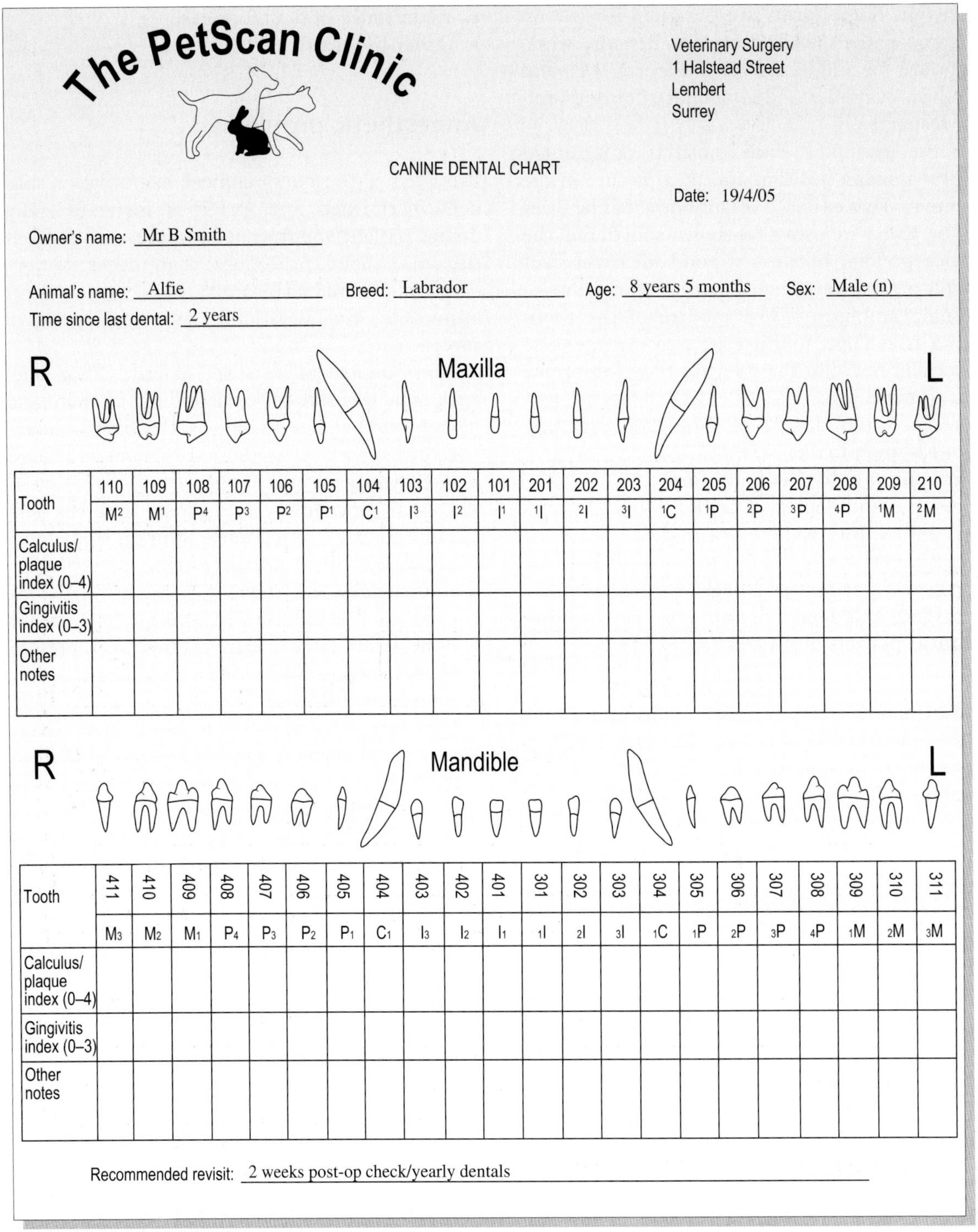

The PetScan Clinic

Veterinary Surgery
1 Halstead Street
Lembert
Surrey

CANINE DENTAL CHART

Date: 19/4/05

Owner's name: Mr B Smith

Animal's name: Alfie   Breed: Labrador   Age: 8 years 5 months   Sex: Male (n)

Time since last dental: 2 years

R — Maxilla — L

Tooth	110	109	108	107	106	105	104	103	102	101	201	202	203	204	205	206	207	208	209	210
	M²	M¹	P⁴	P³	P²	P¹	C¹	I³	I²	I¹	¹I	²I	³I	¹C	¹P	²P	³P	⁴P	¹M	²M
Calculus/ plaque index (0–4)																				
Gingivitis index (0–3)																				
Other notes																				

R — Mandible — L

Tooth	411	410	409	408	407	406	405	404	403	402	401	301	302	303	304	305	306	307	308	309	310	311
	M₃	M₂	M₁	P₄	P₃	P₂	P₁	C₁	I₃	I₂	I₁	₁I	₂I	₃I	₁C	₁P	₂P	₃P	₄P	₁M	₂M	₃M
Calculus/ plaque index (0–4)																						
Gingivitis index (0–3)																						
Other notes																						

Recommended revisit: 2 weeks post-op check/yearly dentals

Figure 9.11 Example of a canine dental record.

The PetScan Clinic

Veterinary Surgery
1 Halstead Street
Lembert
Surrey

FELINE DENTAL CHART

Date: 19/4/05

Owner's name: Mr B Jones

Animal's name: Fifi   Breed: DSH   Age: 11 years 5 months   Sex: Female (n)

Time since last dental: 3 years

R — Maxilla — L

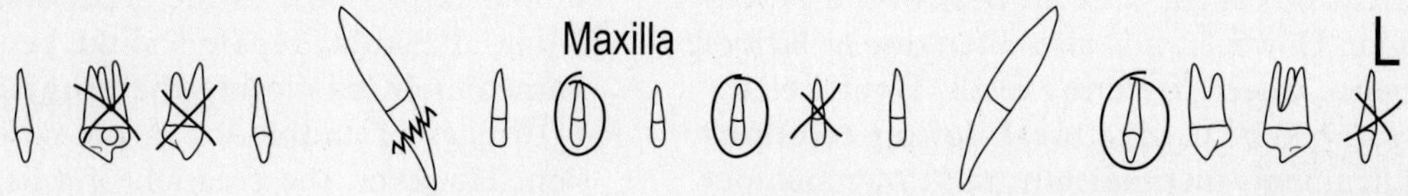

Tooth	109	108	107	106		104	103	102	101	201	202	203	204		206	207	208	209
	M^1	P^3	P^2	P^1		C^1	I^3	I^2	I^1	$_1I$	$_2I$	$_3I$	$_1C$		$_1P$	$_2P$	$_3P$	$_1M$
Calculus/ plaque index (0–4)	1	3	2	1		1	1		1		1	1	2			3	2	2
Gingivitis index (0–3)	1	3	2	1		1	1		2		2	1	2			1	2	2
Other notes	o=ocrl x=extracted					⌇⌇ = crown #		absent	absent		loose x=extracted				0=missing tooth		sub-gingival erosion extracted	

R — Mandible — L

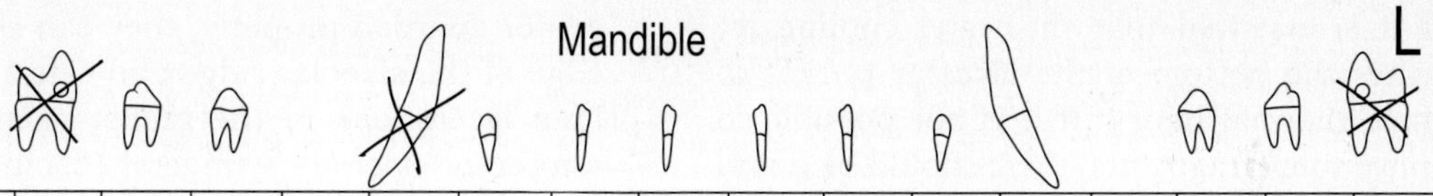

Tooth	409	408	407		404	403	402	401	301	302	303	304		307	308	309
	M_1	P_2	P_3		C_1	I_3	I_2	I_1	$_1I$	$_2I$	$_3I$	$_1C$		$_1P$	$_2P$	$_3M$
Calculus/ plaque index (0–4)	3	2	1		3	2	1			1	1	1		1	2	1
Gingivitis index (0–3)	3	1	1		2	2	1			1	1	2		2	2	3
Other notes	o=ocrl	furcation visible						absent	absent							o=ocrl

Recommended revisit: 2 weeks post-op check/yearly dentals

X = extracted
O = absent

Figure 9.12 Example of (completed) feline dental record.

Iatrogenic damage

It is extremely easy to apply too much force when handling dental instruments or to slip off a tooth or gum margin. There is little sound more concerning during a dental than a sudden sliding noise, usually followed by a muttered oath. Common iatrogenic dental complications include:

- Fracturing teeth during extractions. This may be unavoidable when dealing with severe OCRLs on cat teeth, as the neck becomes very fragile. However, it is also often due to lack of patience when extracting teeth. Dental elevators should be used to break down **periodontal** ligaments methodically, not to wrench out firmly attached teeth by as great a degree of leverage as possible. Any tooth fragments remaining in the alveolus are a potential source of infection. Although in many cases, especially with cats, small fragments may resorb, it is best to attempt to remove them if possible. This may be accomplished by diligent use of a fine dental elevator and fragment forceps, or else by atomising the fragments with a high-speed burr. The latter method works very well, but it is essential that the water-cooling jet reaches the bottom of the alveolar pocket to reduce thermal injury. If it is not possible to remove some fragments, these should be noted and measured on the post dental radiographs and repeat X-rays should be taken a month or so later to confirm resorption
- Fracturing bone during extractions. Although this can be difficult to avoid in cases where **ankylosis** between tooth and **alveolar bone** has occurred, it happens more commonly due to excess force being exerted during extractions. The author has witnessed two accidental **rostral** mandibulectomies on the same day during lower canine removal in dogs! More usually, **alveolar bone** is fractured during extraction. Small fragments may be simply removed and the bony edge resected prior to suturing the gums, but larger fractures may require orthopaedic repair
- Oronasal fistula. This is the worst-case scenario of fracturing **alveolar bone** during extractions. It involves the creation of a permanent communication between the oral cavity and the nasal cavity via the alveolar socket. Although it occurs most commonly following upper canine removal, it is a potential sequel to removal of any maxillary teeth, especially where there is loss of **alveolar bone** during tooth root infections. Dental X-rays may give some indication of likely fistulous teeth and the method of extraction can be adjusted accordingly (i.e. a **buccal** gingival flap approach should be made rather than a simple extraction). In the event of causing an oronasal fistula, repair should be attempted immediately, by closing the **gingiva**, or after 7–10 days of antibiotics in the case of infection. However, the creation of a fistula is not always known immediately, and it may be some days or weeks before clinical signs are seen (nasal discharge, sneezing, discharge into alveolar socket). Treatment of oronasal fistulae can be difficult, with recurrence and persistence of nasal discharge likely. Clients must be made aware of the potential for oronasal fistula prior to any dental extraction
- Damage to gingival tissue by sharp dental instruments. If elevators are held incorrectly or not guarded properly, they can slip off the edge of the alveolar ridge and cause deep and long lacerations in the gums, palate, cheek, tongue or operator's fingers! Placing a finger 1 cm from the tip of the elevator helps to guide the instrument and prevents too much travel if it slips. Although quite nasty lacerations can be made in this way, they are rarely serious and suturing the wound usually suffices. Occasionally, penetration of the sublingual mucosa can result in a large bubble of inflamed and oedematous mucosa 2–3 days postoperatively. This usually resolves spontaneously after 5–7 days, although if severe it can cause discomfort on eating. NSAIDs may help speed up resolution of the inflammation. Very rarely, damage to the salivary ducts can occur and result in a persistent thin-walled swelling (a ranula) or a larger fluid swelling (a sialocele). These conditions may resolve spontaneously, but more usually require specialist soft-tissue intervention

- Thermal injury to teeth and soft tissues. This occurs due to increased contact time with scalers, burrs and polishers and results in necrosis of teeth and gums several days or weeks after dental surgery. Water-coolant jets should be checked frequently during the procedure and instruments should be used carefully, not applying too much pressure and moving the contact area continuously. Thermal injury may cause pain post dental and should be treated with relevant **analgesia** (NSAIDs, opioids)

Recurrence of dental disease

Dental prophylaxis and treatment should not be considered a 'once-in-a-lifetime' event for a patient, nor should it be seen as a cure for dental disease. Rather, it is the first step in controlling **periodontitis** and a treatment for painful or end-stage teeth. Owners should be made aware of the need for ongoing dental care, including repeated dental radiographs, scaling and polishing. However, this does not give one carte blanche to perform an inadequate procedure. Dental disease will recur much more quickly if the subgingival spaces have not been properly scaled and every part of every tooth checked. As discussed above, **plaque**-disclosing solutions are a useful cleaning aid and should be used as a quality control for each dental procedure.

Other problems

Persistent haemorrhage from extraction sites should be dealt with in the same way as haemorrhage in other sites: by applying pressure and using haemostatic packing agents and **cautery** if necessary. If haemorrhage persists from relatively minor wounds, then a coagulation cascade problem should be considered and appropriate steps taken (haematology, clotting profiles, colloids and blood product administration in serious cases).

Problems of septicaemic spread of dental bacteria are occasionally seen. Endocarditis is the most frequently cited example, although nephritis and septic arthritis are also reported. The incidence of distant infection should be anticipated given the high bacterial load of an animal with severe **periodontitis**; antibiotics should be administered for 7–10 days following such dental procedures. As discussed, due to the risk of **haematogenous** and aerosol spread of bacteria, no **sterile** surgery should be performed at the same time as dental surgery.

ONGOING DENTAL CARE

Surgical treatment of **periodontal** disease, including scaling and polishing of teeth, removes **plaque** and **calculus** and reduces gingivitis. It has little in the way of residual effect, though, and without ongoing treatment **periodontal** disease will recur. There are various ways of providing ongoing dental care to cats and dogs:

- Active home care: tooth brushing and dental/oral gels and powders
- Feeding special dental diets
- Regular dental checks
- Repeated scaling and polishing under anaesthesia
- Referral to veterinary dental specialists

Active home care

Encouraging clients to brush their pet's teeth will help to reduce **plaque** build-up and delay the onset and recurrence of **periodontitis**.

- Some pets are simply too excitable or aggressive to brush their teeth safely: personal safety must be stressed to owners to avoid injury
- Any toothbrush may be used; a child's brush is appropriate for most dogs and cats. Motorised toothbrushes are extremely effective, but the noise and vibrations frighten many animals. Rubber toothbrushes that fit on the finger are easy to use, but are not as effective as bristled brushes and pose quite a risk for biting
- It is never too late to start brushing; however, puppy and kitten parties are an ideal time to educate clients in dental care and young animals are often easier to train

- Brushless toothpaste, enzymatic gels and powders are of some use in reducing numbers of **plaque** bacteria, but are usually fairly ineffective at reducing **plaque** build-up and completely ineffective at removing **calculus**
- Regular dental care is important: brushing teeth infrequently (less than every other day) actually hastens **plaque** build-up and gingivitis
- Toothbrushing only cleans parts of some of the teeth: it is unusual to be able to clean the rearmost molars effectively, and almost impossible to clean the **lingual** surface of the teeth

Feeding special dental diets

Many pet food companies produce special dental or oral-care diets. Whilst there is considerable variation in the efficacy of individual diets, some of them seem to work very well indeed.

- Most dental diets rely on the structure of the kibble or pellet: they are usually fairly bulky and require biting to break up into small enough pieces to swallow. The arrangement of fibres in the kibbles has a mild abrasive action on the tooth and gum. It is important, therefore, to feed an appropriately sized diet to the animal, to avoid the possibility of the food being swallowed whole
- Many dogs and cats display laterality: that is, they use one side of the mouth preferentially. This, coupled with the fact that not all teeth will be used to crunch the food, can decrease the overall effectiveness of the diet
- Dietary management may be used as an adjunct to tooth-cleaning and should be strongly recommended for animals that will not allow toothbrushing
- In the last few years many veterinarians have reported a decrease in the incidence of OCRLs in cats. This may be associated with changes in dietary composition over the preceding few years. It remains to be seen whether the incidence of **periodontitis** will be likewise affected
- Dental snacks are, on the whole, less effective at cleaning teeth than complete diets, but may be of some help to pets that will not eat a com-

mercial dental diet. Dental chews and toys may be more effective for dogs and should certainly be used rather than calorie-rich 'junk' treats
- Despite a cosmetic (and aromatic!) improvement in the state of the teeth, it is unlikely that any diets are able to remove subgingival **plaque** and **calculus**. Without regular dental checks this can lead to **periodontal** pocketing and abscessation
- It must be emphasised to clients that home care of teeth is a helpful adjunct, but, as with humans, should not take the place of regular professional dental checks

Regular dental checks

This is the mainstay of dental care in dogs and cats and every effort should be made to educate clients in the importance of such examinations. The ideal interval between checks is uncertain, but at least every 12 months would seem to be reasonable.

- A full dental examination is impossible to perform in a conscious patient, but as much of the oral cavity as possible should be investigated
- The gums should be assessed for gingivitis and any bleeding noted. The degree of **plaque** and **calculus** build-up should be recorded. Unless the patient is amazingly calm, it is not possible to probe the teeth, but any gum recession should be noted
- The client should be asked whether there have been any problems with the pet's appetite, or any signs associated with dental pain (salivating, shuddering of the jaw or pawing at the mouth)
- The mouth should be opened and the **lingual** surfaces of the teeth examined. The tongue and **buccal** mucosa should be examined for any trauma caused by abrasion from maloccluding teeth or contact infection and inflammation
- Any problems should be recorded in the patient's history and the owners advised on the next step (i.e. improved home care or **periodontal** surgery)

- Aggressive or difficult patients should be examined under anaesthesia, especially if they have a history of dental problems
- Remember, **periodontal** disease can cause or worsen disease elsewhere in the body and is a considerable cause of morbidity in many pets. It is the vet's and nurse's responsibility to advise clients of the need for dental treatment

Repeated scaling and polishing under anaesthesia

Some practices advise annual scaling and polishing under general anaesthesia. Since it is only possible to perform a complete dental examination under anaesthesia, it would seem to make sense to combine an examination with prophylactic treatment.

- It is necessary to weigh up the advantages of complete prophylactic dental care with the disadvantages of anaesthesia. However, provided the patient is otherwise healthy, and every precaution is taken to improve anaesthetic safety (preanaesthetic checks, IVFT, good anaesthetic protocols), the risk of anaesthetic injury is minimal. On the other hand, the potential gain in health and well-being of the patient is tremendous
- Any patient will benefit from this, but it may be especially important for animals whose behaviour prevents any sort of home dental care
- Older animals are obviously more likely to require periodontic treatment than younger ones. However, starting regular dental prophylaxis *before* gingivitis is seen is more likely to maintain oral health. Again, excellent client communication is required to promote good veterinary dental care

Referral to veterinary dental specialists

As with any branch of veterinary medicine and surgery, it should be acknowledged that there may be limits to an individual's personal experience, or else limits to the range of treatments available in general practice. Veterinary dentistry is a very specialised subject and there are many new ways of treating various dental diseases that may not be accessible to the general practitioner. For example, endodontic surgery (filling or capping teeth), orthodontic and restorative dentistry are treatment modalities with which the owner may have some experience and may be reasonable alternatives, in expert hands, to extracting teeth. A request for referral should always be considered seriously and with the patient's best interests in mind.

COMMON ORAL TUMOURS

The oral cavity is a very common site for **neoplasia** in the dog and cat, with malignant tumours outnumbering benign ones. Tumours potentially arise from any part of the mouth, but usually originate from the gums in the dog and the gums and tongue in the cat. Table 9.2 lists some of the tumours more commonly encountered.

The term 'epulis' is subject to much confusion. The histological classification of epulides (plural of epulis) has been changed several times in recent years to differentiate between tissue types and **tumour** behaviour, with the result that many texts utilise a variety of names for the same **tumour** type. A good example is the acanthomatous epulis, which is also called a peripheral ameloblastoma. It is probably best referred to now as a basal cell carcinoma, which describes its biological behaviour much better (locally invasive, like many carcinomas). Epulis is also often used wrongly to describe the gingival **hyperplasia** seen in breeds such as the boxer.

Clinical signs of oral tumours

Clinical signs vary tremendously, and include:
- Inappetance
- Weight loss
- Drooling
- Gagging/retching
- Bleeding from the mouth
- Oral pain

Table 9.2 Common oral tumours of dogs and cats

Neoplasia	Benign or malignant	Usual site and behaviour
Odontoma	Benign	**Gingiva**/teeth (not considered neoplastic)
Central ameloblastoma	Benign	Tooth roots. Locally invasive, but does not metastasise
Ameloblastic fibroma	Benign	(Cats only.) **Gingiva**. Locally invasive
Acanthomatous epulis (basal cell carcinoma/ peripheral ameloblastoma)	Malignant	**Gingiva**. Locally invasive and aggressive – does not metastasise, but difficult to remove
Fibroma, papilloma, chondroma, haemangioma	Benign	Various sites around oral cavity, including **gingiva**, buccal mucosa, pharynx and tongue
Squamous cell carcinoma	Malignant	**Gingiva** (dogs), tongue (cats), tonsils. Locally invasive and metastatic
Malignant melanoma	Malignant	**Gingiva**, lips, cheek. Not necessarily pigmented. High metastatic rate
Fibrosarcoma	Malignant	**Gingiva**, palate, buccal mucosa. Locally invasive and aggressive. Rarely metastasise
Lymphosarcoma, osteosarcoma, haemangiosarcoma, mast-cell tumour, adenocarcinoma	Malignant	Various sites around oral cavity, including **gingiva**, buccal mucosa, pharynx and tongue

- Halitosis
- Difficulty breathing
- No clinical signs

Clinical examination may reveal an obvious mass on the gums, lips, **buccal** mucosa or tongue (Figure 9.13). It is more difficult to find masses under the tongue or in the pharyngeal tonsils, unless a meticulous examination is made. The submandibular and retropharyngeal lymph nodes should be palpated for enlargement. A full clinical examination should be made of the rest of the animal to look for other signs of disease. Pyrexia may indicate inflammation, although hyperthermia is a characteristic of many malignancies.

Diagnosis of oral tumours

Oral masses may appear smooth, rounded and similar in appearance to other oral tissues. Alternatively, they may be erosive, ulcerated, bleeding or pigmented. Unfortunately, it is

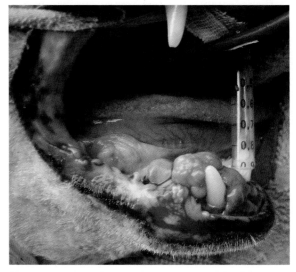

Figure 9.13 Mandibular **tumour** on dog. This large, irregular mandibular mass was noted during routine annual vaccination of a 12-year-old female neutered golden retriever. Fine-needle aspiration biopsy was not rewarding. Wedge biopsy was performed and the histopathologist returned a diagnosis of benign odontoma. A **rostral** hemimandibulectomy proved curative.

usually not possible to tell from the appearance of a mass whether it is neoplastic or inflammatory. Examination of the rest of the oral cavity sometimes gives clues as to the cause of the mass: for example, an ulcerated lesion in an otherwise healthy mouth is more likely to be neoplastic, whereas an inflamed lesion in a mouth with severe chronic **periodontitis** is fairly likely to be inflammatory. A trial course of antibiotics can be used to differentiate between **neoplasia** and inflammation, but there are drawbacks to this:

- Often the neoplasm is secondarily infected and may respond, to some extent, to antibiotics
- Time spent trying a course of antibiotics will increase the delay between diagnosis and treatment of **neoplasia**

There is little correlation between the appearance of an oral **tumour** and its biological behaviour: even the most benign-appearing rounded pink masses can turn out to be squamous cell carcinomas. Thus the *only way* to distinguish between benign and malignant oral masses is to perform biopsy (see below).

In addition to surgical biopsy, radiography of the oral cavity should be performed to investigate the extent of any bony changes associated with the mass. A search for metastases should include radiography of the thorax and abdomen, ultrasonography of the liver and aspiration of enlarged regional lymph nodes (or surgical biopsy of the lymph nodes). Metabolic profiles (haematology and biochemistry, urinalysis) should be carried out to look for signs of concurrent or secondary illness.

Treatment of oral tumours

Treatment will depend on **tumour** type and presence or absence of metastases.

- Benign tumours and locally invading malignant tumours are best treated by surgical excision. In order to gain a suitable margin of excision, it is often necessary to excise bone together with the mass. Depending on the site, this may involve maxillectomy or partial mandibulectomy

- Radiation therapy can be used with some degree of success to treat squamous cell carcinoma and basal cell carcinoma, with or without surgical debulking of the mass
- **Chemotherapy** is usually not successful in treating oral **neoplasia**, although cisplatin, doxorubicin and cyclophosphamide may provide short-term relief for patients with squamous cell carcinoma

In general, tumours towards the front of the mouth have a slightly better prognosis than tumours at the back of the oral cavity.

It must be remembered that many oral tumours are extremely painful, especially sublingual tumours. Pain is often responsible for the hypersalivation and anorexia of these patients (although other factors such as mechanical impairment of the tongue and malignancy-associated nausea are also involved). It is therefore important to provide **analgesia** for dogs and cats with oral **neoplasia,** and to consider humane euthanasia for patients that are non-responsive to treatment.

BIOPSY TECHNIQUES

Although FNAB can be performed on oral masses, its use is best restricted to soft masses under the tongue or in the **buccal** mucosa or the pharynx. Tougher gingival masses tend not to exfoliate (i.e. the yield of cells from FNAB is only very small and usually non-diagnostic). Often the architecture and spatial relationship between neoplastic cells are required to obtain a definitive diagnosis. Surgical biopsy is therefore recommended.

All surgical biopsy procedures require that the animal is anaesthetised, and so routine preanaesthetic checks and blood tests should be carried out. It is usually convenient to perform a surgical biopsy at the same time as thoracic radiography to look for evidence of metastases.

As with biopsies of masses elsewhere in the body, either a sample of tissue may be taken (incisional biopsy) or else an attempt is made to remove the whole mass and submit it for **histopathology** (excisional biopsy).

Incisional biopsy

- Radiographs of the oral cavity should be performed prior to the biopsy, so that the best biopsy site can be chosen. Haemorrhage due to the biopsy can also obscure radiographic changes
- The patient should be placed in sternal or lateral recumbency, so that the mass is uppermost. Sandbags may be placed under the patient's head to facilitate surgery. The pharynx should be packed with dental sponges or damp gauze swabs to prevent aspiration of blood
- A dental gag should be used as necessary to improve access to the mass. It is not possible to perform a proper surgical scrub in the oral cavity, but 0.12% chlorhexidine solution can be used to reduce bacterial counts. It is unusual to have a problem with biopsy wound infection in the mouth, due to the rich blood supply and the specialised immune defences. The surgical area should be draped and hats, masks and **sterile** gowns and gloves worn
- A no. 15 scalpel blade is used to obtain a biopsy: this can be performed in various ways. If the mass lies within the gums then a line of **gingiva** can be cut off (**gingivectomy**); if the mass is larger and deeply seated, then a wedge can be cut out of the gum. The sample should be taken from the edge of the mass, to include normal tissue. Many gingival masses are ossified or calcified and these can be difficult to remove with a scalpel blade. In these situations, bone-cutting forceps or an **osteotome** may be used to remove a section of bone
- There is usually a fair degree of haemorrhage, which can be controlled by pressure. The edges of the biopsy wound should be apposed and closed with simple interrupted sutures of 4/0 (1.5 metric) or 5/0 (1 metric) synthetic absorbable suture material (e.g. Polyglytone 6211 Caprosyn, Vetoquinol). Some masses are fairly **friable** and may not hold sutures. In this case, the wound may be left to granulate
- The biopsy should be placed in 10% formal-saline and sent for **histopathology**. Samples containing bone usually take longer for the histopathologist to examine as the sample needs to be decalcified for several days

Excisional biopsy

Small, well-demarcated masses on the **gingiva** can be removed completely and sent for **histopathology**. The complete removal of larger masses as an initial biopsy procedure is not recommended, as it is not possible to determine the margin of excision until a diagnosis has been reached.

- The patient should be prepared as above and aseptic precautions taken as applicable
- An elliptical incision is made around the mass, and extended to include an excision margin of at least 5 mm on all sides (and deep to the mass, if possible)
- Pressure is used to control haemorrhage and the wound is sutured with 4/0 (1.5 metric) or 5/0 (1 metric) synthetic absorbable suture material (e.g. Caprosyn, Vetoquinol) in a simple interrupted pattern
- The excised tissue is placed in 10% formal-saline and sent for **histopathology**

DENTAL PROCEDURES IN RABBITS

This section is intended to be an overview of rabbit dentistry, which is the main reason for presentation of rabbits at a veterinary practice. Many of the procedures for dealing with rabbits (medicine, anaesthesia, **analgesia**, surgery) require special knowledge and dedicated instrumentation. The interested reader is urged to consult a specialist text.

Normal dentition of the rabbit

Rabbits are hypsodont, meaning that the teeth are not closed at the apical region and continue to grow throughout life.

The dental formula of the rabbit is:

$$\frac{2I\ 0C\ 3P\ 3M}{1I\ 0C\ 2P\ 3M} = 28\ \text{Teeth}$$

There are two pairs of upper incisors, although the second pair are rather vestigial and lie behind the large upper incisors. There is a long, tooth-free space (the diastemer) between the incisors and the premolars (Figure 9.14), which is important for food **prehension** and mastication.

Dental disease in rabbits

Since rabbit teeth are constantly being worn down and replaced by rapid growth, build-up of **plaque** tends not to be a feature of rabbit dentistry. The two main dental/oral problems of rabbits are malocclusion and dental abscesses.

Malocclusion

Malocclusion can affect the incisors, the cheek teeth or both and affects a very high proportion of the pet rabbit population. Diet, genetics, trauma and infection are all known to have a role in the development of malocclusion.

Malocclusion results in lack of wearing of part or the entire occlusal surface of a tooth (Figure 9.15). Since the teeth constantly grow, any lack of wearing causes overgrowth of that tooth (or part of the tooth). This leads to the production of very long, abnormal-shaped teeth (usually

incisors) or sharp spurs (on molars) that rub against the tongue or the cheek and cause painful ulcerations. This in turn leads to inability to prehend (grasp) food or to masticate properly. Another problem is that rabbits fail to groom adequately and become dishevelled, or else are unable to carry out coprophagism, resulting in further nutritional deficiencies.

Depending on the angle of growth, upper and lower incisors may both grow out of the mouth and are often easily seen. Alternatively, they can grow inside the mouth and cause considerable trauma to the palate or mandible, or else interfere with the movement of the tongue.

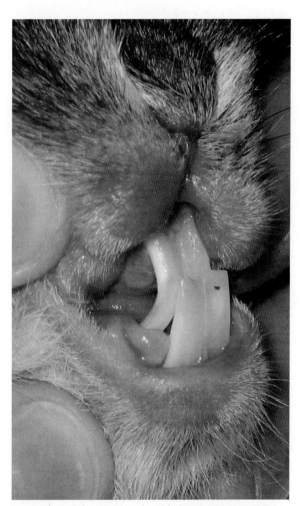

Figure 9.15 Overgrowth of incisors. Examination under anaesthesia demonstrated severe molar malocclusion.

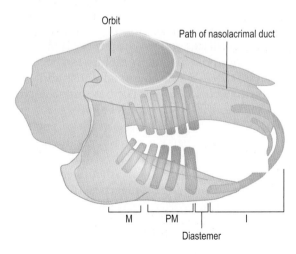

Figure 9.14 Rabbit skull showing normal dentition and path of nasolacrimal duct. M, molars; PM, premolars; I, incisors.

Clinical signs associated with malocclusion in rabbits are:
- Weight loss
- Inappetance, or inability to hold food in the mouth
- Hypersalivation (usually caused by the presence of sharp spurs)
- Patches of fur loss and scabbing on the chin and neck (caused by dribbling)
- Matted or patchy fur, or other evidence of lack of grooming
- Faecal soiling around the perineum (lack of coprophagia)
- Ocular discharge (secondary to blockage of nasolacrimal duct by impacted molars)

Chronic malocclusion is a welfare issue because it is painful, results in malnourishment and predisposes rabbits to eye infections, skin infections, digestive problems and myiasis (fly strike, due to faecal soiling).

Dental abscesses

Tooth abscesses typically occur in the cheek teeth of rabbits and are often secondary to malocclusion:
- Food may become impacted between deranged teeth
- Ulceration and inflammation of the **buccal** or gingival mucosa allows ingress of pyogenic (pus-forming) bacteria
- Tooth-root impaction secondary to malocclusion causes **periodontal** and apical pocketing, giving a site for bacterial colonisation

Pasteurella multocida and *Staphylococcus aureus* are most commonly isolated from rabbit abscesses (see Chapter 8). Clinical signs are usually fairly obvious: a large mass bulging out from the cheek or the jaw. Dribbling and anorexia are also common features. Occasionally, thick, creamy pus can be seen emanating from the **periodontal** space of affected molars.

Treatment of dental disease in rabbits

In every case, the rabbit should have a full clinical examination. It is not possible to examine the oral cavity of a conscious rabbit fully; although a brief glance with an otoscope may reveal molar spurs, if these are not seen on a conscious examination it should not be assumed the molars are healthy.

Rabbits presenting with dental disease may be healthy, and eating well. Many, however, will be malnourished to some extent. Since general anaesthesia is required for most dental interventions, it is important to warn clients that anaesthesia carries a higher mortality rate in rabbits than in cats and dogs, and that this is worsened with dehydration and malnutrition.

IVFT should be instigated, and, if possible, severely malnourished rabbits should be hospitalised and syringe-fed for several days to reduce anaesthetic risks. Dental disease is invariably painful, and most rabbits benefit from **analgesia** (opioids, NSAIDs, e.g. buprenorphine, 0.05 mg/kg subcutaneously (SC), meloxicam 0.2 mg/kg SC).

There are various anaesthesia protocols for rabbits, and the reader is recommended to read a specialist rabbit surgery text. Suggestions are:
- Induction and maintenance with volatile anaesthetic: isoflurane is unpleasant-smelling and often causes breath-holding in rabbits, resulting in a 'messy' induction. Sevoflurane is much better tolerated and rapidly induces anaesthesia. Intubation of rabbits is difficult, due to the long, narrow pharynx, but with practice it is possible with a small (size 2–3-mm non-cuffed) endotracheal tube. If intubation is not possible, many rabbits can be kept anaesthetised by intranasal administration of **volatile agent** (a urinary catheter attached to an endotracheal tube connector is placed in one of the nostrils to the level of the soft palate – rabbits are obligate intranasal breathers and so cannot respire via the oral cavity). Halogenated volatile anaesthetics have no appreciable analgesic properties, so opioids and NSAIDs, or even local **analgesia**, must be used in addition
- Injection of anaesthetic or sedative drugs (Table 9.3). Intramuscular injection can be very painful in rabbits; injection via the SC route appears to result in similar rates of distribution and is often easier to perform. The

Table 9.3 Sedative/anaesthetic combinations for rabbits (all are administered intramuscularly or subcutaneously unless otherwise stated)

Combination	Dose/3-kg rabbit
Medetomidine (Domitor, Pfizer) 0.25 mg/kg	Domitor 0.75 ml
Buprenorphine (Vetergesic, Alstoe Animal Health) 0.05 mg/kg	Vetergesic 0.5 ml
and/or	
Ketamine (Ketaset, Fort Dodge) 15 mg/kg	Ketaset 0.45 ml
Can be partially reversed by atipamezole (Antisedan, Pfizer) 1 mg/kg	Antisedan 0.6 ml
Ketamine 15 mg/kg and diazepam (Phoenix Pharma) 1 mg/kg	Ketaset 0.45 ml Diazepam 0.6 ml

suggested combinations usually provide sufficient **analgesia** and sedation to perform most dental procedures: additional anaesthesia can be provided by the intranasal administration of volatile anaesthesia

Trimming incisors

Incisor overgrowth due to malocclusion can often be managed by regular trimming. Clipping incisors with nail clippers or similar implements is no longer recommended; the teeth can easily shatter, causing pain and predisposing to root abscessation. The teeth can be easily and rapidly sectioned to a normal anatomical length using a high-speed dental drill or burr, or a cutting disc attached to a drill. Provided the rabbit is adequately restrained, there is no need for sedation. The water-cooling jet should be turned off, or down to avoid the risk of aspiration. Provided the cutting tool is sharp and the procedure is performed quickly, there is minimal build-up of heat. Some sort of guard should be used to prevent inadvertent damage to the gums or lips by the burr.

Incisors grow in excess of 2 mm weekly, so the interval between trimmings should be no more than 3–6 weeks.

Incisor removal

In some cases, regular trimming is not possible (either due to the temperament of the rabbit or lack of owner compliance). In these cases, or if regular trimming fails to manage the problem, the incisors can be removed, providing a permanent solution. The procedure is technically more demanding than carnivore incisor removal and is made much easier by correct instrumentation. The **periodontal** ligament is patiently broken down with a small dental elevator and the tooth is removed by rotating in the direction of the curve of the tooth. Incomplete removal of the root will result in regrowth, necessitating repeated surgery. Antibiotics (e.g. enrofloxacin (Baytril, Bayer) 20 mg/kg SC SID) should be administered for 7–10 days following surgery, and analgesics should be continued for 3–5 days.

Molar trimming

Sharp spurs on molars are painful and can result in severe trauma to the tongue and cheeks. As discussed, it is not possible to examine the mouth of a conscious rabbit fully, so if there is a strong index of suspicion for cheek teeth malocclusion, then the rabbit should be sedated or anaesthetised. Spurs should be clipped back using rodent teeth clippers (Figure 9.16) and the edges of all the molars should be brought back to a uniform size and shape using a molar rasp. Alternatively, high-speed burrs and cutting discs may be used and there are a number of commercially available 'hobby' drills available that are suitable. Access to the molar arcades is the main problem: rabbit pouch dilators and dental gags should be used to improve visualisation, and a climber's head torch

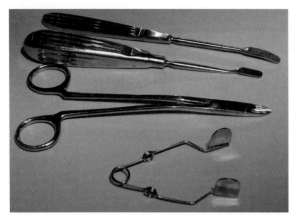

Figure 9.16 Selection of dental instruments for rabbits: top to bottom: diamond-coated tooth rasp, metal tooth rasp, rodent molar clippers, cheek dilators.

is an incredibly useful way of improving illumination.

Molar extraction

Molar extraction is indicated when there is severe impaction or root **abscess**, or if malocclusion results in rapid production of molar spurs. As with incisor extraction, the process is helped by specialised instruments and experience. It may be necessary to remove the molar from the opposite arcade, to avoid overgrowth of that tooth.

Treatment of dental abscesses

As discussed in Chapter 8, the prognosis for abscesses in rabbits is generally poor. Thorough **debridement** of the **abscess** is required, including extraction of the affected tooth or teeth and deep curettage of the **alveolar bone**. The wound

is usually left open and managed by regular flushing and repeated **debridement**. Various packing agents (calcium hydroxide, gentamicin-impregnated beads) have been suggested, but owners should be advised that long courses of antibiotics and repeated surgery are often required.

Prevention of dental disease in rabbits

The incidence of rabbit dental disease, especially malocclusion, has been linked fairly conclusively to badly designed commercial diets. Development of **alveolar bone** is easily disrupted by imbalances in calcium, phosphorus and vitamin D. Most commercial diets claim to have a correct balance of these nutrients, but they rely on rabbits eating all the components of the diet in equal ratios. Unfortunately, many rabbits pick their favourite bits of the diet, and leave other parts. This results in an overall dietary imbalance and abnormal bone growth. **Alveolar bone** growth is affected, softens slightly and allows movement of the tooth root and subsequent deviation of the plane of growth of the tooth.

In addition, the softer texture of the commercial diet requires less grazing and masticating time: this is also important in even wearing of incisor and molar surfaces.

The introduction of pellet diets, where there is no chance to pick and choose has helped: by far the healthiest diet for rabbits is grass and ideally rabbits should be encouraged to graze grass for at least 6 h every day. Good-quality hay should also be provided.

There does appear to be some hereditary nature to dental disease in rabbits, and owners of rabbits with malocclusion should be encouraged to have them neutered, or at least to refrain from allowing them to breed.

10 The postoperative patient

THE RECOVERY PHASE

Monitoring of the patient should not cease once the endotracheal tube has been removed. The precise level of monitoring each patient receives during the recovery period will depend on:

- The age and general health of the patient; in particular, the preoperative condition
- The nature of the surgery performed, and the anaesthetic or sedative used
- Any complications that may have occurred during surgery (e.g. blood loss, anaesthetic problems)
- The presence of any surgical implants (e.g. thoracic drains, Penrose drains, orthopaedic implants)
- The rate of recovery of the patient

In general, the patient should be constantly monitored until it is able to maintain itself in sternal recumbency and raise its head. Most postoperative anaesthetic deaths occur due to airway occlusion (through **emesis**, saliva or occlusion from poor positioning). Once in sternal recumbency, the risk of inadvertent occlusion of the airway due to body position is small. Monitoring may be relaxed a little, but the patient should be checked at least every 5 min and preferably kept in line of vision for some while after.

If the anaesthetic has been correctly administered, most patients will achieve sternal recumbency by about 5 min postsurgery. Elderly animals, or those suffering from debilitating or chronic illness, may take longer to recover to this level. In addition, loss of body temperature during the anaesthetic will prolong recovery time. Regardless of actual loss of body temperature, most animals are likely to benefit from warm blankets on recovery. Shivering, seen during the recovery phase, may indicate cold or pain, or may simply be an anaesthetic effect.

Once a reasonable recovery has been made from the anaesthetic, the owners should be phoned and informed of their pet's progress. If an appointment has not already been made for discharge, it can be done at this time.

Intravenous (IV) fluid therapy should be maintained until the patient is able to drink or eat (or until hydration has been restored in ill patients). Other than supplying fluids, the catheter remains a useful IV access for postanaesthetic emergencies. When removing the catheter, the venepuncture site should be cleaned with water (with disinfectant soap, if desired) and a temporary dressing placed (a pad of cotton wool and a layer of cohesive bandage are usually adequate) to reduce bruising. The dressing should be removed after 2 h, or the client instructed to remove it that evening.

Any surgical drains should be checked regularly to ensure the patient has not removed them and that the level of discharge is not excessive (perhaps indicating internal haemorrhage). Elizabethan collars should be worn to reduce the risk of drain removal. Draining fluids should be cleaned up as soon as possible as they constitute infection hazards. A little petroleum jelly may be smeared on to the skin around a drain to prevent irritation. If dressings are placed over drains then they should be checked at least four times daily and more often if they become rapidly soiled. Active drains should be checked for adequate seal and the suction device recharged as necessary. Due to the risk of pulling out or infection, and due to hygiene considerations, it is not recommended that patients be sent home with wound drains in place. Animals with thoracic drains placed should not be left unattended at any time as death can occur rapidly due to lung collapse following accidental removal of these tubes. Discharge will never cease completely with drains in situ, and so they should be removed (under the veterinary surgeon's instruction) when an acceptable low level of discharge has been reached.

Food and water should be withheld from the patient until it is able to stand. A little water may then be offered: if this is accepted and held down, then a small amount of food may be given. If water is not drunk, but the animal appears alert, it is perfectly acceptable to offer a little food.

Geriatric patients in particular will benefit from receiving nutrition soon after surgery. Animals recovering from gastrointestinal surgery will usually have food withheld for the first 12–24 h, but water should be offered soon after recovery unless otherwise stated.

The surgical wound should be examined soon after surgery, every few hours during the day and immediately before discharging the patient to ensure there is no haemorrhage or self-mutilation of sutures. Haemorrhage should be carefully monitored and quantified. If bleeding is excessive, or if any fresh blood is seen after surgery, the patient's pulse, heart rate, capillary refill time and mucous membrane colour should all be assessed and the blood pressure measured. Any alteration from normal should alert the examiner to the possibility of slipped ligatures. If a **laparotomy** wound is losing fresh blood and there is a drop in blood pressure, increase in capillary refill time or heart rate, and the mucous membranes look pale, then the animal should be reanaesthetised and the wound opened to search for bleeding vascular stumps. Any fresh haemorrhage from a minor surgical wound may be managed by applying a pressure bandage, which may be checked after 1 h, or sooner if blood is seen to be seeping through the dressing. If pressure is insufficient to control haemorrhage, consideration should be given to reanaesthetising the patient and exploring the wound. If this is done, then the surgical site must be fully prepped for aseptic surgery and **sterile** clothing and gloves worn. Antibiotics should be administered.

If no obvious cause is found for the haemorrhage, the wound should be closed and another pressure bandage applied, or **sterile** cotton gauze stents sutured to the wound. Bloods should be taken to investigate disorders of **haemostasis** and a colloidal drip (or transfusion) commenced if severe fluid or blood losses have occurred.

Any sign of nibbling of sutures or excessive interest in the wound site by the patient should be prevented by the use of an Elizabethan collar or wound dressing.

The patient's urine output should be monitored postoperatively. It is usually sufficient to note whether or not the patient has urinated prior to discharge for minor surgical patients.

Box 10.1

Normal urine output (dog and cat) = 1–2 ml/kg per h

So:

A 10-kg dog should produce between 240 ml and 480 ml in 24 h

A 4-kg cat should produce between 96 ml and 192 ml in 24 h

Hospitalised patients should have urine output recorded in as much detail as possible. Cat litter can be weighed before and after urination to provide a fairly accurate measure of urine production. Animals with urinary catheters should have closed-bag systems in place, facilitating urine measurement. It may be possible to measure the urine output of dogs by timely interposition of a measuring jug. What is important, however, is to ensure that the anaesthetic has not reduced urine production. Therefore, if the animal has not urinated by the time of discharge, the owner must be asked to keep an eye on this and report back the following day if no urine has been passed (Box 10.1).

It is unacceptable to discharge patients that are soiled with blood or excrement. Any such soiling reflects poorly on the practice and negates all the hard work that has been done thus far. Any blood from the surgery should be sponged off and the surrounding fur dried and groomed as necessary.

INDICATORS OF PAIN AND POSTOPERATIVE ANALGESIA

As discussed in Chapter 3, attention to recognition of pain and balanced **analgesia** is crucial to minor (indeed, any) surgery. The appropriate and reasoned use of analgesics, before a painful procedure is carried out, dramatically decreases the potential for postoperative pain. However, it is important to realise that there is still likely to be some degree of postoperative pain and it is necessary to keep a tight rein on this to prevent pain worsening beyond our ability to control it.

Table 10.1 Simple postoperative pain-scoring system (the lower the score, the better)

Pain assessment modality	Score
Vocalisation: 1–4 1, quiet; 2, occasional whimpering; 3, frequent crying or yelping; 4, continuous crying or yelping	
Behaviour: 1–4 1, asleep; 2, frightened, hunched; 3, restless, moving frequently; 4, unable to settle, constantly moving	
Reaction to stroking: 1–4 1, purring or responding to stroke; 2, occasional response to stroking; 3, not responding to stroking; 4, becoming aggressive when stroked	
Touching wound site: 1–4 1, no response or change in behaviour when wound touched; 2, stops purring briefly when wound touched; 3, tries to move away when wound touched; 4, becomes aggressive or vocalises when wound touched	
Total (minimum 4, maximum 16)	

Repeating the **opioid** dose prior to the animal waking up is more effective than after waking.

Indicators of pain postoperatively include:

- Shivering
- Vocalisation (this is a certain sign of pain when it happens as a response to moving an injured limb or when touched over the surgical site)
- Panting (or abnormally shallow breathing if thoracic surgery has been performed), or an increased respiratory or heart rate
- Inappetance
- Abnormal behaviour (sudden aggression or fear)
- Hunched posture, restlessness
- Attempts to bite or scratch the surgical site

Pain scoring should be carried out prior to surgery and at regular intervals following surgery. Several systems for scoring exist; some are easier to use than others. A very simple scoring system is shown in Table 10.1. This system is very basic and may need to be modified for some patients (e.g. naturally aggressive patients may not be amenable to stroking assessment!), but it has the benefit of being extremely easy to perform with little extra training in practice. It is more appropriate to monitor individual trends in pain scores than to compare pain scores between patients.

Non-steroidal anti-inflammatory drugs (NSAIDs) are usually administered prior to surgery and then followed by a course of oral medication from 24 h after surgery. Repeating a dose of NSAID before data sheet recommendations risks gastrointestinal damage and kidney or liver toxicity.

The mainstay of postoperative **analgesia** is **opioid** administration. Suggested dose rates and frequency of administration of **opioids** are shown in Table 3.2.

Buprenorphine may be administered every 8 h (or more frequently if required). Morphine does not last as long (4–6 h) and may need to be repeated more frequently, but the dose range is narrower for this drug, so care must be taken not to overdose.

Local analgesics may be administered around a wound site by injection or topically. The most common method of postoperative administration of local anaesthetics is intrapleurally via chest tube following thoracic surgery.

Epidural analgesia, or fentanyl patches (see Chapter 3) should provide several hours (in the case of the former) or several days (for the latter) of **analgesia**. However, **epidural** injections can wear off quicker than expected and fentanyl patches can be absorbed more rapidly or the patches may become dislodged, so it is important not to forget about monitoring these patients for pain.

For most minor surgical procedures, pain is transient and a 3–5-day course of NSAIDs usually provides sufficient **analgesia**. For minor cases, it may be unnecessary to repeat injections of **opioids** prior to waking the patient up from anaesthesia.

DISCHARGING THE PATIENT

- Wherever possible, it is recommended that a specific appointment be made for a patient's discharge. This ensures that time is made available to brief the owner fully about the surgery and any relevant aftercare, and for the owner to ask any questions. It is preferable to perform the discharge consultation in a separate room to reduce distractions

- It is a good idea to talk to the owner before the pet is given back. The reason for this is that quite often the reunion between animal and owner may well prove distracting and the client is unlikely to be paying full attention to the advice given

- It is also a good idea to issue the owner with written postoperative instructions. These serve as an aide-mémoire for the owner and may be referred to if the client is anxious about any aspect of the pet's recovery later. Written instructions may also be helpful if there is any argument at a later date about postoperative instructions (Figure 10.1)

- In addition to general postoperative instructions, bandage care sheets may be given, with instructions about when to return for a dressing change, how to ensure the bandage remains clean, what the allowed level of exercise is and what to do if the patient manages to remove the dressing (Figure 5.10)

- Remember that some clients may be squeamish. It may be wise to warn clients about the size of wounds (if they haven't already been informed) and about large shaved areas.

- The administration of any ongoing medication should be explained, together with any caveats (whether the medicine should be given with food, or on an empty stomach and whether it is safe to administer several drugs together)

- Prior to returning the patient, a final check is made of the wound to ensure no sutures have loosened and no bleeding has occurred

- When the patient is returned to the client, the wounds, if not obvious, should be pointed out and relevant aftercare or monitoring reiterated. If an Elizabethan collar has not been fitted, the owner should be informed what to do if the patient tries to mutilate the sutures (collect a collar, apply a dressing (sock, stocking, T-shirt), bitter apple spray or Viatop anti-itch cream (Boehringer Ingelheim))

The PetScan Clinic

Veterinary Surgery
1 Halstead Street
Lembert
Surrey

Anaesthesia _____ Alfie's _____ **Convalescence**

_____ Alfie _____ has had an anaesthetic today, and, just as we would, will be feeling a little strange. Anaesthetic is given into the vein in the foreleg, so you will see that a patch of hair has been clipped away to give a clean area to inject into.

It is quite common for animals to have a slight cough after an anaesthetic – this is because a tube is passed into the trachea (windpipe) during the procedure to ensure a clear airway at all times, and to administer the anaesthetic gas mixture.

When you arrive home, please keep_____ Alfie _____ warm and quiet. It is best if young children or other pets are kept away for the first evening, to avoid unintentional excitement, or even possible damage to the wound.

Pain relief after an operation

_____ Alfie _____ will have received pain-killing medication before, during and after the operation. If necessary, you will be supplied with pain-killing tablets to give at home – details will appear under medication and _____ Alfie's _____ veterinary nurse will explain their use to you.

Exercise

Keep dogs on a lead and cats indoors for the first 24 hours, as the anaesthetic can leave them feeling a little disorientated. Even if your cat appears entirely normal, its coordination will not be as good and so it would be at risk when running across roads, jumping fences, etc. The amount of exercise suitable for _____ Alfie _____will vary according to the procedure that has been carried out, and its own rate of recovery. _____ Alfie's _____ vet will advise you.

Feeding

It is not uncommon for animals to feel queasy after an anaesthetic, just as we would ourselves. However, the body needs food to be able to recover and repair itself. You should offer_____ Alfie _____ half_his_ normal amount of food on the evening after the operation, but do not be too concerned if _he_ does not eat very much. If _he_ is not eating normally the day after the operation, please telephone and speak to one of our veterinary nurses who will be able to advise you.

Wound care

You should make regular checks on_____ Alfie's _____ wound to ensure there is no redness, swelling, discharge or other problems. If you are at all concerned about the wound, please feel free to telephone and speak to one of our veterinary nurses. They are all trained to advise you and will not hesitate to refer you to _____ Alfie's _____ veterinary surgeon if they feel it is necessary.

Stitches

Not all wounds will have visible stitches, but _____ Alfie's _____ nurse will advise you about this on collection from the hospital. Normally, stitches are removed after about 10 days.

_____ Alfie's _____ Veterinary Surgeon: _____ Ivor Scalpel _____

_____ Alfie's _____ Veterinary Nurse: _____ Anna Baric _____

Medication: _Synulox 250mg tablets: one tablet twice daily – start tomorrow_

Rimadyl 20mg tablets: one tablet twice daily – start tomorrow

Date and time of next appointment: _____ Thursday 20th, 9.30am _____

Special instructions: _____ Do not allow Alfie to bite the postman's leg again _____

Figure 10.1 Example of a postoperative care sheet.

- An itemised bill should be presented to the client and any unforeseen costs explained. In most practices it is usual for the account to be settled straightaway
- An appointment should be made for postoperative check and/or dressing change

POSTOPERATIVE CHECKS

The purpose of the postoperative check is:
- To check that the patient has suffered no ill-effects from the anaesthetic
- To ensure the wound is progressing well and there is no sign of complication
- To change dressings/bandages if necessary
- To allow the client to voice any queries regarding the surgery

It also acts, importantly, to improve or reinforce bonds between the client and the practice. Postoperative checks are usually carried out 48–72 h after surgery, though the timing should be adjusted to take into account dressing changes.

The animal should be given a brief clinical examination, to include temperature, pulse, respiration and colour of mucous membranes. The owner should be asked whether the animal has eaten, drunk, passed urine and defecated. The dressing should be changed and the wound inspected.

A fresh dressing should be placed, if necessary. As a matter of good hygiene, gloves should be worn when removing dressings and the old dressings should be examined for signs of infected discharge and disposed of immediately into clinical waste. A clean pair of gloves should be worn to place the fresh dressing. Dressings covering open wounds should be placed aseptically following the guidelines in Chapters 5 and 6.

Some sort of pain assessment should be carried out (this may simply involve palpating the wound, noting response and asking the owner whether the pet has been showing any signs of pain). Any problems administering medication should be addressed and the dosing frequency should be confirmed. Any concerns the owner may have should be noted on the patient records and dealt with, if possible.

POSTOPERATIVE COMPLICATIONS FOLLOWING MINOR SURGERY

Postoperative complications following minor surgery tend to fall into several categories:
- Postanaesthetic complications
- Wound infections or breakdown
- Suture reactions
- Seroma/haematoma formation
- Self-trauma of surgical site
- Patient discomfort/pain

Postanaesthetic complications

Provided a thorough preanaesthetic examination was performed, fluid balance was attended to (preferably with IV fluid therapy) and the anaesthetic monitoring was excellent, the risk of postanaesthetic complications should be very small. The most serious postoperative complication arising from anaesthesia is acute renal failure or exacerbation of borderline chronic renal failure. Diagnosis is dependent on blood biochemistry and urine specific gravity measurement. Treatment is aimed at restoring fluid balance and using diuretics to attempt to reverse acute renal failure.

Wound infections or breakdown

Wound infections typically, but not always, result from a failure of aseptic technique (Figure 10.2). **Haematogenous** spread of bacteria and self-trauma result in the remainder of cases. Diagnosis of wound infection is usually based on the appearance of the wound (discharge, inflammation and breakdown) and presence of pyrexia and pain. Swabs should be taken for culture and sensitivity (if not already done: see Chapter 7) and antibiotic treatment instigated, using a broad-spectrum antibiotic (e.g. clavulanate-potentiated amoxicillin (Synulox, Pfizer) 8.7 mg/kg subcutaneously SID or 12.5–25 mg/kg orally BID). The wound should be cleaned and dressed; any sutures involved in the infection should be removed (see Chapter 7). Any wound that breaks down despite proper wound management should

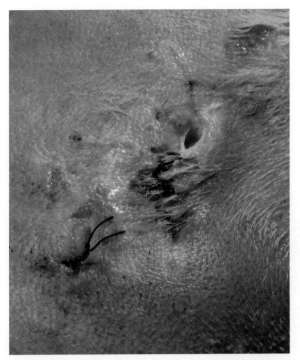

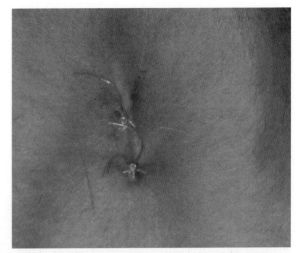

Figure 10.3 This small seroma following midline ovariohysterectomy in a cat was left to resolve spontaneously.

Figure 10.2 Wound breakdown following inappropriate primary closure of an infected wound. The wound was managed by **debridement** and delayed primary closure.

be debrided and the tissue submitted for **histopathology**: occasionally underlying **neoplasia** results in poor wound-healing.

Suture reactions

Provided synthetic absorbable or non-absorbable sutures have been placed, suture reactions are unusual. However, when they do occur they tend to occur several days postoperatively, usually when the wound is almost healed. Diagnosis is made on the basis of inflammation overlying individual sutures, with or without discharge. Pyrexia tends to suggest infection rather than reaction and it is more common to see the knots acting as reservoirs for infection than true suture reactions. If the wound is healed and the reaction is to the skin sutures, treatment involves simply removing the sutures. If, however, the subcutaneous sutures are involved, there may be no alternative but to anaesthetise and open the wound

under aseptic conditions and remove all the suture material, suturing with a different type of material or leaving the wound to heal by secondary intention. The removed suture material should be submitted for culture and sensitivity: most often the suture reaction is in fact caused by bacterial sequestration around the suture material.

Seroma/haematoma formation

Seroma occurs when dead space has been insufficiently closed during wound repair. Fluid accumulates in this dead space and causes bulging of the skin surface. Haematoma occurs when there is potential dead space coupled with bleeding into the wound, usually by inadequate attention to **haemostasis** or a particularly bouncy patient.

Haematoma and seroma formation results in increased healing time and increased risk of infection. Small seromas (1 cm in diameter) may be left to resolve spontaneously (Figure 10.3). Larger seromas and haematomas may be emptied by aspiration with a 22 G needle and application of a pressure bandage to prevent reformation. It is occasionally necessary to drain them by removing the sutures and allowing the wound to heal by secondary intention or to treat surgically by placement of a drain.

Self-trauma of surgical site

Although some patients are notorious bandage worriers and suture chewers, most cases of post-surgical wound self-trauma are caused by inadequate **analgesia**, inflammation or infection (Figure 10.4). Therefore these should be ruled out if self-trauma is seen. Provided the patient has not reopened the wound or allowed infection to gain entry, the wound may be cleaned with a dilute skin disinfectant (e.g. 0.5% chlorhexidine) and a dressing placed to protect the wound. An Elizabethan collar may be fitted. If the patient is scratching the wound with fore- or hind-limb claws, then padded foot bandages may be placed.

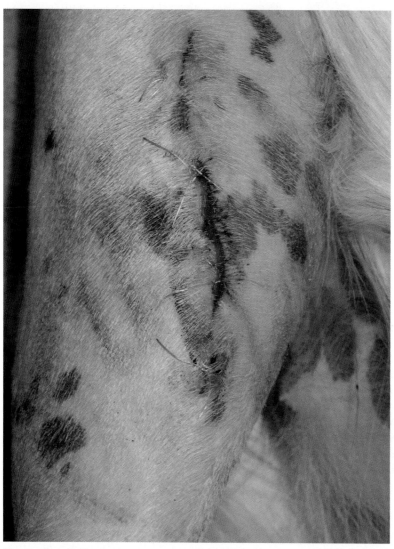

Figure 10.4 Self-trauma: the central wound edges have been displaced and there is a noticeable ridge of exposed skin edge. Self-trauma was most likely due to pain and irritation from the clipper rash. A buster collar was placed and anti-inflammatories administered. The wound healed uneventfully.

If the patient has opened the wound or caused infection, then the wound should be treated as a **contaminated** or infected wound and allowed to heal by delayed primary or secondary intention healing (see Chapter 7).

Patient discomfort/pain

This may be due to inflammation, infection or pulling of sutures. Any tension on the wound edges is a bad thing and will delay healing. Tight sutures with attendant inflammation and discomfort should be removed and the wound managed appropriately (as an open wound if a large number of sutures need to be removed). Any discomfort caused by over-tight subcutaneous sutures will tend to ease after a few days due to elastic accommodation of the tissues. Stents may cause irritation and should be removed 3–5 days postoperatively.

Inflammation and infection causing postoperative pain should be dealt with appropriately (see above) and the level of **analgesia** reappraised.

MRSA

Methicillin-resistant *Staphylococcus aureus* (MRSA) is now one of the most common – and certainly the most notorious – **nosocomial** infections in human surgery. MRSA presents a problem since resistance to various antibiotics has developed, there now being few antibiotics to which the bacterium is sensitive. The mainstay of treatment used to be gentamicin, but resistance to this antibiotic developed in the 1980s. The most effective drug at the moment is vancomycin, although resistance has developed in Japan and it is likely that this resistance will spread to other countries.

At the time of writing, a handful of veterinary cases of MRSA postoperative infections have occurred in the UK, though this number is sure to rise. Many factors have been blamed for the emergence of multiply resistant bacteria in hospitals, the main ones being the widespread overuse (and misuse) of antibiotics, a general reduction in standards of hygiene in hospitals, high theatre caseloads and the poor funds available to the health services.

Whatever the causes, the danger is a very real and growing one to the veterinary profession. With the emergence of multiply resistant other bacteria (vancomycin-resistant enterococci, multidrug-resistant tuberculosis, increasing resistance in *Escherichia coli* and *Salmonella* spp.), it becomes more and more important to act sensibly to reduce the risk in veterinary practice and to make the public aware of the commitment of the profession to deal with the problem.

Potential sources of infection for MRSA include the patient itself, the owner, the surgeon and other members of the surgical and nursing team, and other patients. In addition, clinical waste, poorly disinfected surfaces, cages and instruments may all aid transmission of infection.

There are four main components to tackling the MRSA problem:
1. Preventing infection in the first place (see below)
2. Finding new drugs to treat the infection: research is ongoing to find new classes of antibiotics to which otherwise resistant bacteria are susceptible
3. Limiting the development of further resistance in this and other bacteria, really by promoting sensible and appropriate use of antibiotics. This involves reducing the use of antibiotics to those cases that really need them (and relying more on aseptic technique to prevent infection), using antibiotics on the basis of culture and sensitivity wherever possible (reserving newer antibiotics for the treatment of resistant bacteria only) and using the correct dose and duration of treatment to eliminate targeted bacteria
4. Tracing the source of MRSA infection wherever possible and adjusting cleaning and nursing protocols accordingly

The key to preventing infection with MRSA is hygiene and strict attention to aseptic technique:

- Regular and effective cleaning of the practice; disinfection of all surfaces (including walls, floors and ceilings)
- Ensuring that **sterile** gloves and gowns, hats and masks are worn for every surgical intervention
- Hand-washing between patients (preferably using a combination alcohol and chlorhexidine soap)
- Immediate disposal of soiled dressings and other clinical waste; always wearing disposable gloves to change dressings; wearing disposable aprons and gloves to handle bedding

HANDLING CLIENT CONCERNS AND COMPLAINTS

We live in a litigious society, and are constantly bombarded by advertisements telling us to claim for damages and get compensation for accidents, negligence or misfortune. Fortunately, the veterinary profession has a reputation for honesty and integrity that its members work hard to maintain. Unfortunately, things do not always go according to plan: accidents happen, mistakes occur. Hopefully, this should be rare in any practice. What happens more commonly is that poor communication between the practice and the client leads to misunderstanding or incorrect expectations of treatment in one form or another (Box 10.2).

Client concerns may simply be that: concern. It usually just takes a few minutes to talk to owners to allay any fears or answer any questions they may have about the treatment of their pet. It is all too easy to forget that owners often have little medical knowledge and may be genuinely frightened for their pet. Client concerns often come down to several factors: cost, prognosis, concern for the well-being (pain, illness) of their

pet, or other concerns not necessarily to do with their pet.

Cost

Cost is one of the main reasons for client concerns and complaints. Most of these complaints can be prevented through proper communication about charges prior to any procedure being done. Most practices are computerised now, making the production of printed estimates relatively easy. It is up to us to suggest the best options for treatment; it is up to the clients to see whether that is within their budget. If it looks as though treatment is going to exceed the estimate, the owners should be informed as soon as possible and given a more realistic estimate for costs. It is not acceptable simply to let costs increase and to present the client with an unexpected bill at the end of treatment. The consent form for anaesthetic or hospitalisation should make it clear that the client has understood the charges and is also consenting to payment of those charges. Any changes to the estimate should be annotated in the client records: it may even be appropriate to request the client to sign a new consent form.

Talking frankly about money is something a lot of people find difficult. The main thing is to be comfortable about the pricing policy of the practice. If you consider a certain procedure is costly, it is much more difficult to convince a client that it is fairly priced. Costs of treatment are calculated in a very complex way that must take into account drugs and consumables, purchase price of equipment, building rent/rates, staff salaries, utilities bills and many other running costs. Rather than being embarrassed about charging a client so much for a procedure, you should feel proud about charging a substantial amount of money because a substantial amount of effort, technique and care has gone into the treatment.

Owners often buy pets before they have considered the financial implications of aftercare. They may be unaware of necessary or recommended prophylactic treatment for them and are likely to be unaware of probable costs should any accident or illness befall them. Advising clients

Box 10.2

Most client complaints are due to poor communication, often regarding money.

to make some sort of provision for illness is a very good idea, and may form part of a new pet check or a puppy party. Pet insurance should be encouraged.

Prognosis, concern for the well-being of the pet; informed consent

Naturally enough, many clients may well be concerned as to whether their pet will make a good recovery after surgery, whether it will be a painful procedure or whether there will be any ongoing problems. Clients do not always take in all the information given by the vet. It is worthwhile taking time in the admission consultation to allow owners to ask questions regarding the surgery and make sure they are aware of any postoperative care (e.g. bandages, cage rest, medication). A common question asked by clients is: 'am I doing the right thing?' This sort of question should always be addressed carefully. It is important not to give rash promises regarding the success of a surgical procedure, both from a legal and also from a compassionate point of view. Nor should one be overly pessimistic.

It is important to fulfil the criteria of informed consent. Without the detailed knowledge of all aspects of medicine and surgery that vets and nurses have, it is difficult to be fully informed about a surgical procedure. There is thus great potential for informing a client about a procedure in a biased way. It is therefore crucial that clients are as fully informed as possible and have time to consider the options and to ask any questions that may come to them.

Clients may have justifiable cause for concern if a procedure that they requested was not performed. A more serious cause for complaint is performing a procedure without consent. This latter may constitute surgical trespass and highlights the importance of a signed consent form. Animals are often admitted for multiple procedures (e.g. dental descale, dematting and nail-clipping under the same anaesthetic) and it is frustrating for the owner if one of the ancillary procedures is omitted, especially if the temperament of the animal precludes a conscious nail clip. Some owners are unaware that clipping of

hair may be necessary for procedures and may become annoyed upon seeing various shaved patches. It is not our role to judge owners for what may seem to us to be petty concerns; it is our responsibility to ensure the owners are made aware of procedures like clipping beforehand (Box 10.3).

As discussed in Chapter 2, the owner should be aware of who is performing the procedure. In human hospitals, it is accepted as routine that a nurse sutures wounds. That is not yet the case in veterinary practice and it will take time to educate clients that veterinary nurses are both qualified and competent to carry out various procedures. This will not be helped by misinforming clients or allowing them to assume that the vet will perform the procedure when, in fact, the nurse will do it. Again, the crucial term is client communication.

Dealing with a complaint

Any concerns a client may have should be dealt with as quickly as possible. Individual practices may have specific policies for dealing with client complaints, but regardless of the individual policy, clients must be allowed to air their grievance as soon as possible. Otherwise, a mild concern may fester and turn into a full-blown complaint. If a client is clearly angry and is likely to shout, it is a good idea to attempt to direct the client to an area of the practice away from the waiting room or reception area, where this may create a bad impression on other clients. However, wherever possible, a second member of the practice should be around to serve as witness if necessary.

Inviting the client to sit is a good way of reducing tension and defusing belligerent clients.

Box 10.3

Any client concern should be dealt with as soon as possible, before it has a chance to escalate to a complaint.

Listen to what the client has to say: it may just be a simple misunderstanding that has caused concern, or it may be more than that, but in any case the client should be heard out.

It may be possible to defuse the situation relatively easily if it is a case of misunderstanding, in which case a few well-chosen words should be used. If the situation cannot be instantly remedied, or appears more complex, then reassure the client that the matter will be looked into as soon as possible. If there is no one appropriate available to deal with the problem then explain that to the client: most people understand that there is some sort of hierarchy or complaints procedure. The final resolution of any complaint will depend on the nature of the complaint, but it is far better to be familiar with the procedure for dealing with problems before they occur rather than after.

There are courses designed for improving client communication skills, and these courses are money well spent for any practice. Role-playing exercises to practise problem scenarios are also a good idea and can provide useful practice for dealing with awkward situations as well as being very good for team-building.

Glossary

Abscess pus-filled cavity associated with inflammation. Usually caused by bacteria

Adduction movement of a body part towards the centre

Agonist drug that mimics the action of a naturally occurring hormone or neurotransmitter

Alveolar bone the bone surrounding the tooth roots

Analgesia reduction of pain

Angiogenesis the stimulation and production of new blood vessels

Ankylosis fusion of bones or joints as a result of disease (cf. arthrodesis)

Antagonist drug that opposes or blocks the action of a naturally occurring hormone or neurotransmitter

Apnoea period of cessation or suspension of breathing

Appose to place next to each other; bring into alignment

Autolysis destruction and dissolution of cells by lysosomal enzymes

Brachycephalic breeds with short skulls and noses (e.g. bulldogs, persians): all brachycephalic breeds suffer from respiratory compromise (see brachycephalic obstructive airway disease)

Bradycardia abnormally low heart rate

Buccal relating to the mouth

Calculus hard deposit on teeth, caused by mineralised plaque

Caudal towards the tail

Cautery use of heat to cut or seal tissues and blood vessels

Chemotherapy the use of drugs to treat medical disorders. The term has become restricted to the treatment of (malignant) neoplasia by various agents that slow or stop cell replication

Cicatrisation/cicatrix scar formed by wound contracture

Circuit factor the increase in minute volume required for each anaesthetic circuit to ensure sufficient delivery of oxygen

Coagulopathy disease or condition affecting the clotting pathways

Contaminated indicating the presence of microorganisms within a wound. The wound is not termed infected until the microorganisms are reproducing

Cytokine protein produced by the lymphoid cells which affects production and chemotaxis of other inflammatory cells (e.g. interleukin-2, tumour necrosis factor)

Debridement removal of necrotic tissue from a wound

Dehiscence (of wounds) wound breakdown resulting in the wound splitting open

Dolicocephalic breeds with long skulls and noses (e.g. rough collie)

Dominant hand the writing hand; the hand favoured for most coordinated tasks

Emesis vomiting

Enamel extremely hard outer layer of carnivore (and primate) teeth. Consists of 96% mineral (calcium hydroxyapatite), 2% protein (enamelin) and 2% water

Epidural the space surrounding the spinal cord within the vertebral canal

Eschar dried necrotic tissue (or scab) covering a wound. Usually associated with wound breakdown

Friable fragile or brittle

Gingiva mucosa surrounding the teeth (otherwise known as gums)

Gingivectomy excision of excess gingiva

Haematogenous spread (of infectious agents, chemicals or tumour cells) via the blood stream

Haemostasis control of bleeding

'Heath Robinson' slang term used to denote a repair by unorthodox methods

Histopathology microscopic examination and study of diseased tissue

Hypercapnia abnormally high level of carbon dioxide in the blood

Hyperplasia overgrowth of tissue

Hypoplasia failure of an organ or tissue to grow or develop properly

Iatrogenic caused unintentionally by the veterinary surgeon (or nurse)

IgE class of immunoglobulin associated with the immunological response to parasites and allergens

Intraocular pressure internal pressure of the eyeball (or globe). Persistent increased intraocular pressure is termed glaucoma and causes retinal and optic nerve damage

Keratoconjunctivitis sicca immune-based (autoimmune) disease in which the production of aqueous tear film is severely reduced (otherwise called 'dry eye')

Laparotomy surgical incision through the abdominal wall to allow visualisation of abdominal organs

Lavage washing or flushing of a wound or body cavity

Lingual relating to the tongue

Lumpectomy (see Chapter 8) removal of a small, well-demarcated benign cutaneous or immediately subcutaneous mass

Lymphopenia abnormally low lymphocyte count

Manometer instrument used to measure pressure

Metastatic ability of a malignant tumour to spread to remote parts of the body

Minute volume the volume of air moved in 1 min by the patient (minute volume = tidal volume × respiratory rate)

Neoplasia abnormal, uncontrolled growth of tissue. In other words, cancerous growth. May be benign or malignant

Nosocomial disease or condition acquired in hospital

Onychomycosis fungal infection of the claws or nails

Opioid any drug having a similar effect to opium

Osteotome surgical instrument used to cut or shave bone

Otitis externa/media inflammation and infection of the external/internal ear canals

Palmigrade, plantigrade stance in which the entirety of the paw (fore and hind respectively) is in contact with the ground. This is the way bears walk

Parasympatholytic drug which antagonises the parasympathetic system (e.g. atropine)

Perineal around the anus

Periodontal area surrounding the teeth and roots

Periodontitis inflammation of the periodontal tissues

Periosteum membrane surrounding the bone

Phlebitis inflammation of veins: usually associated with intravenous catheterisation or intravenous injection of irritating drugs

Plaque cellular and organic debris build-up on the surface of teeth

Plasmatic imbibition method by which skin grafts obtain nutrition during the first 2–3 days. The graft absorbs serum, becoming oedematous and dark in appearance

Pneumothorax/pneumoperitoneum presence of air within the thoracic cavity/abdomen

Prehension taking firm hold of something

Psychotropic any drug that affects the mind or targets mental activity

Rebreathing system anaesthetic system with carbon dioxide absorber, so that air may be recycled through the system

Rostral towards the nose

Soporific causing drowsiness or sleepiness

Sphygmomanometer blood pressure cuff with built-in manometer

Status epilepticus severe presentation of epilepsy, where the seizure is maintained for a prolonged period of time

Sterile absence of any microorganisms (bacteria, fungi, viruses or spores)

Stomatitis inflammation of the soft tissues within the mouth

Strike-through the transfer of fluids and microorganisms from one side of a barrier to the other by a process of capillary action

Tranquilliser drug used to reduce anxiety

Tumour literally, a growth or swelling. Usually, but not necessarily, neoplastic

Ulcer wound involving loss of a basal epidermis

Uraemia presence in the blood stream of abnormally high levels of urea. Causes may be prerenal, renal or postrenal. Determination of urine specific gravity helps to distinguish renal from pre- or postrenal causes

Volatile agent anaesthetic agent requiring a vaporiser (e.g. isoflurane)

SURGICAL SUFFIXES

-ectomy to remove all or part of an organ (e.g. splenectomy, colonectomy)

-ostomy to make a permanent surgical entrance into a hollow organ (e.g. tracheostomy, urethrostomy)

-otomy suffix meaning to effect surgical entry into a hollow organ (e.g. cystotomy, tracheotomy)

Further reading

Easton S (2002) Practical radiography for veterinary nurses. Oxford: Butterworth-Heinemann.

Fossum TW, Hedlund CS, Hulse DA et al. (2002) Small animal surgery, 2nd edn. St Louis, MO: Mosby.

Fowler D, Williams JM (eds) (1999) BSAVA manual of canine and feline wound management and reconstruction. Cheltenham: BSAVA.

Gorrel C (2004) Veterinary dentistry for the general practitioner. Oxford: Saunders.

Gorrel C, Derbyshire S (2005) Veterinary dentistry for the nurse and technician. Oxford: Butterworth-Heinemann.

Hillyer EV, Quesenberry KE (1997) Ferrets, rabbits, and rodents: clinical medicine and surgery. Philadelphia, PA: WB Saunders.

Holmstrom SE, Fitch PF, Eisner ER (2004) Veterinary dental techniques for the small animal practitioner, 3rd edn. Philadelphia, PA: Saunders.

Hotston Moore A (1999) BSAVA manual of advanced veterinary nursing. Cheltenham: BSAVA.

King L, Hammond R (1999) BSAVA manual of canine and feline emergency and critical care. Cheltenham: BSAVA.

McCurnin DM, Bassert JM (2002) Clinical textbook for veterinary technicians, 5th edn. Philadelphia, PA: Saunders.

Orpet H, Welsh P (2002) Handbook of veterinary nursing. Oxford: Blackwell.

Tighe MM, Brown M (1998) Mosby's comprehensive review for veterinary technicians, 2nd edn. St Louis, MO: Mosby.

Tracy DL (2000) Small animal surgical nursing, 3rd edn. St Louis, MO: Mosby.

Veterinary Surgeons' Act 1066 (schedule 3 amendment) order 2002/2004. London: HMSO.

Useful addresses

Professional bodies

British Small Animal Veterinary Association
Woodrow House
1 Telford Way
Waterwells Business Park
Quedgeley
Gloucester GL2 4AB
Tel: 01452 726700
Fax: 01452 726701
E-mail: adminoff@bsava.com
Website: www.bsava.com

British Veterinary Association
7 Mansfield Street
London W1G 9NQ
Tel: 020 7636 6541
Fax: 020 7436 2970
E-mail: bvahq@bva.co.uk

British Veterinary Nursing Association
Suite 11, Shenval House
South Road
Harlow
Essex CM20 2BD
Tel: 01279 450567
Fax: 01279 420866
E-mail: bvna@bvnaoffice.plus.com
Website: www.bvna.org.uk

Royal College of Veterinary Surgeons
Belgravia House
62–64 Horseferry Road
London SW1P 2AF
Tel: 020 7222 2001
Fax: 020 7222 2004
E-mail: membership@rcvs.org.uk
Website: www.rcvs.org.uk

Veterinary Defence Society
4 Haig Court
Parkgate Estate
Knutsford
Cheshire WA16 8XZ
Tel: 01565 652737
Fax: 01565 751079

Nursing journals

Veterinary Nursing Journal
Lion Lane
Needham Market
Ipswich
Suffolk IP6 8NT
Tel: 01449 723800
Fax: 01449 723801
E-mail: enquiries@jcagroup.com

VN Times
Olympus House
Werrington Centre
Peterborough
Cambridgeshire PE4 6NA
Tel: 01733 325522
Fax: 01733 325512
E-mail: vntimes@vetsonline.com
Website: www.vetnurse.co.uk

Poisons, toxicology

Veterinary Poisons Information Service (VPIS)
  (London)
Medical Toxicology Unit
Avonley Road
London SE14 5ER
Tel: 020 7635 9195
Fax: 020 7771 5309
E-mail: vpis@gstt.sthames.nhs.uk

Laboratories, equipment and services

Abbott Animal Health
Abbott Laboratories
Queenborough
Kent ME11 5EL
Tel: 01795 580303
Fax: 01628 644183

Alstoe
Animal Health
Sheriff Hutton Industrial Park
Sheriff Hutton
Yorkshire YO60 6RZ
Tel: 01347 878606
Fax: 01347 878333
E-mail: info@alstoe.co.uk

AnimalCare
Common Road
Dunnington
York YO19 5RU
Tel: 01904 487687
Fax: 01904 487611
Website: www.animalcare.co.uk

Arnolds Veterinary Products
Cartmel Drive
Harlescott
Shrewsbury SY1 3TB
Tel: 01743 441632
Fax: 01743 462111
E-mail: technical@arnolds.co.uk
Website: www.arnolds.co.uk

Astrazeneca Pharmaceuticals
Mereside
Alderley Park
Macclesfield
Cheshire SK10 4TG
Tel: 01625 582828
Website: www.astrazeneca.com

Axiom Veterinary Laboratories
George Street
Teignmouth
Devon TQ14 8AH
Tel: 01626 778844
Fax: 01626 779570
E-mail: admin@axiomvetlab.co.uk

Bayer
Bayer HealthCare
Animal Health Division
Bayer House
Strawberry Hill
Newbury
Berkshire RG14 1JA
Tel: 01635 563000
Fax: 01635 563622
Website: www.bayer.co.uk

Boehringer Ingelheim Vetmedica
Ellesfield Avenue
Bracknell
Berkshire RG12 8YS
Tel: 01344 424600
Fax: 01344 741349
E-mail: vetmedica.uk@boehringer-ingelheim.
  com
Website: www.boehringer-ingelheim.com

B Braun Medical
Thorncliffe Park
Sheffield S35 2PW
Tel: 0114 2259000
Fax: 0114 2259111
Website: www.braun.com

Burtons Medical Equipment
Units 1–4 Guardian Industrial Estate
Pattenden Lane
Marden
Kent TN12 9QD
Tel: 01622 834300
Fax: 01622 834330
E-mail: info@burtons.uk.com
Website: www.burtons.uk.com

Cytopath Veterinary Pathology
PO Box 24
Ledbury
Herefordshire HR8 2YD
Tel: 01531 630063
Fax: 01531 630033

Elanco Animal Health
Eli Lilly and Company
Kingsclere Road
Basingstoke
Hants RG21 6XA
Tel: 01256 353131
Fax: 01256 315081
E-mail: elanco.uk.info@lilly.com
Website: www.elanco.com

Ellman International (UK)
16 Ryehill Court
Lodge Farm
Northampton NN5 7EU
Tel: 01604 589928
Fax: 01604 759098
E-mail: ellmanintuk@aol.com

Feline Advisory Bureau (FAB)
Taeselbury
High Street
Tisbury
Wiltshire SP3 6LD
Tel: 01747 871872
Fax: 01747 871873
E-mail: fab.fab@ukonline.co.uk
Website: www.fabcats.org

Finn Pathologists
The Veterinary Laboratory
One Eyed Lane
Weybread
Diss
Norfolk IP21 5TT
Tel: 01379 854180
Fax: 01379 852424
E-mail: finnpathologists@vetpathology.com

Fort Dodge Animal Health
Flanders Road
Hedge End
Southampton SO30 4HQ
Tel: 01489 781711
Fax: 01489 788306
Website: www.ahp.com

Greendale Veterinary Diagnostics
Lansbury Estate
Lower Guildford Road
Knaphill
Woking
Surrey GU21 2EW
Tel: 01483 797707
Fax: 01483 797552
E-mail: lab@greendale.co.uk

Hills Pet Nutrition
Suite 8 Sherbourne House
Croxley Business Park
Hatters Lane
Watford
Hertfordshire WD18 8WY
Tel: 01923 652800
Fax: 01923 652801
Website: www.hillspet.com

HSE Books
PO Box 1999
Sudbury
Suffolk CO10 2WA
Tel: 01787 881165
Website: www.hsebooks.com
www.hse.gov.uk

Idexx Laboratories
Grange House
Sandbeck Way
Wetherby
West Yorkshire LS22 7DN
Tel: 01937 544000
Fax: 01937 544001
Website: www.idexx.co.uk

Intervet UK
Walton Manor
Walton
Milton Keynes
Buckinghamshire MK7 7AJ
Tel: 01908 665050
Fax: 01908 664778
Website: www.internet.co.uk

Janssen Veterinary
PO Box 79
Saunderton
High Wycombe
Buckinghamshire HP14 4HJ
Tel: 01494 567555
Fax: 01494 567556
E-mail: ahealth@jacgb.jnj.com

Kruuse UK
14a Moor Lane Industrial Estate
Sherburn in Elmet
North Yorkshire LS25 6ES
Tel: 01977 681523
Fax: 01977 683537
E-mail: kruuse.uk@kruuse.com
Website: www.kruuse.com

Leo (Vetxx) Animal Health
Longwick Road
Princes Risborough
Buckinghamshire HP27 9RR
Tel: 01844 347333
Fax: 01844 274832
E-mail: ah.ukenquiries@leo-pharma.com

JM Loveridge
Southbrook Road
Southampton
Hampshire SO15 1BH
Tel: 023 8022 8411
Fax: 023 8063 9836
E-mail: admin@jmloveridge.com
Website: www.jmloveridge.com

Medichem International
PO Box 237
Sevenoaks
Kent TN15 0ZJ
Tel: 01732 763555
Fax: 01732 763530
E-mail: info@medichem.co.uk
Website: www.medichem.co.uk

Menarini Diagnostics
Wharfedale Road
Winnersh
Wokingham
Berkshire RG41 5RA
E-mail: menavet@menarinidiag.co.uk
Website: www.menarinidiag.co.uk

Novartis Animal Health UK
New Cambridge House
Littlington
Nr Royston
Hertfordshire SG8 0SS
Tel: 01763 850500
Fax: 01763 850600
E-mail: uk.info@novartis.com

Pharmacia Animal Health
Hatton House
Hunters Road
Weldon North Estate
Corby
Northamptonshire NN17 5JE
Tel: 01536 276400
Fax: 01536 263365
Website: www.pharmaciaah.com

Pfizer
Walton Oaks
Dorking Road
Tadworth
Surrey KT20 7NS
Tel: 01304 616161
Fax: 01304 656221
Website: www.pfizer.com

Royal Canin
25 Brympton Way
Yeovil
Somerset BA20 2JB
Tel: 0800 717800
Fax: 01935 414446
Website: www.royalcanin.co.uk

RVC Diagnostic Laboratories
Hawkshead Lane
North Mymms
Hatfield
Hertfordshire AL9 7TA
Tel: 01707 666208
Fax: 01707 661464
E-mail: rdouthwaite@rvc.ac.uk
Website: www.rvc.ac.uk

Schering-Plough Animal Health
Breakspear Road South
Harefield
Uxbridge
Middlesex UB9 6LS
Tel: 01895 626000
Website: www.spah.com

Shor-Line
Unit 39A
Vole Business Park
Llandow
Vale of Glamorgan CF71 7PF
Tel: 0800 616770
Fax: 01446 773668
Website: www.shor-line.co.uk

Veterinary Instrumentation
Broadfield Road
Sheffield S8 0XL
Tel: 0845 1309596
Fax: 0845 1308687
E-mail: info@vetinst.com
Website: www.vetinst.com

Vetlab Supplies
Unit 13 Broomers Hill Park
Broomers Hill Lane
Pulborough
West Sussex RH20 2RY
Tel: 01798 874567
Fax: 01798 874787
E-mail: info@vetlabsupplies.co.uk
Website: www.vetlabsupplies.co.uk

Vetoquinol UK
Wedgwood Road
Bicester
Oxfordshire OX26 4UL
Tel: 01869 355000
Fax: 01869 320145
Website: www.vetoquinol.co.uk

Woodley Equipment Company
St Johns Street
Horwich
Bolton
Lancashire BL6 7NY
Tel: 01204 669033
Fax: 01204 669034
E-mail: sales@woodleyequipment.com

Appendix 1
Suggested contents of emergency box

Drugs (see Table A1 for drug dosages)

Atropine	0.6 mg/ml
Dexamethasone	2 mg/ml
Calcium gluconate	10%
Doxapram hydrochloride	20 mg/ml
Dobutamine hydrochloride	50 mg/ml
Dopamine hydrochloride	40 mg/ml
Adrenaline (epinephrine)	1 : 1000
Adrenaline (epinephrine)	1 : 10 000
Heparin	1000 IU/ml
Propranolol	1 mg/ml
Furosemide	40 mg/ml
Lidocaine	2%
Naloxone	0.4 mg/ml

Methylprednisolone sodium succinate 125 mg, 500 mg

Crystalloid (e.g. saline 0.9% 1 l)
Mannitol
Colloid (e.g. Haemaccel)
Heparinised saline (for flush)

Equipment
Variety of intravenous catheters
Variety of sterile syringes and needles
Three-way taps
Scissors
Giving sets (and burette)
Curved haemostats
Range of endotracheal tubes
Surgical tape
Sterile lubricant
3/0 monofilament nylon suture with straight needle
Laryngoscope with large and small blade
Tracheostomy kit

Larger equipment (which should be checked and charged weekly)
Electrocardiograph machine with leads and connectors
Defibrillator with paddles (internal and external)

Table A1 Emergency drug dosages

Drug and concentration supplied (or kept)	Dose (mg/kg)	Dose: 10-kg dog (ml)	Dose: 4-kg cat (ml)
Atropine 0.6 mg/ml	0.02–0.04 mg/kg IV	0.33–0.66	0.13–0.26
Dexamethasone 2 mg/ml	Shock: 5 mg/kg IV	25	10
Calcium gluconate 10%	0.5–1.5 ml/kg IV over 20–30 min	5–15	2–6
Doxapram hydrochloride 20 mg/ml	5–10 mg/kg IV	2.5–5	1–2
Dobutamine hydrochloride 50 mg/ml	Add 0.5 ml to 1 l sterile saline. Infuse at: Dogs: 1–20 µg/kg per min Cats: 0.5–10 µg/kg per min Both IV	(Diluted) 0.4–8 ml/min	(Diluted) 0.08–1.6 ml/min
Dopamine hydrochloride 40 mg/ml	Add 1 ml to 1 l sterile saline. Infuse at: Dogs: 2–10 µg/kg per min Cats: 1–5 µg/kg per min Both IV	(Diluted) 0.1–0.5 ml/min	(Diluted) 0.02–0.1 ml/min
Adrenaline (epinephrine) 1:1000 (1000 µg/ml)	Add 1 ml of 1:1000 to 9 ml sterile saline (= 1:10 000, or 100 µg/ml) 10–20 µg/kg IV	(Diluted) 0.1–0.2	(Diluted) 0.04–0.08
Heparin 1000 IU/ml	100–200 IU/kg IV	1–2	0.4–0.8
Propranolol 1 mg/ml	Dogs: 0.02–0.08 mg/kg Cats: 0.04–0.06 mg/kg Slow IV	0.2–0.8	0.12–0.24
Furosemide 40 mg/ml	1–2 mg/kg IV	0.2–0.4	0.1–0.2
Lidocaine 2%	Dogs: 2–8 mg/kg IV Cats: 0.25–1 mg/kg slow IV	1–4	0.05–0.25
Naloxone 0.4 mg/ml	0.015–0.4 mg/kg	0.37–1	0.15–0.4
Methylprednisolone sodium succinate 125 mg, 500 mg	20–30 mg/kg	3.2–4.8	1.28–1.92

Appendix 2
Emergency procedure – cardiopulmonary arrest

N_2O, nitrous oxide; ET, endotracheal; O_2, oxygen; IV, intravenously; IT, intratracheally; IPPV, intermittent positive-pressure ventilation; ECG, electrocardiogram.

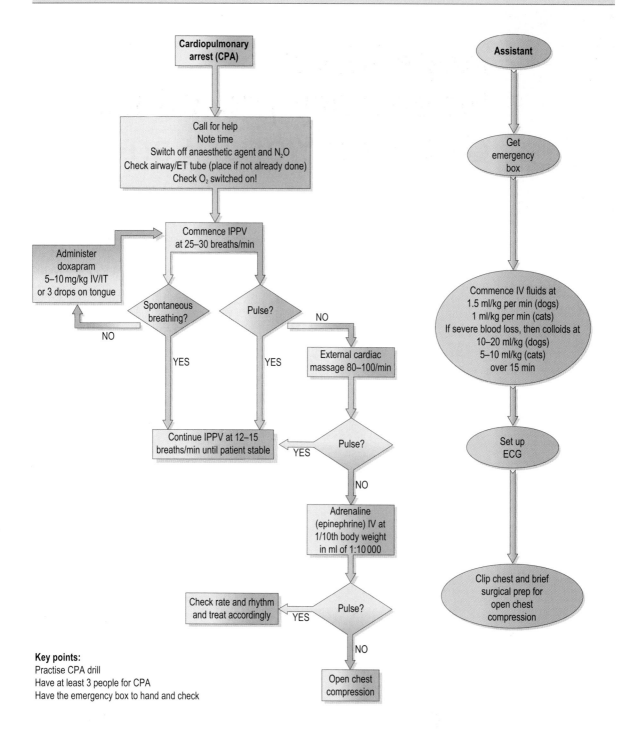

Cardiopulmonary arrest (CPA)

Call for help
Note time
Switch off anaesthetic agent and N$_2$O
Check airway/ET tube (place if not already done)
Check O$_2$ switched on!

Commence IPPV
at 25–30 breaths/min

Administer
doxapram
5–10 mg/kg IV/IT
or 3 drops on tongue

Spontaneous breathing?

Pulse?

NO

External cardiac
massage 80–100/min

YES

YES

Continue IPPV at 12–15
breaths/min until patient stable

Pulse?

YES

NO

Adrenaline
(epinephrine) IV at
1/10th body weight
in ml of 1:10 000

Check rate and rhythm
and treat accordingly

Pulse?

YES

NO

Open chest
compression

Assistant

Get
emergency
box

Commence IV fluids at
1.5 ml/kg per min (dogs)
1 ml/kg per min (cats)
If severe blood loss, then colloids at
10–20 ml/kg (dogs)
5–10 ml/kg (cats)
over 15 min

Set up
ECG

Clip chest and brief
surgical prep for
open chest
compression

Key points:
Practise CPA drill
Have at least 3 people for CPA
Have the emergency box to hand and check

Appendix 3
Emergency procedure –
status epilepticus

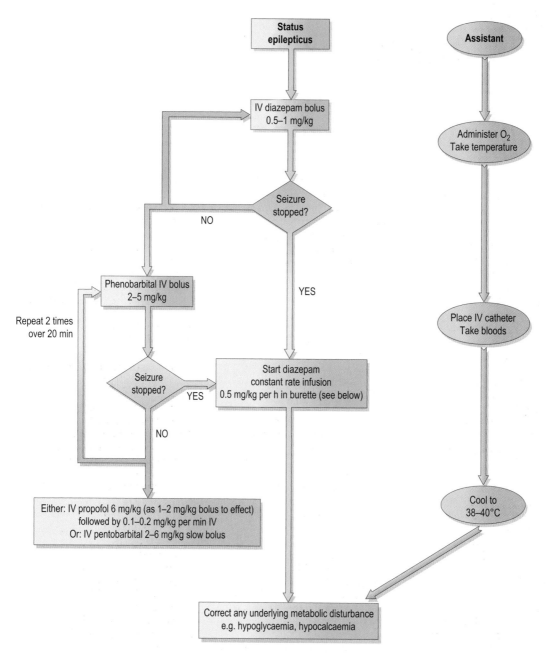

N.B.:

To make a constant infusion of diazepam, work out how much fluid the patient will need at maintenance rate over 2 h, add that to the burette and then add diazepam at 0.5 mg/kg/h (x 2).

Example: 10 kg dog: IV fluids = 50 ml/kg/24h = 2 ml/kg/h = 20 ml/h (40 ml in burette). Diazepam = 0.5 mg/kg/h = 5 mg/h (10 mg in burette).

Note: diazepam is denatured by light and adheres to the plastic of IV tubing, so do not make up more than a 2-h supply at one time.

Index

Gowns, 93
  disposable/reusable, 94
Granulation tissue, 74
  secondary wound closure, 81
  skin grafting, 86
Grass awns removal, 102,
    148–149
Grazes, 72
Greyhounds, 16, 27, 32, 33
Gunshot wounds, 73
  first aid, 77
Gutter splint, 83, 87

H
Haematoma
  aural, 145–146
  postoperative, 201–202
Haemorrhage, 50
  dental extractions, 184
  recovery phase care, 196
  wound first aid, 76
Haemostasis, 116–118
  cautery, 117–118
  haemostats, 116
  ligatures, 116–117
  principles, 109
  scrubbed assistant's role
    during major surgery,
    160
  surgical staples, 108
  swabbing, 116
  tissue adhesives, 107
  wound care
    debridement, 79–80
    dressings, 55
    first aid, 76
  wound healing, 74
Haemostatic forceps, 103, 116
Hair removal, 10
  consent, 205
  intravenous cannula
    placement, 22
  intravenous drug
    administration, 22
  surgical site preparation, 98
  transdermal patch application,
    28
  wound first aid, 76–77
Halothane, 35
Halstead's principles of tissue
    handling, 109
Hand disinfectants, 92
Hand ties, 112, 113–114
Hand-drying, 93
Hand-scrubbing, 92–93
Hanging-limb technique, 99
Hartmann's solution
  burns first aid, 77

wet-to-dry dressings, 56
wound infection management,
  67
wound lavage, 77
Histopathology, 132, 133
Horizontal mattress sutures, 111
  tension-relieving sutures, 119
  walking sutures, 119
Horner's syndrome, 147
Humphrey ADE system, 43, 44
Hydroactive dressings, 57
Hydrocolloid dressings, 57, 67,
  81
Hydrofoam dressings, 81
Hydrogel dressings, 57, 67, 85
Hyperadrenocorticism, 84
Hypercalcaemia, 45
Hypercapnia, 45
Hyperkalaemia, 45
Hyperthyroidism, dental patients,
  171, 172
Hypothermia, 50, 172
Hypoxia monitoring, 45

I
Iatrogenic complications
  bandage wounds, 73
  burns, 98
  dental, 183–184
Incisional wounds, 71–72, 77
Incisions, relaxing, 120
Infiltration anaesthesia, 28–29
Inflammation, wound healing,
  74
Information for owners, 5
  bandage care, 67–68, 198
  informed consent, 205
  postoperative care, 123, 198,
    199
Inhalant (volatile) anaesthetic
    agents, 32, 34–36
  administration, 34
  minimum alveolar
    concentration (MAC),
    35
  overdosage, 50
  respiratory gas analysis, 47
  scavenging, 35, 37, 39
  solubility, 34, 35
Injectable anaesthetic agents,
    32–34
  advantages/disadvantages,
    32–33
  antagonists, 49
  constant infusion anaesthesia,
    32, 34
  drugs, 33–34
  methods of use, 32

overdosage, 49–50
Instruments, surgical, 100–105
  cleaning/maintenance,
    104–105
  dental surgery, 167–171
  markers, 105
Insulin-like growth factor, 88
Intercostal nerve block, 29
Intermittent positive pressure
    ventilation (IPPV), 37,
    41, 42, 43
  anaesthetic agent overdosage
    management, 49, 50
  emergencies management, 50,
    51
Interosseous catheter placement,
    155, 157–158
  needles, 156
Interrupted sutures, 109
  cruciate, 111
  horizontal mattress, 111, 119
  removal, 123
  simple, 111
  skin, 110
  subcutaneous/subcuticular
    tissues, 110
Intralesional antibiotics, 30
Intramuscular administration,
  22
Intraocular pressure elevation,
  16
Intratracheal administration, 50
Intravenous administration, 22
Intravenous cannulas
  care, 23–24
  placement, 22–23
  problems, 23
Intravenous fluids, 12, 24–27,
    172
  administration rate, 24, 26
  blood loss replacement, 118
  burns first aid, 77
  circulatory arrest prevention,
    50
  rationale for use, 24
  recovery phase, 196
  selection, 24
  urine production monitoring,
    24
Intravenous regional anaesthesia,
    29
Isoflurane, 35, 36, 37, 52, 53,
    192

J
Jellyfish stings, 74
Job satisfaction, 5
Joint surgery, 30

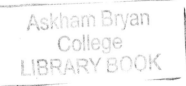